Operative Techniques in Orthopedic Surgery

Operative Techniques in Orthopedic Surgery

Edited by Markus Wagner

hayle medical
New York

Hayle Medical,
750 Third Avenue, 9th Floor,
New York, NY 10017, USA

Visit us on the World Wide Web at:
www.haylemedical.com

ISBN: 978-1-64647-104-1

Cataloging-in-Publication Data

Operative techniques in orthopedic surgery / edited by Markus Wagner.
p. cm.
Includes bibliographical references and index.
ISBN 978-1-64647-104-1
1. Orthopedic surgery. 2. Orthopedics. 3. Surgery, Operative. I. Wagner, Markus.
RD731 .O64 2022
617.3--dc23

Table of Contents

Preface

Orthopedic surgery is the branch of surgery that is concerned with the surgical management of musculoskeletal conditions. The treatment of musculoskeletal trauma, degenerative diseases, tumors, spine diseases, congenital disorders and sports injuries come under the scope of this field. Orthopedic surgical procedures may fall under the categories of total joint replacement, spine surgery, total joint reconstruction, foot and ankle surgery, etc. Some of the common orthopedic procedures are knee arthroscopy, knee replacement, hip replacement, shoulder arthroscopy, repair of femoral neck fracture, laminectomy, low back intervertebral disc surgery, lumbar spinal fusion, etc. Modern orthopedic surgery is often less invasive and involves implanted components that are better and more durable. The objective of this book is to give a general view of the different operative techniques in orthopedic surgery. The ever growing need of advanced surgical interventions is the reason that has fueled the research in this domain in recent times. This book is a vital tool for all researching or studying orthopedics as it gives incredible insights into emerging trends and concepts.

Various studies have approached the subject by analyzing it with a single perspective, but the present book provides diverse methodologies and techniques to address this field. This book contains theories and applications needed for understanding the subject from different perspectives. The aim is to keep the readers informed about the progresses in the field; therefore, the contributions were carefully examined to compile novel researches by specialists from across the globe.

Indeed, the job of the editor is the most crucial and challenging in compiling all chapters into a single book. In the end, I would extend my sincere thanks to the chapter authors for their profound work. I am also thankful for the support provided by my family and colleagues during the compilation of this book.

Editor

1

Influence of change of tunnel axis angle on tunnel length during double-bundle ACL reconstruction via the transportal technique

Joon Ho Wang[1,2,3], Do Kyung Lee[4], Sung Taek Chung[5] and Byung Hoon Lee[5*]

Abstract

Background: Commercially available flexible reamer and curved guide systems allow a certain degree of control over intra-articular tunnel orientation, therefore allows a wide range of intra-osseous femoral tunnel orientations, contrary to the femoral tunneling technique using a straight guide pin, which are determined by knee flexion angle. We sought to find the clinical relevance of intra-osseous femoral tunnel orientations in the respect of tunnel length. To evaluate the relationship between the tunnel axis angle in three orthogonal planes and tunnel length in the anteromedial (AM) and posterolateral (PL) femoral tunnels in patients who underwent anatomic double-bundle anterior cruciate ligament reconstruction (DB-ACLR) using the transportal (TP) technique with a 42° curved guide.

Methods: A total of 40 patients who underwent primary DB-ACLR with the TP technique using a curved guide were evaluated retrospectively. The tunnel axis angle in three orthogonal planes were evaluated on a three-dimensional surface model constructed using an axial computed tomography scan obtained after reconstruction. Then, correlations with tunnel length were analyzed.

Results: In the AM tunnel, tunnel axis angles in the coronal ($\beta = 0.0252$, $p = 0.022$) and sagittal ($\beta = 0.0168$, $p = 0.029$) plane showed significant correlations with tunnel length, while the axial plane did not ($p = 0.493$) (adjusted $R^2 = 0.801$). In the PL tunnel, only tunnel axis angles in the axial plane ($\beta = 0.0262$, $p = 0.008$) showed a significant relationship with tunnel length (adjusted $R^2 = 0.700$).

Conclusion: Drilling at a higher angle in the coronal and sagittal planes in AM tunnels and at a higher angle in the axial plane in PL tunnels decreases the incidence of short femoral tunnels.

Keywords: Anterior cruciate ligament reconstruction, Transportal, Femoral tunnel orientation, Quadrant method

Background

Recently, anterior cruciate ligament (ACL) surgical techniques with a primary focus on anatomic reconstruction have been considered to restore normal knee anatomy, kinematics, and stability more thoroughly [1–3]. This is provided by placing tunnels in the center of native ACL insertion sites on the tibia and femur using either the single- or double-bundle technique [4]. To achieve anatomic ACL femoral tunnel positions more easily, transportal drilling has been proposed as an alternative to the transtibial technique [5–8]. However, more horizontal or oblique femoral tunnel positions result in a shorter distance between the notch and the lateral femoral cortex, which results in shorter overall tunnel length, iatrogenic damage to the medial femoral condyle cartilage [9], and a higher chance of posterior wall blowout from tunneling toward the posterior femoral condyle compared to the traditional transtibial technique [10–12].

Therefore, there are increasing interests to attain an adequate tunnel length and prevent posterior wall breakage [11–13]. Recently, commercially available flexible reamer and curved guide system was made to decrease the chance

* Correspondence: oselite@naver.com
[5]Department of Orthopaedic Surgery, Kang-Dong Sacred Heart Hospital, Hallym University Medical Center, Gil-dong, Seoul 134-701, South Korea
Full list of author information is available at the end of the article

of injuring the medial femoral condyle cartilage. Furthermore, it has been suggested to achieve longer femoral intraosseous tunnel lengths than with a straight guide pin [14].

During femoral tunneling procedure using curved guide, we noticed changeable intra-articular tunnel orientations could be allowed by the certain degrees of guide's movement within the intercondylar notch space. Meanwhile, in the femoral tunneling technique with a straight guide pin, the intra-articular tunnel orientation is mainly determined by the knee flexion angle because it involves the fixed intra-articular tunnel orientation from two points: the portal, and a femoral tunnel center within the anatomic femoral footprint (Figs. 1 and 2). Controllable intra-articular tunnel orientation can assure a wide range of tunnel axis angles in three-dimensional planes. We became interested in the interosseous tunnel orientation in three dimensional planes, the extension of the intra-articular tunnel orientation.

The purpose of this study was to evaluate the relationship between tunnel axis angle in the three orthogonal planes and tunnel length using in vivo imaging data. The following research question was addressed: In which plane is the tunnel axis angle correlated to the tunnel length in both anteromedial (AM) and posterolateral (PL) femoral tunnels after anatomic double-bundle ACLR? Our hypothesis is that intra-osseous femoral tunnel orientations depending on the entrance angle of the guide pin influence tunnel length, which can be useful for the acquisition of longer tunnel length with use of commercially available flexible reamer and curved guide systems.

Methods

Demographic data

Between October 2013 to May 2014, 83 patients underwent primary anatomic double-bundle ACL reconstruction with the transportal (TP) technique using a curved guide and flexible reamer (Clancy Anatomic Cruciate Guide System; Smith & Nephew, Andover, MA, USA) (Table 1).

Inclusion criteria were a primary unilateral ACL injury with or without meniscus injury that was treated by double-bundle ACL reconstruction with the TP (accessory AM) technique, as well as patient age ranging from 15 to 60 years. Of the 83 patients, 43 were excluded because they (1) had undergone ACL reconstruction using a rigid guide because there was no flexible reamer size option for either AM or PL grafts less than 6 mm in diameter (n = 19), (2) had undergone ACL reconstruction using another technique (outside-in) (n = 15), (3) had any combined multiple-ligament injury (n = 2), or (4) they had undergone a single bundle reconstruction for open physis (n = 2) and simultaneous reconstruction of the ACL and PCL (n = 4) combined with HTO (n = 1). Finally, 40 patients who underwent anatomic double-bundle ACL reconstruction by the TP technique were retrospectively evaluated in the present study. Institutional Review Board approval (2015-05-085) was obtained from our institution (Samsung Medical Center, Seoul, South Korea) before the study, and the protocol was approved. All patients provided informed consent prior to participation in this study.

Surgical technique

A single surgeon (J.H.W.) experienced in ACL reconstruction performed all operations using the TP arthroscopic-assisted technique. Femoral and tibial tunnels were created in the centers of their respective anatomic insertions. Grafts were fixed with a cortical suspension system using the shortest possible loop (10 to 15 mm) to ensure maximal contact between the grafts and tunnel walls on the femoral side. Bio-absorbable interference screws with a post tie were used on the tibial side for all cases.

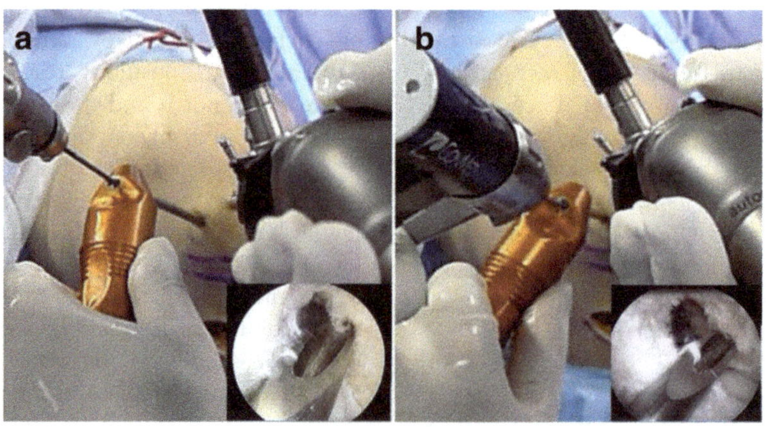

Fig. 1 During femoral tunneling procedure using curved guide, the change of intra-articular tunnel orientations could be allowed by the certain degrees of guide's movement within the intercondylar notch space. **a** First, curved guide is positioned for targeting the intended tunnel position. **b** Then, the guide can be rotated within the intercondylar notch space

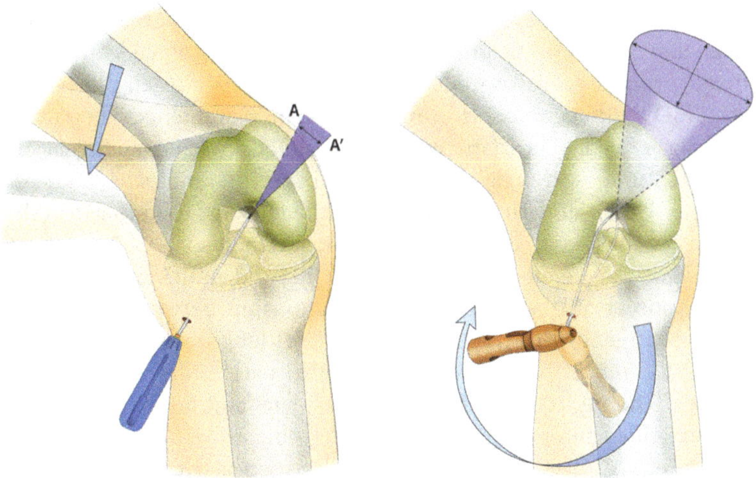

Fig. 2 The curved guide system allows a certain degree of control over intra-articular tunnel orientation regardless of the knee flexion angle due to the rotational freedom of the guide in the intercondylar notch space. This is contrary to tunneling with a straight guide pin, which has fixed intra-articular tunnel orientation from two points, the AM or AAM portal and the femoral tunnel center

Portal formation was conducted in the usual manner. An anteromedial (AM) portal was placed in a slightly more proximal position than usual, with the distal extent of the portal ending at the level of the inferior pole of the patella. An accessory anteromedial (AAM) portal was made approximately 1.5 cm medial from the standard AM portal and just above the medial meniscus anterior horn. The arthroscope was inserted into the AM portal, and another working device was inserted into the AAM portal. After the ACL rupture was confirmed and remnant tissue was debrided, the femoral footprints of both the AM and PL bundles were carefully defined in reference to the ACL remnants and bony ridges [13]. Centers of both footprints were then indicated with a curved microfracture awl. The center of the AM bundle footprint was 6–7 mm distal (shallow) to the posterior cartilage margin, 2 mm from the posterior bony ridge of the lateral femoral condyle [15, 16], and 3–4 mm posterior (low) to the extended line of the posterolateral corner of the intercondylar notch, which was verified at 90° of knee flexion. The center of the PL bundle footprint was positioned 5 mm anterior (high) to the edge of the joint cartilage on an imaginary line perpendicular to the tangent of the lowermost portion of the lateral femoral condyle at 90° of knee flexion [17]. Our considerations in placement of femoral tunnel were 1) to prevent slippage on the medial wall of the lateral femoral condyle while placing guide wires within the anatomical footprint of the ACL 2) to secure appropriate tunnel length of 20 mm or more 3) to prevent of posterior cortical breakage. After creating the femoral tunnel, its length was measured with a ruler. The required EndoButton size (Smith & Nephew Endoscopy, Andover, MA) for the TP technique was then determined. A femoral guide was inserted through the AAM portal, and a 2.4-mm guide pin was advanced 2 to 3 mm to engage the guide to the center of the AM and PL bundle femoral footprints. The knee joint was then bent as fully as possible and the guide was advanced until the pin passed the cortex and skin. After changing the viewing portal from AM to anterolateral, the tibial footprints of both the AM and PL bundles were carefully defined in reference to the ACL remnants and bony ridges. The anterior margin of the ACL footprint was described as the ACL ridge, and the posterior margin was defined as the retro-eminence of the tibial spine [18, 19].

Table 1 Patient demographics and baseline characteristics[a]

	Data
Age, y, mean ± SD (range)	32.3 ± 10.9 (15–57)
Sex, male/female, n^a	28 / 10
BMI, kg/m^2	25.4 ± 4.1 (17.6–36.3)
Femoral condyle size	
M-L epicondylar distance (mm)	82.2 ± 5.8 (69.8–95.7)
LPC offset distance (mm)	25.3 ± 2.4 (20.2–29.3)
Time from injury to reconstruction (Log[b])	1.6 ± 1.9 (−1.6–4.8)

BMI body mass index, *M-L* medial to lateral, *LPC* lateral posterior condyle
[a]Values are expressed as mean ± standard deviation (range) except for sex
[b]Time was log-transformed because it showed abnormal distribution

Measurement of tunnel axis angle using three-dimensional computed tomography

Computed tomography (CT) scans were performed on all knees after ACL reconstruction. The knee was placed in full extension. Digital Imaging and Communications in Medicine data were extracted from the picture archiving and communication system. Data were segmented by Mimics software (Materialise, Leuven, Belgium), a commercially available image processing software used to create three-dimensional (3D) surface models from stacks of two-dimensional image data. The data were then imported into Geomagic Studio software, version 12.0 (Geomagic, Rock Hill, SC, USA), and the 3D surface model was projected into coronal, axial, and sagittal planes to measure the tunnel axis angle in each plane (Fig. 3). As described by Basdekis et al. [20], the angle between the tunnel and the line tangent to the distal and posterior aspects of the femoral condyles was measured in the coronal and axial planes. The sagittal plane angle between the tunnel and the extended intersectional line of the femoral shaft was measured. A lower tunnel angle in the sagittal plane indicated that the tunnel orientation is extended compared with the femoral shaft, while a higher tunnel angle in the sagittal plane indicated that tunnel orientation is flexed compared with the femoral shaft.

To measure the femoral tunnel length, the plane in which the entire length of the femoral tunnel showed the maximal width was selected. The distance between the centers of the intra-articular and extra-articular tunnel apertures was measured [21]. To evaluate its correlation with distal femoral anatomy, the lateral posterior condyle (LPC) AP size (LPC offset distance) and medial-to lateral (M-L) epicondylar distance were measured [21]. The incidence of posterior cortical damage was evaluated by 3D CT scan. Cases with posterior cortical damage or in which the tunnel center was not placed within the anatomical footprint boundary would have been excluded, but none occurred in this study.

Reliability and statistical analysis

Two orthopedic surgeons (independent observers) together developed and agreed to the measurement methods. They were blinded to each other's measurements and their own prior measurements. They measured the tunnel axis angle in sagittal, coronal, and axial planes, and tunnel length for AM and PL bundles of all knees. The intra-class correlation coefficient was used to assess the interobserver reliability of measurements.

Uni- and multivariate regression analyses evaluated the relationship between independent influential factors and tunnel length using the SigmaStat software package. Influential factors were considered demographic factors (sex, age, and body mass index), LPC offset distance, and M-L epicondylar distance. Significance was set at $P < 0.05$. All statistical analyses were performed using SAS ver. 9.3 (SAS Institute, Cary, NC, USA).

Results

The interobserver and intraobserver reliability ranged from 0.83 to 0.96 and 0.85 to 0.95, respectively (Table 2). The mean AM tunnel length was 33.5 ± 4.3 mm (range, 21.6 to 42.9), and the mean PL tunnel length was 35.4 ± 4.0 mm (range, 24 to 41.0).

Influence of tunnel Axis angle change in 3-D planes on tunnel length in AM and PL femoral tunnels

Tables 3 and 4 show data regarding measured variables.

In the AM femoral tunnel, the mean tunnel axis angle was 44.5° ± 5.7° in the coronal plane, 40.9° ± 6.4° in the sagittal plane, and 32.9° ± 7.2° in the axial plane. Univariate regression analyses identified that the patient factors related to longer femoral tunnel length include male gender ($\beta = 0.5212$, $p = 0.001$), age ($\beta = 0.0145$, $p = 0.023$),

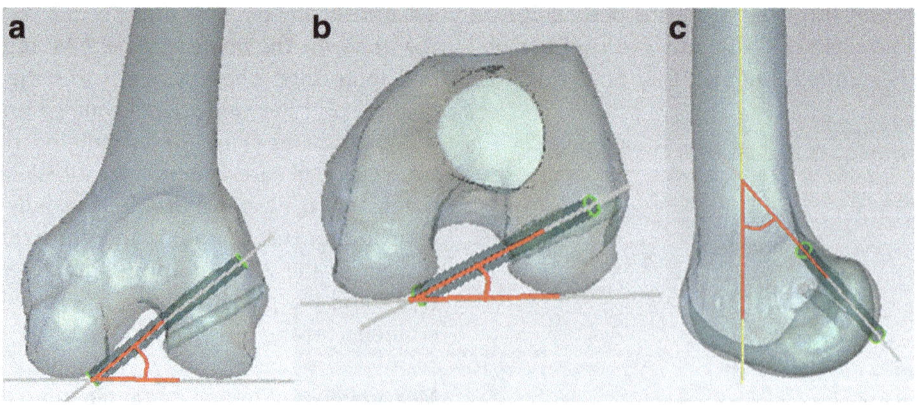

Fig. 3 Angle in each plane projected from a three-dimensional surface model. **a** The angle between the tunnel and a line tangent to distal aspects in the coronal plane was measured. **b** The angle between the tunnel and a line tangent to the posterior aspects of the femoral condyles was measured in the axial plane. **c** The angle between the tunnel and the extended intersectional line of the femoral shaft in the sagittal plane was measured

Table 2 Results of Intraclass Correlation Coefficient (ICC) value of each measurement

	AM tunnel			PL tunnel		
	Tunnel Axis Angle in			Tunnel Axis Angle in		
	Coronal plane	Sagittal plane	Axial plane	Coronal plane	Sagittal plane	Axial plane
Intertester						
ICC	0.81	0.85	0.86	0.85	0.91	0.90
Lower ICC	0.67	0.73	0.76	0.74	0.83	0.82
Upper ICC	0.90	0.92	0.93	0.92	0.95	0.95

height (β = 0.0375, p < 0.001), weight (β = 0.0119, p = 0.008), femoral condyle size (M-L epicondylar distance) (β = 0.4473, p < 0.001), and greater femoral tunnel axis angle in the coronal (β = 0.0465, p < 0.001) and axial (β = 0.0285, p = 0.003) planes.

In the PL femoral tunnels, the mean tunnel axis angle was 30.5° ± 6.3° in the coronal plane, 51.7° ± 16.4° in the sagittal plane, and 25.1° ± 6.1° in the axial plane. Univariate regression analyses identified that the patient factors related to longer femoral tunnel length include male gender (β = 0.6471, p < 0.001), height (β = 0.0399, p < 0.001), weight (β = 0.0136, p = 0.001), femoral condyle size (M-L epicondylar distance) (β = 0.4751, p < 0.001), and greater femoral tunnel axis angle in all three planes: coronal (β = 0.0326, p = 0.001) sagittal (β = −0.0087, p = 0.038), and axial (β = 0.0224, p = 0.038).

Multivariate regression analysis (Table 4) identified a disparate result between the AM and PL tunnels. In the AM tunnel, coronal (β = 0.0252, p = 0.022) and sagittal (β = 0.0168, p = 0.029) angles showed a significant correlation with AM femoral tunnel length, while this was not identified in the axial plane (p = 0.493) (adjusted R^2 = 0.801). In the PL tunnel, only the axial angle (β = 0.0262, p = 0.008) showed a significant relationship with PL femoral tunnel length (adjusted R^2 = 0.700).

Discussion

The principal findings of our study are that tunnel length is correlated with tunnel axis angle in the three-dimensional planes, but differently in AM and PL tunnels. In AM tunnels, tunnel length was related to tunnel axis angle in the coronal and sagittal planes (p = 0.022, 0.029 respectively), whereas PL tunnel lengths were related only to the tunnel axis angle in the axial plane (p = 0.008).

Several authors have recommended appropriate tunnel lengths. The ideal or minimal tunnel length remains unclear, but most surgeons anecdotally prefer to have 20 mm or more of graft to allow strong tendon healing to the bone within the tunnel. The lack of graft incorporation is a common cause of surgical failure [14]. Greis et al. reported that the length of a tendon placed within a bone tunnel influences tendon pullout strength, and advocated maximizing the tendon length inside the bone tunnels [22]. Previous cadaveric and clinical studies reported that the mean femoral tunnel length drilled through AM portals ranges from 15.7 – 34.2 mm [23, 24]. Moreover, extra length is required to flip and subsequently seat a suspensory fixation button device on the outside of the femoral cortex.

Table 3 Univariate analysis for correlation between femoral tunnel length and independent variables including patient factors[a]

	AM Femoral Tunnel			PL Femoral Tunnel		
Variables	Beta coefficient (β)	Standard error β	*p*-value	Beta coefficient (β)	Standard error β	*p*-value
Age	0.015	0.006	**0.023**	0.005	0.006	0.420
Sex	0.521	0.135	**0.001**	0.647	0.106	**<0.001**
Height	0.038	0.007	**<0.001**	0.040	0.006	**<0.001**
Weight	0.012	0.004	**0.008**	0.014	0.004	**0.001**
Femoral condyle size						
M-L epicondylar distance	0.447	0.100	**<0.001**	0.475	0.086	**<0.001**
LPC offset distance	0.468	0.288	0.112	0.497	0.267	0.072
Tunnel axis angle in						
Coronal plane	0.047	0.010	**<0.001**	0.033	0.009	**0.001**
Sagittal plane	0.001	0.0112	0.933	−0.009	0.004	**0.038**
Axial plane	0.029	0.0088	**0.003**	0.022	0.010	**0.038**

M-L medial-to lateral, *LPC* lateral posterior condyle
[a]Values <0.05 are displayed in bold

Table 4 Multivariate linear regression analysis for correlation between femoral tunnel length and tunnel axis angle in three dimensional planes[a] (Entry criteria *p*-value <0.05)

	AM Femoral Tunnel			PL Femoral Tunnel		
Variables	Beta coefficient (β)	Standard error β	*p*-value	Beta coefficient (β)	Standard error β	*p*-value
Tunnel axis angle in						
Coronal plane	0.025	0.010	**0.022**	−0.001	0.012	0.909
Sagittal plane	0.017	0.007	**0.029**	−0.004	0.004	0.331
Axial plane	0.007	0.009	0.493	0.026	0.009	**0.008**

AM anteromedial, *PL* posterolateral
[a]Values <0.05 are displayed in bold. Adjusted R square: 0.8012 in AM, 0.6996 in PL femoral tunnel

To attain adequate tunnel length with the AM portal technique and prevent posterior wall breakage, many researchers have investigated femoral tunnel orientation and intraosseous length changes with knee flexion angle. Basdekis et al. [20] and Bedi et al. [25] noted that increasing knee flexion increases the tunnel length and decreases the risk of posterior cortical breakage. Iyyampillai et al. suggested that femoral tunnel drilling with maximal knee hyperflexion in ACL reconstruction consistently produced tunnel lengths greater than 30 mm with no posterior wall fractures [26]. However, others have suggested that increased sagittal inclination or reduced guide wire axial angles have little effect on tunnel length [20, 25, 27]. Some have refuted the correlation of knee flexion angle with tunnel length because maximum flexion varies from one subject to another. In addition, tunnel lengths might be affected by patient height, weight, leg size, operative positioning, and larger lateral femoral condyle dimensions [14, 26].

However, previous studies have been based on fixed intra-articular tunnel orientation by drilling with a straight guide pin. We thought it was necessary to investigate tunnel configurations made using curved guides with a three-dimensional approach because it allows a certain degree of control over intra-articular tunnel orientation. Few previous studies have investigated the ideal tunnel axis angle for longer tunnel lengths [22, 28]. These studies were limited because they were experimental studies using a bone saw or cadaver, and the results are difficult to reproduce in a practical surgical situation. To our knowledge, no in vivo studies have been conducted with respect to the potential correlation between femoral tunnel length and guide pin entrance angle after anatomic ACLR with the TP technique.

Regression analyses confirmed our hypothesis that tunnel length is influenced by changes in the tunnel axis angle, and the AM and PL tunnels were significantly correlated with changes in the tunnel axis angle for each different plane.

For AM tunnels, multivariate regression showed that tunnel length had significant correlations with tunnel orientation in the sagittal and coronal planes (p = 0.022, p = 0.029, respectively) with high reliability (adjusted R^2 = 0.801), while there was no significant correlation in the axial plane (p = 0.493). We interpreted this result as 1) longer tunnel lengths can be achieved when the sagittal tunnel angle is increased because outer orifice of the tunnel on the globular-shaped lateral condyle would be made further from the tunnel placement position, 2) the increased coronal tunnel angle provides tunnels with longer hypotenuses, and 3) there was no significant correlation in axial tunnel angle with tunnel length because the inner orifice of the AM tunnels is located in the posterior side of the anatomic ACL footprint, making it technically difficult to create a tunnel outlet oriented near the lateral epicondyle or the apex of lateral femoral condyle, due to abrupt tunnel bending angles. Contrary to the AM tunnels, for the PL tunnels, only the axial tunnel angle showed a significant correlation to tunnel length (p = 0.008, adjusted R^2 = 0.700). We explained this result as 1) the PL tunnel can made easily in the outer orifice near the apex of the lateral femoral condyle, lateral epicondyle, and nearer to the lateral epicondyle, which would increase the axial tunnel angle and lengthen the tunnel, and 2) significant correlations with the tunnel axis angle in the sagittal and coronal planes were not identified due to restricted changes in the tunnel axis angle in the sagittal and coronal planes by its more intra-articular horizontal tunnel orientation even though the curved guide was used.

Recently, the CLANCY 42° curved guide (Clancy Anatomic Cruciate Guide System; Smith & Nephew, Andover, MA) has been utilized with the TP technique to access native femoral ACL insertion. This method achieves longer tunnel lengths with straight, rigid instrumentation that does not require hyperflexion, but is associated with the loss of visualization, fat pad ingress, poor arthroscopic inflow, inability to seat instrumentation, and the bending of rigid guide wires [14]. Andrew et al. noticed that commercially available flexible reamers and curved guides result in longer femoral interosseous tunnel lengths than those achieved with a straight guide pin [14, 29]. Furthermore, the rotational freedom of the intra-articular portion of a curved guide can assure a wide variability of tunnel angle orientation (Fig. 1) (video clip is available as a Additional file 1: Movie S1).

Our results provide a technical consideration for the acquisition of longer tunnel lengths, combined with the use of commercially available flexible reamer and curved guide systems. This study also indicates that three-dimensional tunnel orientations should be stressed for appropriate femoral tunnel length in anatomic ACL reconstruction.

This study has several limitations. At first, there may be a certain degree of variability in the AM and PL femoral tunnel center locations. However, every efforts were put to standardize the starting position of femoral tunnels according to anatomic landmarks of the lateral femur and the knee flexion angle, described in previous literature from our team [15, 24]. And the individual data in the present study has been controlled for patient factors and anatomic variables that may affect tunnel length, and this study was performed using 3D virtual models constructed by applying reverse engineering software with high reliability and accuracy. Several authors have stressed the limitations of two-dimensional radiographic assessment [30, 31]. Khalfayan et al. [32] included inadequate radiographic data as one of the exclusion criteria in their study. Sommer et al. [33] were concerned with tunnel invisibility on the tunnel view and inaccurate projection on the lateral view. Seconds, we are not able to be sure that all femoral tunnels in this study provide the best configuration of tunnels. However, our considerations at femoral tunneling should be common agreements to other surgeons for anatomic ACL reconstruction.

Conclusion

Drilling at a higher angle in the coronal and sagittal planes in AM tunnels and at a higher angle in the axial plane in PL tunnels decreases the incidence of short femoral tunnels.

Abbreviations

AAM: Accessory anteromedial; ACLR: Anterior cruciate ligament reconstruction; AM: Anteromedial; CT: Computed tomography; HTO: High tibial osteotomy; LPC offset distance: Lateral posterior condyle (LPC) AP size; M-L: From medial to lateral; PL: Posterolateral; TP: Transportal

Acknowledgements

The authors thank all members of the Sports Medicine Center, Samsung Medical Center for their great scientific debates.

Funding

This research was supported by a grant of the Korea Health Technology R&D Project through the Korea Health Industry Development Institute (KHIDI), funded by the Ministry of Health & Welfare, Republic of Korea (grant number: HI15C2424) and by the National Research Foundation of Korea(NRF) grant funded by the Korea government(MSIP) (NO.2012R1A1A2044586). The funding sources were not involved in the study design, collection, analysis or interpretation of the data, writing of the manuscript, or in the decision to submit the manuscript for publication.

Authors' contributions

JHW and BHL participated in the study design and helped to draft the manuscript. DKL as a consultant for statistical analysis performed the statistical analysis. STC conceived of the study, and participated in its design and coordination and helped to draft the manuscript. All authors read and approved the final manuscript.

Competing interests

The authors declare that they have no competing interests.

.Consent for publication

The authors have received written consent from all patients to publish this study

Author details

[1]Department of Orthopaedic Surgery, Samsung Medical Center, Sungkyunkwan University School of Medicine, Seoul 06351, South Korea. [2]Department of Health Sciences and Technology, SAIHST, Sungkyunkwan University, Seoul 06351, South Korea. [3]Department of Medical Device Management and Research, SAIHST, Sungkyunkwan University, Seoul 06351, South Korea. [4]Department of Orthopaedic Surgery, Konyang University Hospital, 158, Gwanjeodong-ro, Seo-gu, Daejeon, South Korea. [5]Department of Orthopaedic Surgery, Kang-Dong Sacred Heart Hospital, Hallym University Medical Center, Gil-dong, Seoul 134-701, South Korea.

References

1. Bedi A, Maak T, Musahl V, Citak M, O'Loughlin PF, Choi D, et al. Effect of tibial tunnel position on stability of the knee after anterior cruciate ligament reconstruction: is the tibial tunnel position most important? Am J Sports Med. 2011;39:366–73.
2. Debandi A, Maeyama A, Hoshino Y, Asai S, Goto B, Smolinski P, et al. The effect of tunnel placement on rotational stability after ACL reconstruction: evaluation with use of triaxial accelerometry in a porcine model. Knee Surg Sports Traumatol Arthrosc. 2013;21:589–95.
3. Zantop T, Diermann N, Schumacher T, Schanz S, Fu FH, Petersen W. Anatomical and nonanatomical double-bundle anterior cruciate ligament reconstruction: importance of femoral tunnel location on knee kinematics. Am J Sports Med. 2008;36:678–85.
4. Yasuda K, van Eck CF, Hoshino Y, Fu FH, Tashman S. Anatomic single- and double-bundle anterior cruciate ligament reconstruction, part 1: basic science. Am J Sports Med. 2011;39:1789–99.
5. Bernard M, Hertel P, Lais E, Gomez F. Reconstruction of the proximal insertion of the anterior cruciate ligament. Studies on the accuracy of a non-instrumental method. Unfallchirurg. 1990;93:565–9.
6. Giron F, Buzzi R, Aglietti P. Femoral tunnel position in anterior cruciate ligament reconstruction using three techniques. A cadaver study. Arthroscopy. 1999;15:750–6.
7. Arnold MP, Kooloos J, van Kampen A. Single-incision technique misses the anatomical femoral anterior cruciate ligament insertion: a cadaver study. Knee Surg Sports Traumatol Arthrosc. 2001;9:194–9.
8. Pastrone A, Ferro A, Bruzzone M, Bonasia DE, Pellegrino P, D'Elicio D, et al. Anterior cruciate ligament reconstruction creating the femoral tunnel through the anteromedial portal. Surgical technique. Curr Rev Musculoskelet Med. 2011;4:52–6.

9. Lubowitz JH. Anteromedial portal technique for the anterior cruciate ligament femoral socket: pitfalls and solutions. Arthroscopy. 2009;25:95–101.
10. Rupp S, Muller B, Seil R. Knee laxity after ACL reconstruction with a BPTB graft. Knee Surg Sports Traumatol Arthrosc. 2001;9:72–6.
11. Scopp JM, Jasper LE, Belkoff SM, Moorman CT 3rd. The effect of oblique femoral tunnel placement on rotational constraint of the knee reconstructed using patellar tendon autografts. Arthroscopy. 2004;20:294–9.
12. Howell SM, Gittins ME, Gottlieb JE, Traina SM, Zoellner TM. The relationship between the angle of the tibial tunnel in the coronal plane and loss of flexion and anterior laxity after anterior cruciate ligament reconstruction. Am J Sports Med. 2001;29:567–74.
13. Ferretti M, Ekdahl M, Shen W, Fu FH. Osseous landmarks of the femoral attachment of the anterior cruciate ligament: an anatomic study. Arthroscopy. 2007;23:1218–25.
14. Silver AG, Kaar SG, Grisell MK, Reagan JM, Farrow LD. Comparison between rigid and flexible systems for drilling the femoral tunnel through an anteromedial portal in anterior cruciate ligament reconstruction. Arthroscopy. 2010;26:790–5.
15. Kim JG, Wang JH, Lim HC, Ahn JH. Femoral graft bending angle and femoral tunnel geometry of transportal and outside-in techniques in anterior cruciate ligament reconstruction: an in vivo 3-dimensional computed tomography analysis. Arthroscopy. 2012;28:1682–94.
16. Fu FH, Jordan SS. The lateral intercondylar ridge–a key to anatomic anterior cruciate ligament reconstruction. J Bone Joint Surg Am. 2007;89:2103–4.
17. Yasuda K, Kondo E, Ichiyama H, Kitamura N, Tanabe Y, Tohyama H, et al. Anatomic reconstruction of the anteromedial and posterolateral bundles of the anterior cruciate ligament using hamstring tendon grafts. Arthroscopy. 2004;20:1015–25.
18. Purnell ML, Larson AI, Clancy W. Anterior cruciate ligament insertions on the tibia and femur and their relationships to critical bony landmarks using high-resolution volume-rendering computed tomography. Am J Sports Med. 2008;36:2083–90.
19. Ziegler CG, Pietrini SD, Westerhaus BD, Anderson CJ, Wijdicks CA, Johansen S, et al. Arthroscopically pertinent landmarks for tunnel positioning in single-bundle and double-bundle anterior cruciate ligament reconstructions. Am J Sports Med. 2011;39:743–52.
20. Basdekis G, Abisafi C, Christel P. Influence of knee flexion angle on femoral tunnel characteristics when drilled through the anteromedial portal during anterior cruciate ligament reconstruction. Arthroscopy. 2008;24:459–64.
21. Wang JH, Kim JG, Ahn JH, Lim HC, Hoshino Y, Fu FH. Is femoral tunnel length correlated with the intercondylar notch and femoral condyle geometry after double-bundle anterior cruciate ligament reconstruction using the transportal technique? An in vivo computed tomography analysis. Arthroscopy. 2012;28:1094–103.
22. Iyyampillai G, Raman ET, Rajan DV, Krishnamoorthy A, Sahanand S. Determinants of femoral tunnel length in anterior Cruciate ligament reconstruction: CT analysis of the influence of tunnel orientation on the length. Knee Surg Relat Res. 2013;25:207–14.
23. Chang CB, Choi JY, Koh IJ, Lee KJ, Lee KH, Kim TK. Comparisons of femoral tunnel position and length in anterior cruciate ligament reconstruction: modified transtibial versus anteromedial portal techniques. Arthroscopy. 2011;27:1389–94.
24. Lubowitz JH, Konicek J. Anterior cruciate ligament femoral tunnel length: cadaveric analysis comparing anteromedial portal versus outside-in technique. Arthroscopy. 2010;26:1357–62.
25. Bedi A, Raphael B, Maderazo A, Pavlov H, Williams RJ 3rd. Transtibial versus anteromedial portal drilling for anterior cruciate ligament reconstruction: a cadaveric study of femoral tunnel length and obliquity. Arthroscopy. 2010;26:342–50.
26. Tompkins M, Milewski MD, Carson EW, Brockmeier SF, Hamann JC, Hart JM, et al. Femoral tunnel length in primary anterior cruciate ligament reconstruction using an accessory medial portal. Arthroscopy. 2013;29:238–43.
27. Hamilton SC, Jackson ER 2nd, Karas SG. Anterior cruciate ligament femoral tunnel drilling through anteromedial portal: axial plane drill angle affects tunnel length. Arthroscopy. 2011;27:522–5.
28. Lubowitz JH, Akhavan S, Waterman BR, Aalami-Harandi A, Konicek J. Technique for creating the anterior cruciate ligament femoral socket: optimizing femoral footprint anatomic restoration using outside-in drilling. Arthroscopy. 2013;29:522–8.
29. Park SH, Moon SW, Lee BH, Chae SH, Ahn JH, Chang M, et al. The sagittal plane angle and tunnel-related complications in double-bundle anterior cruciate ligament reconstruction using the transportal technique: an in vivo imaging study. Arthroscopy. 2015;31:283–92.
30. Golish SR, Baumfeld JA, Schoderbek RJ, Miller MD. The effect of femoral tunnel starting position on tunnel length in anterior cruciate ligament reconstruction: a cadaveric study. Arthroscopy. 2007;23:1187–92.
31. Hoser C, Tecklenburg K, Kuenzel KH, Fink C. Postoperative evaluation of femoral tunnel position in ACL reconstruction: plain radiography versus computed tomography. Knee Surg Sports Traumatol Arthrosc. 2005;13:256–62.
32. Khalfayan EE, Sharkey PF, Alexander AH, Bruckner JD, Bynum EB. The relationship between tunnel placement and clinical results after anterior cruciate ligament reconstruction. Am J Sports Med. 1996;24:335–41.
33. Sommer C, Friederich NF, Muller W. Improperly placed anterior cruciate ligament grafts: correlation between radiological parameters and clinical results. Knee Surg Sports Traumatol Arthrosc. 2000;8:207–13.

2

Biomechanical evaluation of an arthroscopic transosseous repair as a revision option for failed rotator cuff surgery

Felix Dyrna[1], Andreas Voss[1], Leo Pauzenberger[2], Elifho Obopilwe[2], Augustus D. Mazzocca[2], Alessandro Castagna[3] and Cory Edgar[2*]

Abstract

Background: The number of revision rotator cuff cases is increasing. The literature is lacking guidance or biomechanical evaluation for fixation strength in a revision case scenario. Therefore, the aim of the study was to provide biomechanical data investigating primary fixation strength of a transosseous technique after anchor pullout failure of a single row reconstruction. It was hypothesized that an arthroscopic transosseous repair system as a procedure for rotator cuff revisions is providing equivalent stability compared to a primary single row suture anchor fixation due to change of fixation site.

Methods: Eight matched pairs ($n = 16$) of fresh frozen human shoulders were tested. The paired specimen shoulders were randomly divided into two repair groups (**A** single row and **B** primary transosseous repair). The potted specimens were mounted onto the Servohydraulic test system. Both groups were tested under cyclic loading followed by load to failure testing. Suture anchor repair shoulders (group A) that were tested to failure underwent a revision transosseous repair and were subsequently tested again using the same setup and protocol (group C).

Results: The mean native footprint areas did not show a significant difference between groups. The reconstructed footprint area showed a significantly greater coverage in favor of the transosseous repair. Ultimate load to failure of reconstructions with the primary anchor fixation (344.73 N ± 63.19) and the primary transosseous device (375.36 N ± 70.27) was not significantly higher compared to the revision repair (332.19 N ± 119.01 $p = 0.45$, $p = 0.53$).

Conclusion: The tested transosseous anchor device is a suitable option to widely used suture anchors, providing equivalent fixation properties even in a revision case scenario.

Level of evidence: Basic Science Study, Biomechanics.

Keywords: Rotator cuff, Cuff repair, Revision, Transosseous repair, Arthroscopic repair

* Correspondence: coedgar@uchc.edu
[2]Department of Orthopaedic Surgery, University of Connecticut, Farmington, CT, USA
Full list of author information is available at the end of the article

Background

Despite promising results in biomechanical studies, the clinical re-tear rate of rotator cuff repairs is still high. In the literature the incidence of recurrences has been reported of over 30% for small injuries [1, 2] and may extend to 90% in cases of massive tears [3–6]. Reasons for failure of reconstruction are variegated [7]. Rotator cuff revision surgery is always challenging and results are often inferior to primary repairs [8, 9]. Arthroscopic repair may present advantages compared to historical open transosseous repairs, such as minimal infraction of the deltoid muscle, the ability to dynamically inspect the entire glenohumeral joint for associated pathologies, characterize tear patterns, and decrease postoperative pain and stiffness [10, 11].

The quest for improved methods of rotator cuff repair led to the development of all-arthroscopic transosseous rotator cuff repair techniques [12], which could potentially combine the biomechanical strengths of open transosseous repairs with all of the advantages of arthroscopic techniques. Recent studies, that have compared traditional transosseous equivalent techniques with modern single- and double-row anchor-based configurations, showed superior load to failure strength in transosseous repairs [13, 14].

The purpose of the present study was to compare displacement under cyclic loading, load-to-failure, and footprint coverage of rotator cuff reconstructions performed with a new, all-arthroscopic transosseous repair (TOR) system and an established single row suture anchor repair configuration, as (a) a primary repair technique and (b) in case of failed anchor based initial repair. Our primary hypothesis was that an arthroscopic transosseous repair system as a procedure for rotator cuff revisions is providing equivalent stability compared to a primary single row suture anchor fixation due to change of fixation site.

Methods

Preparation

The test involved the use of eight matched pairs ($n = 16$) fresh frozen human shoulders without macroscopic evidence of rotator cuff pathology. The mean age of specimens was 69,9 years with a range from 74 to 66 years including 8 female and 8 male specimens. All specimens were obtained from Medcure Inc. (Portland, OR). The study was reported via Human Research Determination Form to the institutional review board (IRB) of the University of Connecticut and it was documented, that no IRB approval was required (de-identified specimen do not constitute human subjects research). Specimens were thawed for 24 h at room temperature prior to dissection. Bone Density via micro-CT (Lunar DXE, Madison, Wis) was performed to ensure consistent bone quality among tested specimens at the greater tuberosity in a consistent manner at a 1 × 1-cm area.

Selected specimens were prepared by removing all soft tissues, but leaving the supraspinatus, infraspinatus, and teres minor tendons intact. The native supraspinatus footprint was measured with digital calipers for linear measurements (Absolute Digimatic; Mitutoyo, Kawasaki, Japan). While the supraspinatus muscle was held in a superior direction, the width of the footprint at its greatest dimension was measured by placing 1 limb of the digital caliper precisely on the articular edge of the intact supraspinatus tendon and the other arm of the caliper on the lateral bursal-side edge of the insertion. The anterior and posterior insertions of the supraspinatus were measured likewise. This procedure allowed an estimated contact area to be calculated. Although the supraspinatus footprint does not represent a true rectangle, these measurements provided a consistent means to compare the contact areas of the intact and repaired supraspinatus tendons. To ensure correct measurements, results were compared with a measured area using a MicroScribe digitizer (Immersion, San Jose, CA) by lifting the supraspinatus muscle and tracing the outline of the attachment [15], before creating the tear. The same investigator performed all footprint measurements. The next step involved the sharp dissection of the supraspinatus tendon from its footprint to create a uniform 20x10mm full-thickness tendon tissue defect approximately 5 mm proximally to the humeral insertion of the tendon, as previously described [16].

Prior to the repair the footprint area was macroscopically completely decorticated to mimic a revision case scenario and weaken the bone quality. The paired specimen shoulders were randomly divided into two groups. A total of 8 specimens per group were tested.

Repair configurations

Group A Single Row

The single-row repair was performed using two double loaded titanium corkscrew anchors (Arthrex, Naples, FL) placed lateral to the cartilage margin in the greater tuberosity 12 mm apart. The anchors were placed at the "dead man's angle" to maximize pullout strength [17]. Both strands of No. 2 FiberWire (Arthrex, Naples, FL) in each anchor were then shuttled in a typical fashion using a Suture Lasso (Fig. 1a). Knot tying was performed in arthroscopic fashion using a standard knot pusher with overhand throws, alternating half hitches and posts to maximize loop and knot security [18].

Group B primary TOR

The transosseous repair was performed with the Sharc-FT® system (NCS Lab, Medical Devices Factory),

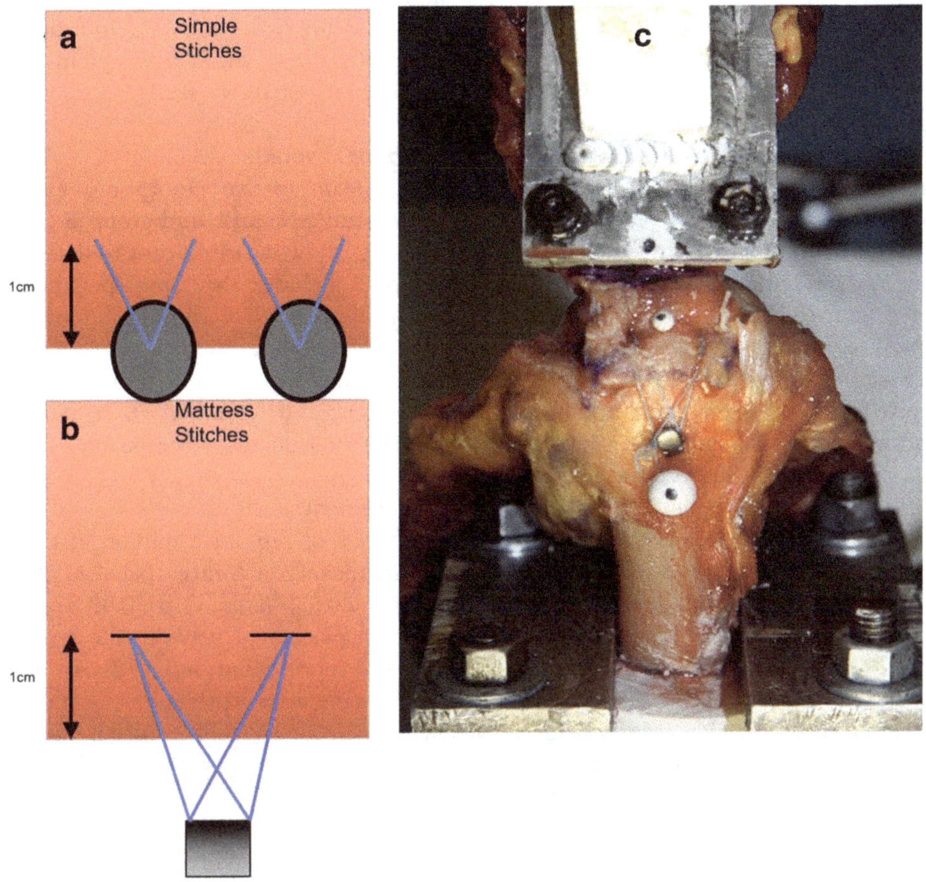

Fig. 1 shows (**a**) single row repair, (**b**) TOR with Sharc-FT, (**c**) TOR repair final set-up

which is based on diverging canals created by a drill guide the Taylor stitcher® (NCS Lab, Medical Devices Factory) through the great tuberosity of the humerus consisting of one lateral entering and - depending on tear size - multiple medial exit tunnels. The transosseous configuration involved the creation of a lateral entry hole centered laterally from the lesion and two medial exit holes, one anterior and one posterior with a distance of 10-12 mm in between. Therefore, the first medial exit tunnel, a 2 mm hole in the ventral third of the footprint was punched with the guidance of the Taylor stitcher® device (NCS Lab, Medical Devices Factory). Furthermore, this guide was used to place the lateral 2 mm hole 3 cm from the greater tuberosity edge. The posterior medial exit tunnel was created in the same manner while keeping the guide in the lateral exit hole. Once the canals were placed, the Sharc-FT (NCS Lab, Medical Devices Factory) device preloaded with two internal sutures was used to shuttle the definite sutures, No. 2 FiberWire (Arthrex, Naples, FL). These sutures were arranged to obtain two mattress stitches over the tendon (Fig. 1b), then the four suture limbs were used to close the suture loop passing them through the eyelet on the device to function as a second row increasing the footprint coverage and area of compression [19].

Group C revision Transosseous repair with Sharc-FT

After load-to-failure testing of the single-row group, shoulders, which showed a sufficiently intact footprint and tendon after initial testing, underwent a revision procedure with the Sharc-FT(R) (NCS Lab, Medical Devices Factory) system following the before mentioned technique. Hence, comparing transosseous refixation with this device as a suitable revision technique. Again the aiming device (Taylor stitcher) was used to place as previously descripted the two converging tunnels at the spot of the removed anchors and the revision repair was completed.

Biomechanical testing

All samples were tested in air at room temperature. The humerus was cut 20 cm from the joint, centered in a polyvinylchloride pipe, and potted with plaster of Paris. The potted cadaveric specimen was then mounted on the testing apparatus with the tendons oriented in line with the anatomic pull of the myo-tendinous unit The medial portion of the supraspinatus tendon was freeze-clamped and attached to a MTS, Eden Prairie, MN) as described in previous studies [18, 20]. In this setup, the specimens were tested under cyclic load, while measuring gap formation. To quantify gap formation one marker was placed laterally below the greater tuberosity and one in line centric on the musculotendinous junction of the supraspinatus.

A video digitizing system that involved video recording and computer digitization of the markers, creation of centroids representing the center of the markers, and the calculation of distances between them with MaxTRAQ 2D (Innovision Systems, Inc., Columbiaville, Michigan) software was used (Fig. 1c).

After a preload phase with 10 N for 1 min and ten initial cycles, the load was set to change from a minimum value of 10 N to a maximum of 180 N at a velocity of 33 mm/s [21–24] for a total of 200 cycles [21, 25–27]. In the event of gap formation greater than 5 mm, the test was stopped and the number of completed cycles was noted. After a preload phase samples that reached 200 cycles with a gap variation less than 5 mm were then tested to load-of-failure at a rate of 33 mm/s.

Shoulders from the anchor repair group A that were tested to failure underwent a revision transosseous repair and were subsequently tested regarding gap formation under cyclic loading and load-to-failure using the same setup and protocol group C.

Statistical analyses

Given the exploratory nature of this study, an a priori power analysis was difficult. We anticipated a medium effect size (30–45% difference in load to failure or about 100 N) between the primary suture anchor and revision transosseous repair with an estimated variability of ±50 N. A sample size of 6 per group will provide 80% power to detect a difference of 100 N an alpha value of 0.02 between the repair groups. Descriptive statistics were calculated using mean and standard deviation for the repair groups. Both independent and pair t test were used to compare differences in load to failure, slope, displacement, and footprint reconstruction. The revision trans-osseous repair group included the same shoulders tested in primary suture group creating dependency within the data which necessitated the use of separate t tests as opposes to a global ANOVA. To avoid inflating our Type I error rate, a Bonferroni adjusted p value of 0.02 was used as the threshold for statistical significance. All statistical analysis was performed using Stata 12 (StataCorp. 2011. *Stata Statistical Software: Release 12.* College Station, TX: StataCorp LP.).

Results

The results for footprint reconstruction, displacement during cyclic loading, load to failure and stiffness were summarized in Fig. 2 a-d. The bone quality (BMD) was measured for each specimen and did not differ between groups (group A mean 0.361 g/cm^2 ± 0.05 and group B 0.435 g/cm^2 ± 0.09 $p = 0.094$).

Footprint coverage

The mean native footprint areas in group **A** 264.91 mm^2 ± 103.12, and group **B** 307.68 mm^2 ± 116.13 did not show a significant difference $p = 0.48$. Since group **C** includes the same specimens as group **A** the native footprints are equal. The covered footprint areas after the repair in group **A** 192.48 mm^2 ± 59.55, group **B** 246.25 mm^2 ± 61.16, and group **C** 259.93 mm^2 ± 43.28 were compared A vs. B $p = 0.01$ and A vs. C $p = 0.12$ in favor of the transosseous repair.

Displacement

200 cycles of repetitive motion at time zero resulted in no significant differences between the three groups (A vs. B $p = 0.57$, A vs. C $p = 0.98$ and B vs. C $p = 0.47$). Mean displacement between the groups was not significant and represented in Fig. 2b An overall displacement over 5 mm was considered as a failure. This occurred once in group **A** and group **B** as the anchor already pulled out but not in group **C**. (Fig. 2b).

Ultimate Load to Failure

Ultimate load to failure of reconstructions with the primary anchor fixation (344.73 N ± 63.19 group A) and the primary Sharc-FT device (375.36 N ± 70.27 group B) was not significantly higher compared to the revision repair (332.19 N ± 119.01 group C, A vs. B $p = 0.45$, A vs. C $p = 0.53$). There were also no significant differences comparing the slope of the constructs, and yield loads. (Fig. 2c, d). The failure modes were 5/8 (63%) anchor pullouts and 3/8 (37%) suture pull through in group A. For group B the main failure was suture cutting through tendon 5/8 (63%) and 3/8 (37%) bony suture pullouts. Group C showed 6/8 (75%) anchor pullouts and 2/8 (25%) suture tendon interface failures.

Discussion

The purpose of this study was to evaluate the load to failure, stiffness, displacement under cyclic loading, and footprint reconstruction of two different fixations at time zero. The number of suture passages through the tendon was equal ($n = 4$) between the groups to focus on bony fixation strength. Generated results did confirm the original hypothesis that the transosseous fixation technique restores similar fixation strength in a revision case scenario compared to primary single row anchor fixation. We found no significant difference in the biomechanical properties of the compared techniques. The rotator cuff repair represents one of the most frequently

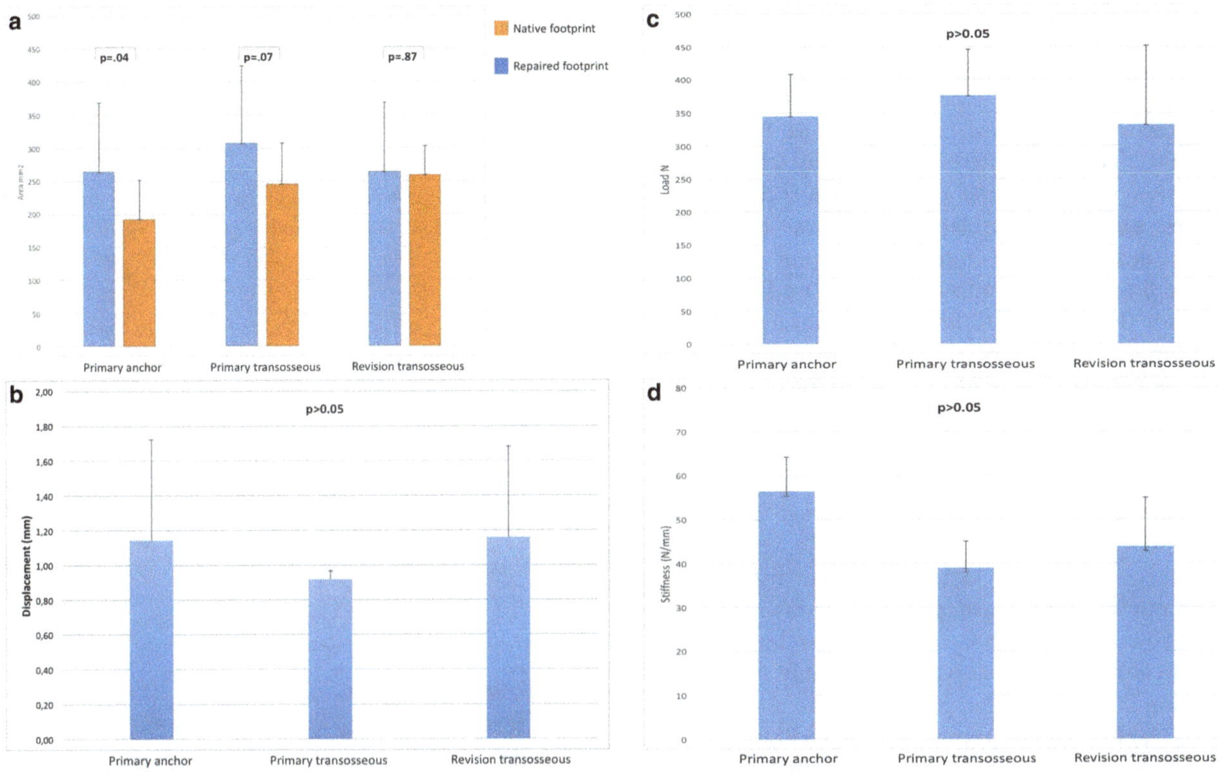

Fig. 2 (**a**) displaces the native and repaired footprint data for each repair technique, (**b**) represents displacement data after cyclic loading, (**c, d**) shows ultimate load to failure results and stiffness of the repair constructs

performed orthopedic surgical intervention [28]. Hence of numerous technological innovations, the re-tear rate is still unsatisfactory high [3, 4, 7, 10] .With a raising number of surgeons performing their arthroscopic rotator cuff repairs with suture anchors our attention has been placed on a possible revision fixation technique. To our mind the TOR serves as a reasonable option to fulfill this task preserving similar biomechanical parameters by changing the fixation site. McLaughlin was the first one describing a transosseous rotator cuff repair back in 1944 [29]. Since then a progress of technological improvements established a save and reproducible technique that can even be performed arthroscopically [19]. According to Gerber et al. [30], in theory a perfect repair should combined high fixation strength, minimal gap formation, and sufficient mechanical stability for tendon-bone healing. The existing literature consist of studies demonstrating that transosseous techniques have equivalent biomechanical properties relative to suture anchor fixation [21, 31–33]. Lately, Behrens et al. [34] showed that traditional transosseous suture construct without anchors can even provide an initial fixation strength equivalent to suture bridge repairs. The stress load is distributed wider in the bone tunnel of the transosseous repair, whereas in suture anchor repair, resulting in less local stress loads [35]. In addition, the pressure is more homogenously assigned in transosseous sutures in opposite to the anchor repair, where high values may be a risk factor for ischemic tissue damage [36]. To evaluate the Gap-formation and displacement two optical markers were positioned centric on either side of the repair as shown in Fig. 1c. This position was chosen to analyze the average displacement since Tashjian et al. [32] found that gapping significantly increased from the anterior to posterior region. The gap formation observed in our three groups did not differ significantly and approached similar values as previously reported in literature [34]. Hence, we had two failures in groups A and B and no failure in group C during cyclic loading due to anchor pull outs caused by weak bone quality. The bone quality (BMD) was measured for each specimen and did not differ between groups (group A mean 0.361 g/cm^2 ± 0.05 and group B 0.435 g/cm^2 ± 0.09 $p = 0.094$). The macroscopically decortication was performed after the BMD measuring and prior to the repairs to mimic poor bone quality. In regarding to Tingart et al. [37] who published that a successful rotator cuff repair highly depends the bone density at the greater tuberosity we expected to weaken our primary suture anchor repair by this decortication process but we still reached comparable anchor pull out values compared to the literature [31]. Pointing out that we may did not weaken the bone significantly even if macroscopically a full removal of cortical bone was performed. Pointing out that the suture anchors mainly rely on the trabecular, not the cortical bone [38]. During our ultimate load to failure testing, anchor pullout was the main failure mode in all groups A-C. The most interesting factor is that we were able to show that even after pulling out a suture anchor repair the subsequent implanted TOR was not significantly weaker than the initial anchor nor the initial TOR. Leading to the assumption that after a failed single row anchor repair the TOR is a possible revision option.

Knowing the initial strength characteristics of different rotator cuff repair techniques may influence surgical decision-making and may ultimately improve patient outcomes. Traditionally, the TOR technique was performed open and later modified to mini-open procedures. Apreleva et al. [39] demonstrated that TOR provides superior supraspinatus footprint coverage compared to suture anchor systems. Similar results were found in our study comparing a transosseous repair with a single row suture anchor.. The primary limitation of this study is that it is an in-vitro study only incorporating fixation strength at time point zero and a small sample size. The results cannot be extrapolated to the potential impact of tendon healing. Further the study specimens had intact rotator cuff tendons that do not replicate normal tendon and joint degeneration. We also created an isolated supraspinatus defect, which does not necessarily replicate the clinical situation. We try to include specimens with comparable age and bone quality. Lastly, the repairs in our study were performed under the ideal condition of being open procedures. Finally, the results of our study suggest that the initial fixation strength of single row suture anchor and TOR for rotator cuff repair at time point zero with comparable tendon and bone is equivalent. Both reconstructions prevented Gap-formation and early failure but preserved good footprint coverage. The revision TOR proved its biomechanical properties to be fully capable as an option for primary and secondary repairs. The clinical relevance of this study showed that there is no difference when comparing a current used arthroscopic single row suture anchor repair with a novel arthroscopic transosseous technique, supporting its use as a revision option.

Conclusion

The tested transosseous anchor device is a suitable option to widely used suture anchors, providing equivalent fixation properties even in a revision case scenario for single row reconstructions.

Abbreviations

ANOVA: Analysis of variance; BMD: Bone mineral density; TOR: Transosseous repair

Funding

The University of Connecticut Health Center / UConn Musculoskeletal Institute has received direct funding and material support for this study from NCS Lab s.r.l. (Carpi, Italia). The company had no influence on study design, data collection, interpretation of the results, or the final manuscript.
Augustus D. Mazzocca has received research support from Arthrex, Inc., Naples, Florida.
This work was supported by the German Research Foundation (DFG) and the Technische Universität München within the funding programme Open Access Publishing.

Consent to publish

No consent for publication was needed, because of the de-identified data.

Authors' contributions

Felix Dyrna, M.D. Principle investigator, data analysis, biomechanical testing.
Andreas Voss, M.D. Biomechanical testing and data analysis.
Leo Pauzenberger, M.D. Revising the work critically for important intellectual content.
Elifho Obopilwe, M.S. Biomechanical support for testing and setup.
Augustus D. Mazzocca Data analysis, native language corrections.
M.S., M.D.
Alessandro Castagna M.D. Major contribution to discussion.
Cory Edga M.D., Ph.D. Surgical procedure and final approval of manuscript to be published.
The authors attest that the manuscript has been read and approved by all authors, and each author believes that the manuscript represents honest work.

Competing Interests

The following authors declare that they have no competing interests: AV, LP, EO, AC.
The following authors declare that they have competing interests:
- FD received finical support from the German Research Foundation (DFG) and the Technische Universität München for publication of this manuscript (processing fee).
- ADM received research funding from Arthrex Inc., (Naples, Fl, USA).
- CE received direct funding and material support for this study from NCS Lab s.r.l. (Carpi, Italia).
None of the authors have non-financial competing interests.

Author details

[1]Department of Orthopaedic Sports Medicine, Technical University, Munich, Germany. [2]Department of Orthopaedic Surgery, University of Connecticut, Farmington, CT, USA. [3]Department of Shoulder and Elbow IRCCS Humanitas Institute, Milan, Italy.

References

1. Gazielly DF, Gleyze P, Montagnon C. Functional and anatomical results after rotator cuff repair. Clin Orthop Relat Res 1994;&NA;:43???53.
2. Boileau P, Brassart N, Watkinson DJ, Carles M, Hatzidakis AM, Krishnan SG. Arthroscopic repair of full-thickness tears of the supraspinatus: does the tendon really heal? J Bone Joint Surg Am. The American Orthopedic Association. 2005;87:1229–40.
3. Galatz LM, Ball CM, Teefey SA, Middleton WD, Yamaguchi K. The outcome and repair integrity of completely arthroscopically repaired large and massive rotator cuff tears. J Bone Joint Surg. 2004;86-A:219–24.
4. Heuberer PR, Smolen D, Pauzenberger L, Plachel F, Salem S, Laky B, et al. Longitudinal long-term magnetic resonance imaging and clinical follow-up after single-row arthroscopic rotator cuff repair: clinical superiority of structural tendon integrity. Am J Sports Med. 2017;45:1283–8.

5. Charousset C, Grimberg J, Duranthon L-D, Bellaiche L, Petrover D. Can a double-row anchorage technique improve tendon healing in arthroscopic rotator cuff repair?: a prospective, nonrandomized, comparative study of double-row and single-row anchorage techniques with computed tomographic arthrography tendon healing assessment. Am J Sports Med. 2007;35:1247–53.
6. Park J-Y, Siti HT, Keum J-S, Moon S-G, Oh K-S. Does an arthroscopic suture bridge technique maintain repair integrity?: a serial evaluation by ultrasonography. Clin Orthop Relat Res. Springer-Verlag. 2010;468:1578–87.
7. Spennacchio P, Banfi G, Cucchi D, D'Ambrosi R, Cabitza P, Randelli P. Long-term outcome after arthroscopic rotator cuff treatment. Knee Surg Sports Traumatol Arthrosc. Springer Berlin Heidelberg. 2015;23:523–9.
8. Kilinc AS, Giarreti R, Diaz L, Sauzières P, Valenti P. Recurrent rotator cuff tears: an evaluation of open re-surgery results. Eur J Orthop Surg Traumatol. 2010;20:373–80.
9. Parnes N, DeFranco M, Wells JH, Higgins LD, Warner JJP. Complications after arthroscopic revision rotator cuff repair. Arthroscopy. Elsevier. 2013; 29:1479–86.
10. Piasecki DP, Verma NN, Nho SJ, Bhatia S, Boniquit N, Cole BJ, et al. Outcomes after arthroscopic revision rotator cuff repair. Am Orthop Soc Sports Med. 2010;38:40–6.
11. Wilson F, Hinov V, Adams G. Arthroscopic repair of full-thickness tears of the rotator cuff: 2- to 14-year follow-up. Arthroscopy. 2002;18:136–44.
12. Garofalo R, Castagna A, Borroni M, Krishnan SG. Arthroscopic transosseous (anchorless) rotator cuff repair. Knee Surg Sports Traumatol Arthrosc. 2012; 20:1031–5.
13. Lavery KP, Rasmussen JF, Dhawan A. Arthroscopic transosseous-equivalent rotator cuff repair. Arthrosc Tech. 2013;2:e183–5.
14. Lee TQ. Current biomechanical concepts for rotator cuff repair. Clin Orthop Surg. 2013;5:89–97.
15. Curtis AS, Burbank KM, Tierney JJ, Scheller AD, Curran AR. The insertional footprint of the rotator cuff: an anatomic study. Arthroscopy. 2006;22:603–609.e1.
16. Lee S, Mahar A, Bynum K, Pedowitz R. Biomechanical comparison of bioabsorbable sutureless screw anchor versus suture anchor fixation for rotator cuff repair. Arthroscopy. 2005;21:43–7.
17. Burkhart SS. Reprint of: the deadman theory of suture anchors: observations along a South Texas fence line. Arthroscopy. 2014;30:895–9.
18. Mazzocca AD, Millett PJ, Guanche CA, Santangelo SA, Arciero RA. Arthroscopic single-row versus double-row suture anchor rotator cuff repair. Am J Sports Med. 2005;33:1861–8.
19. Baudi P, Rasia Dani E, Campochiaro G, Rebuzzi M, Serafini F, Catani F. The rotator cuff tear repair with a new arthroscopic transosseous system: the Sharc-FT(®). Musculoskelet Surg Springer Milan. 2013;97(Suppl 1):57–61.
20. Beitzel K, Chowaniec DM, McCarthy MB, Cote MP, Russell RP, Obopilwe E, et al. Stability of double-row rotator cuff repair is not adversely affected by scaffold interposition between tendon and bone. Am J Sports Med. 2012;40: 1148–54.
21. Bisson LJ, Manohar LM. A biomechanical comparison of transosseous-suture anchor and suture bridge rotator cuff repairs in cadavers. Am J Sports Med. 2009;37:1991–5.
22. Burkhart SS, Johnson TC, Wirth MA, Athanasiou KA. Cyclic loading of transosseous rotator cuff repairs: tension overload as a possible cause of failure. Arthroscopy. 1997;13:172–6.
23. Meier SW, Meier JD. The effect of double-row fixation on initial repair strength in rotator cuff repair: a biomechanical study. Arthroscopy. 2006;22: 1168–73.
24. Zheng N, Harris HW, Andrews JR. Failure analysis of rotator cuff repair: a comparison of three double-row techniques. J Bone Joint Surg Am. 2008;90: 1034–42.
25. Kim DH, ElAttrache NS, Tibone JE, Jun B-J, DeLaMora SN, Kvitne RS, et al. Biomechanical comparison of a single-row versus double-row suture anchor technique for rotator cuff repair. Am J Sports Med. 2006;34:407–14.
26. Barber FA, Drew OR. A biomechanical comparison of tendon-bone interface motion and cyclic loading between single-row, triple-loaded cuff repairs and double-row, suture-tape cuff repairs using biocomposite anchors. Arthroscopy. 2012;28:1197–205.
27. Anderl W, Heuberer PR, Laky B, Kriegleder B, Reihsner R, Eberhardsteiner J. Superiority of bridging techniques with medial fixation on initial strength. Knee Surg Sports Traumatol Arthrosc. 2012;20:2559–66.
28. Iyengar JJ, Samagh SP, Schairer W, Singh G, Valone FH III, Feeley BT. Current trends in rotator cuff repair: surgical technique, setting, and cost. Arthroscopy. 2014;30:284–8.
29. McLaughlin HL. Lesions of the musculotendinous cuff of the shoulder. The exposure and treatment of tears with retraction. 1944. Clin Orthop Relat Res. 1994;304:3–9.
30. Gerber C, Schneeberger AG, Beck M, Schlegel U. Mechanical strength of repairs of the rotator cuff. J Bone Joint Surg Br. 1994;76:371–80.
31. Pietschmann MF, Fröhlich V, Ficklscherer A, Hausdorf J, Utzschneider S, Jansson V, et al. Pullout strength of suture anchors in comparison with transosseous sutures for rotator cuff repair. Knee Surg Sports Traumatol Arthrosc. Springer-Verlag. 2008;16:504–10.
32. Tashjian RZ, Levanthal E, Spenciner DB, Green A, Fleming BC. Initial fixation strength of massive rotator cuff tears: in vitro comparison of single-row suture anchor and transosseous tunnel constructs. Arthroscopy. 2007;23: 710–6.
33. Frank JB, ElAttrache NS, Dines JS, Blackburn A, Crues J, Tibone JE. Repair site integrity after arthroscopic transosseous-equivalent suture-bridge rotator cuff repair. Am J Sports Med. 2008;36:1496–503.
34. Behrens SB, Bruce B, Zonno AJ, Paller D, Green A. Initial fixation strength of transosseous-equivalent suture bridge rotator cuff repair is comparable with transosseous repair. Am J Sports Med. 2012;40:133–40.
35. Sano H, Yamashita T, Wakabayashi I, Itoi E. Stress distribution in the supraspinatus tendon after tendon repair: suture anchors versus transosseous suture fixation. Am J Sports Med. 2007;35:542–6.
36. Tuoheti Y, Itoi E, Yamamoto N, Seki N, Abe H, Minagawa H, et al. Contact area, contact pressure, and pressure patterns of the tendon-bone interface after rotator cuff repair. Am J Sports Med. 2005;33:1869–74.
37. Tingart MJ, Apreleva M, Lehtinen J, Zurakowski D, Warner JJP. Anchor design and bone mineral density affect the pull-out strength of suture anchors in rotator cuff repair: which anchors are best to use in patients with low bone quality? Am J Sports Med. 2004;32:1466–73.
38. Mahar A, Allred DW, Wedemeyer M, Abbi G, Pedowitz R. A biomechanical and radiographic analysis of standard and intracortical suture anchors for arthroscopic rotator cuff repair. Arthroscopy. 2006;22:130–5.
39. Apreleva M, Ozbaydar M, Fitzgibbons PG, Warner JJP, et al. Arthroscopy. 2002;18:519–26.

3

Radiological changes do not influence clinical mid-term outcome in stemless humeral head replacements with hollow screw fixation: a prospective radiological and clinical evaluation

Philipp R. Heuberer[1,2], Georg Brandl[1], Leo Pauzenberger[1], Brenda Laky[1,2], Bernhard Kriegleder[1] and Werner Anderl[1,2*]

Abstract

Background: Stemless shoulder arthroplasty is a fairly new concept. Clinical and radiological follow-up is essential to prove implant safety and concept. This prospective single-centre study was performed to evaluate the influence of radiological changes on clinical mid-term outcome following stemless humeral head replacement with hollow screw fixation.

Methods: Short- and mid-term radiological and clinical evaluations were performed in 73 consecutive shoulders treated mainly for idiopathic and posttraumatic osteoarthritis with stemless humeral head arthroplasty including 40 hemi- (HSA) and 33 total shoulder arthroplasties (TSA). Operating times of stemless implantations were compared to 110 stemmed anatomical shoulder prostheses. Appearances of humeral radiolucencies or radiological signs of osteolysis or stress shielding were assessed on standardized radiographs. Patients' clinical outcome was evaluated using the Constant score and patients' satisfaction was documented.

Results: Radiological changes, detected in 37.0%, did not affect clinical outcome. Constant scores significantly improved from baseline to short and mid-term follow-up ($p < 0.001$). The majority of patients (96.2%) were satisfied with the procedure. No loosening of the humeral head component was detected during a mean follow-up of 58 months. Operating times were significantly shorter with stemless compared to stemmed implants ($p < 0.001$).

Conclusions: Clinical mid-term outcome after stemless humeral head replacement was not affected by radiological changes.

Keywords: Stemless shoulder arthroplasty, Mid-term outcome, Radiological and clinical results, Hemiarthroplasty, Anatomic shoulder arthroplasty

* Correspondence: werner.anderl@kh-herzjesu.at

[1]St. Vincent Shoulder and Sports Clinic Vienna, Baumgasse 20A, 1030 Vienna, Austria

[2]Austrian Research group for Regenerative and Orthopedic Medicine (AURROM), Vienna, Austria

Background

Shoulder arthroplasty is the standard treatment for patients with severe shoulder osteoarthritis with numbers continually rising. Modern anatomically designed shoulder arthroplasty systems have proven to provide significant pain relief and improvement of function over time [1]. Long-term survivorship is mostly affected by implant related complications [2]. Although loosening of the glenoid component is more common than stem related problems [3], given the growing number of shoulder replacements and revision surgeries, the humeral side becomes increasingly clinically relevant. Loosening is not the only indication for revision, as removal of the humeral stem is also required for implant unrelated complications such as infection or secondary rotator cuff tear. In revision surgery, complications commonly arise with difficulty of stem removal, cement extraction, bone loss or osteolysis due to polyethylene wear debris, and intraoperative fracture associated with potentially longer operating times, increased risk of infection, nerve injuries, and worse outcome [1, 4–6]. Shaft malunion after fracture, where the deformity does not allow an anatomic positioning of the humeral stem [7, 8], is another challenging situation to treat.

An expedient alternative is humeral head resurfacing. Nevertheless, humeral resurfacing is a technically challenging procedure requiring at least 60% of intact humeral head [9]. Firstly, it is mandatory to find the correct centre of rotation to avoid overstuffing and secondly with the remaining head in situ correct glenoid component implantation may be difficult [10].

A contemporary, promising alternative are stemless anatomic shoulder implants, which generally rely on metaphyseal or meta- and epiphyseal fixation, combining the advantages of humeral head resurfacing and common shoulder replacement. Potential benefits are (1) the possibility of anatomic shoulder reconstruction regardless of medial and posterior offset of the proximal humerus, caput-collum-diaphyseal angle, and retrotorsion of the humeral head; (2) the ability to perform implantation in fracture sequelae with shaft malunion and secondary post-fracture situations with humeral head deformities; (3) good glenoid exposure; (4) bone stock preservation; and (5) facilitating further revision surgery.

The main purpose of this prospective study was to evaluate radiological changes around the humeral component of a stemless shoulder implant with hollow screw fixation and their influence on clinical outcome. We hypothesized that clinical mid-term outcome after stemless humeral head replacement would be affected by radiological changes. Secondary objectives were to compare operating times between stemless and stemmed hemi- and total shoulder arthroplasty and to report short and mid-term clinical outcome after stemless hemi- and total shoulder arthroplasty.

Methods

Between September 2005 and December 2011, a total of 136 shoulder arthroplasties using a stemless humeral head implant were performed by two experienced surgeons (W.A., B.K.) at our clinic. The stemless humeral head replacement (Eclipse™ Shoulder Prosthesis, Arthrex Inc., Naples, FL, USA) consists of an anatomical humeral head, which is mounted on a baseplate (trunion) for cortical support at the anatomical neck (epiphyseal fixation) and fixated to the cancellous metaphyseal bone over a screw-in mechanism with a hollow screw (Fig. 1).

Indications for surgery included primary or secondary osteoarthritis of the shoulder with severe pain and limited function. Patients with any kind of rotator cuff tears, cuff tear arthropathies, axillary nerve lesions, or revision arthroplasty were not suitable for this procedure. HSA was indicated, when the glenoid presented without erosion and macroscopically fairly intact cartilage. Included were all patients between 40 and 85 years of age at the time of surgery, who were scheduled for primary anatomical shoulder replacement for the treatment of degenerative, rheumatic, posttraumatic osteoarthritis and fracture sequelae. Institutional review board approval (201212_EK01) was obtained. The trial is registered at ClinicalTrials.gov (NCT02754024).

A total of 95 eligible patients with 100 stemless humeral head implants signed the written informed consent and were enrolled in the prospective trial. Patients

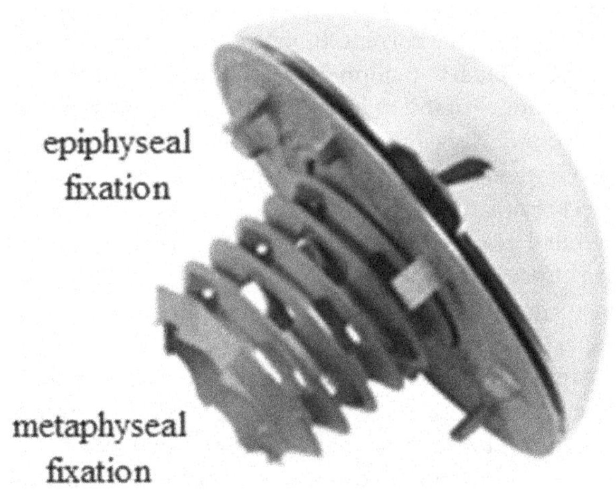

Fig. 1 The stemless humeral head Eclipse prosthesis consists of three components: the anatomical humeral head; the trunion for epiphyseal fixation; and the hollow cage screw for metaphyseal fixation. Published with permission from (Arthrex Inc., Naples, FL, USA)

who died or withdrew before the mid-term follow-up were excluded. During the study period 11 patients died from unrelated causes (five before and six after the short follow-up) and one patient with bilateral implants withdrew from the study before the short follow-up due to an unexpected comorbidity. A complete, prospectively collected data set before, two years (short follow-up) and at least 48 months (mid-term follow-up) after surgery, or until indicated revision surgery was required for inclusion of radiographic and clinical evaluation.

Additionally, operating times of a consecutive cohort of 93 patients (100 implants), who underwent anatomical shoulder arthroplasty with a stemmed anatomical shaft prostheses (Anatomical Shoulder™ System, Zimmer Inc., Warsaw, IN, USA) by the same two experienced surgeons (W.A., B.K.) at our clinic were obtain.

Surgical procedure

Patients were operated under general anaesthesia combined with an interscalene block. Through a standard deltopectoral approach after tenotomy of the subscapularis tendon and exposition of the humeral head, a resection at the anatomical neck was performed.

Thereafter, for the stemless procedure, the humeral head size was determined using templates and the best fitting length of a hollow screw, which allows trabecular ingrowth into the bone and fixation to the trunion, was assessed with a measure pin. A hole for the cage screw was prepared with a hand coring reamer. In case of glenoid replacement, a standard cemented all-polyethylene glenoid component (Arthrex Inc., Naples, FL, USA) was implanted. Again the humeral head was exposed and with a centering device, the trunion of the previously determined head size was impacted for epiphyseal fixation. Thereafter, the appropriate hollow screw was advanced until the screw head was flush with the neck of the trunion. Finally, the correct humeral head was mounted. The subscapularis tendon was reattached with two suture anchors (titanium Corkscrew FT-III, Arthrex) and the wound was closed. Immediately postoperative, fluoroscopic images in two planes were taken to confirm correct implant positioning. Routine follow-ups were scheduled two weeks, three months, one, two, and five years after the procedure. The operating time from incision to final closure for each shoulder replacement was prospectively recorded.

Postoperatively, the arm was secured with an abduction cushion (UltraSling, Breg MDSS GmbH, Hannover, Germany). The physiotherapy regimen included immediate passive motion and passive assisted motion with closed chain exercises to work scapula-thoracic muscles after up to seven days. After six weeks patients were allowed to remove sling; active movements and strengthening exercises started six weeks after implantation.

Clinical evaluation

Pre- and postoperative clinical and functional investigations included the Constant Score [11] adjusted for age and gender [12]. All clinical evaluations were performed by orthopaedic fellows. A single subjective question categorized into very satisfied, satisfied, and unsatisfied was asked to evaluate patient satisfaction. Complications and necessity of revision surgery were recorded. Clinical outcome before revision surgery was recorded, but not included in short- and mid-term analyses.

Radiographic evaluation

Pre-, peri-, two- and five-year postoperative radiographs of the humeral head in anteroposterior and axial view using a fully-digital 2-in-1 system (AXIOM Luminos dRF, Siemens, Munich, Germany) were assessed by one experienced radiologists (rater 2) and two experienced orthopaedic surgeons (rater 1 and 2). Differences in radiological ratings were discussed to find a consensus. In case no consensus could be reached, the final decision was made by the senior author (rater 1). This grading was used for data analysis.

In the event of revision surgery, radiographs obtained before the second procedure were evaluated. Presence of or progression of radiolucency, especially around the bone-implant interface, was recorded. Five radiographic zones including the superior and inferior interface (zone 1 and 5) and the interface around the hollow screw (zones 2, 3, and 4) were assessed for radiolucent areas or osteolysis (Fig. 2).

A radiologic classification system for this specific implant was established using allocations for radiolucent lines similar to Cil et al. [13], and for osteolysis and internal stress shielding similar to Raiss et al. [14]. Radiological findings were grouped into three groups: (group1) no lucency or osteolysis with minor radiolucent lines in one or more zones; (group2) minor radiological findings including major radiolucent lines or partial osteolysis in one or more zones; and (group3) major radiological findings and complete osteolysis in one or more zones. Humeral head implants were considered to be at risk of loosening, if complete osteolysis was detectable in two or more zones. Possible internal stress shielding (loss in bone density around the hollow screw) was also described.

Statistical analysis

For sample size calculation, we assumed that 20% of implants will present with radiological changes and that postoperative Constant scores of those patients will be approximately 70 (60–80) %. Thus, we assume that those patients without radiological changes (80% of patients) will have significantly better Constant scores (approximately 80 (70–90) %). If the true difference in mean

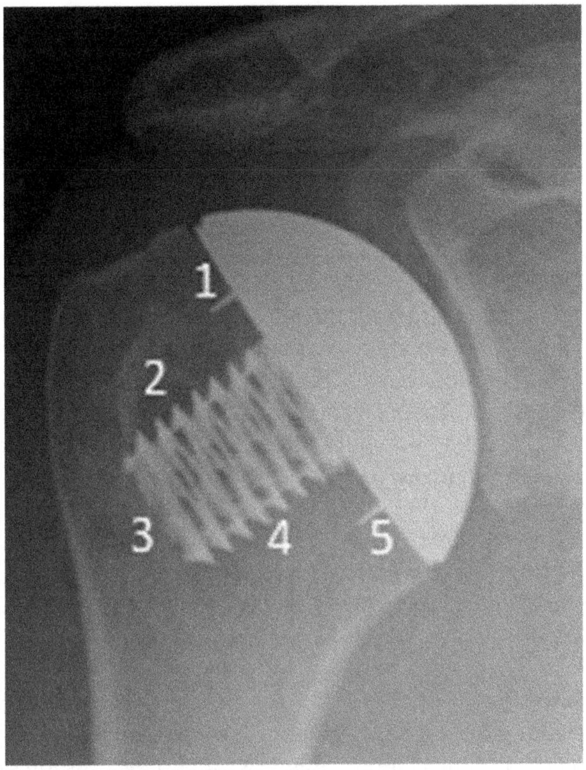

Fig. 2 Anteroposterior radiographs of the stemless humeral head implant showing five radiographic zones including the superior and inferior interface (zone 1 and 5) and the interfaces around the hollow screw (zones 2, 3, and 4), which were used for the assessment of radiolucency and osteolysis

Constant scores is 10% (independent *t*-test), we planned to study 10 patients with and 42 without radiological changes to be able to reject the null hypothesis that the population means of the two groups are equal with probability (power) 0.8. The Type I error probability associated with this test of this null hypothesis is 0.05. To account for exclusions and loss to follow-up we enrolled 100 cases.

Descriptive statistic was used to present patient characteristics. Data distribution was assessed by a visual inspection of histograms and the Kolmogorov-Smirnov-test. Categorical data were assessed using Fisher's exact tests. Differences regarding age- and gender-adjusted Constant scores as well as operating times between two independent groups were calculated using independent t-tests. Paired t-tests were used to compare age- and gender-adjusted Constant scores between pre- and postoperative assessments. Kappa statistic was performed to determine consistency regarding radiographic gradings among raters. All data were analysed using SPSS software (PAWS Statistics 21; SPSS Inc., Chicago, IL). Statistical significance was set at a p-value of < 0.05 (two-sided).

Results

Of the 83 patients (87 shoulders) who met inclusion criteria, 11 patients (three with bilateral implants) were lost to follow-up or had incomplete data (follow-up rate: 86.7%). Demographics of 72 patients (73 shoulders; Table 1) were comparable between stemless HSA (n = 40) and TSA ($n = 33$) regarding age (68.0 ± 10.1 range, 44–84; vs. 67.2 ± 10.5 range, 40–83; $p = 0.752$); gender (female: 75.0% vs. 54.5%, $p = 0.085$); and indication (idiopathic osteoarthritis: 75.0% vs. 87.9%, posttraumatic osteoarthritis: 15.0% vs. 9.1%, humeral head necrosis: 7.5% vs. 3.0%, and instability arthritis: 2.5% vs. 0%, respectively; $p = 0.500$).

A comparison of the duration of the surgical procedure between stemless and stemmed HSA as well as TSA showed significantly shorter operating times for stemless shoulder arthroplasty (Table 2).

Postoperative clinical assessment was performed after an average of 27.7 (22 to 37) months (short follow-up; n = 53) and 58.1 (48 to 87) months (mid-term follow-up; $n = 53$). Radiographs of patients with an indication for revision surgery ($n = 7$) or with revision surgery ($n = 13$) were assessed 38.3 (4 to 99) months postoperatively. The reasons for revision surgery and those with an indication for a further procedure are listed in Table 3. Revision surgery was mainly indicated for secondary glenoid erosion in patients with HSA (61.5%) and secondary rotator cuff tendon tear for patients with TSA (71.4%). Not significant, but more patients with HSA (32.5%) compared with TSA (21.2%) were revised ($p = 0.306$). None of the patients required revision surgery for humeral implant loosening. Patients not requiring revision surgery showed no signs of glenoid erosion (HSA), stable glenoid components (TSA), and intact rotator cuff situations at final follow-up.

Rater agreements for radiologic gradings were very good (rater 1 and 2: $\kappa = 0.871$, 95% confidence interval (CI): 0.764–0.978; rater 1 and 3: $\kappa = 0.920$, 95% CI: 0.833–1.000; rater 2 and 3: $\kappa = 0.898$, 95% CI: 0.802–

Table 1 Patient demographics

	Stemless humeral head replacement ($n = 73$)
Gender (n)	48 female (65.8%) / 24 male (1 bilateral; 34.2%)
Mean age at surgery (years)	67.6 (SD 10.2; range, 40–84)
Indications	
idiopathic osteoarthritis (n)	59 (80.8%)
posttraumatic osteoarthritis (n)	9 (12.3%)
humeral head necrosis (n)	4 (5.5%)
instability arthritis (n)	1 (1.4%)

Abbreviation: *HSA* hemi shoulder arthroplasty, *SD* standard deviation, *TSA* total shoulder arthroplasty

Table 2 Comparison of operating times between stemless and stemmed shoulder arthroplasties

Operating Time[a] (minutes)	Stemless	Stemmed	*p*-value
HSA	73.2 (SD, 17.8; range, 42–129)	95.1 (SD, 23.0; range, 35–143)	< 0.001
TSA	95.7 (SD, 20.3; range, 67–163)	120.7 (SD, 36.4; range, 53–249)	< 0.001

Abbreviation: *HSA* Hemi Shoulder Arthroplasty, *TSA* Total Shoulder Arthroplasty
[a]The values are given as the mean and standard deviation and range in parenthesis

0.994). While humeral implant loosening was not the reason for any revision surgery, according to radiological findings, 11.0% (8 of 73) of humeral head implants were found to be at risk of loosening considering complete osteolysis in two or more zones. Only three of the 12 revised implants were radiologically at risk of humeral head loosening. However, radiological loosening could not be confirmed intraoperatively in those three TSA cases, which were revised for secondary rotator cuff tears. All other implants showed an uneventful progress over time (Figs. 3 and 4).

Radiological changes (group 2 and 3) were detected in 37.0% (HSA: 17.8%; TSA: 19.2%). Partial osteolysis or major radiolucencies (group 2) were detected in 4.1% with HSA and in 2.7% with TSA, while complete osteolysis in one or more zones (group 3) was present in 13.7% in the HSA and 16.4% in the TSA-group (Table 3).

Patients with revision surgery did not have significantly more complete osteolysis in one or more zones than those without revision surgery (30.0% vs. 30.2%, $p = 1.000$; HSA: 15.4% vs. 29.6%, $p = 0.451$; TSA: 57.1% vs. 30.8%, $p = 0.377$, respectively). Internal stress shielding, defined as reduced bone mineral density around the hollow screw, was seen in 42.5% of patients. The number of implants showing internal stress shielding did not differ between patients with and without a revision procedure (25.0% vs. 47.2%, $p = 0.112$; HSA: 30.8% vs. 48.1%, $p = 0.333$; TSA: 14.3% vs. 46.2%, $p = 0.202$, respectively). Further details regarding radiological outcome are provided in Table 4.

Table 3 Reasons for Revision Surgery

	HSA ($n = 13$)	TSA ($n = 7$)
Implant loosening of the humeral head component	0	0
Secondary glenoid erosion or	8	n.a.
Loosening of the glenoid component	n.a.	0
Secondary rotator cuff tendon tear (SSP or SSC)	4	5
Postoperative SNOH fracture	0	1
others	1	1

Abbreviation: *HSA* Hemi Shoulder Arthroplasty, *n.a.* not applicable, *TSA* Total Shoulder Arthroplasty, *SNOH* surgical neck of humeral, *SSC* Subscapularis, *SSP* Supraspinatus

Clinical outcome was not significantly affected by radiological changes (Table 5).

Clinical outcome has significantly improved from pre- to both postoperative follow-ups (37.7 ± 15.4% range, 2.4–80.5 vs. 78.8 ± 16.1% range, 40.2–104.9; $p < 0.001$; and vs. 78.7 ± 15.6% range, 30.5–101.2; $p < 0.001$), but no significant changes ($p = 0.947$) were detectable between the follow-ups (Fig. 5). TSA showed significantly better clinical outcome than HSA at short and mid-term follow-up (Fig. 5). Furthermore, at the mid-term follow-up 96.2% of the patients were very satisfied (15 HSA, 20 TSA) or satisfied (10 HSA, 6 TSA).

Discussion

Previous studies have been reporting radiological and clinical findings after stemless anatomical shoulder arthroplasty; however, to our knowledge we are the first to compare radiological findings to clinical mid-term outcome in a prospective single-centre trial. We were not only able to show that clinical and radiological results with the stemless shoulder prosthesis showed favourable improvements from pre- to short and mid-term outcome with no revision surgery due to humeral component loosening, we also had to reject our hypothesis that radiological changes would negatively impact clinical outcome. Constant scores were not significantly different between patients with and without radiological changes in the mid-term follow-up.

Recently, comparable Constant scores were detected by Habermeyer et al. [15]. In accordance to the literature for stemmed shoulder arthroplasty, TSA showed significantly higher relative Constant Scores than HSA in this study, and values remained stable over time [16, 17]. As the present study and current literature [18, 19] demonstrated, stemless shoulder arthroplasty provides similar clinical results as established stemmed arthroplasty systems. The main focus of our study was the radiologic behaviour of the implant and its influence on clinical outcome. Interestingly, the present results regarding radiolucencies and osteolysis are rather different to the findings of Habermeyer et al. [15], who reported an osteolysis rate of not more than 4%. Such variations could be explained by the fact that radiographs were assessed and classified differently. While we adapted a rather concise nomenclature, Habermeyer did not provide detailed

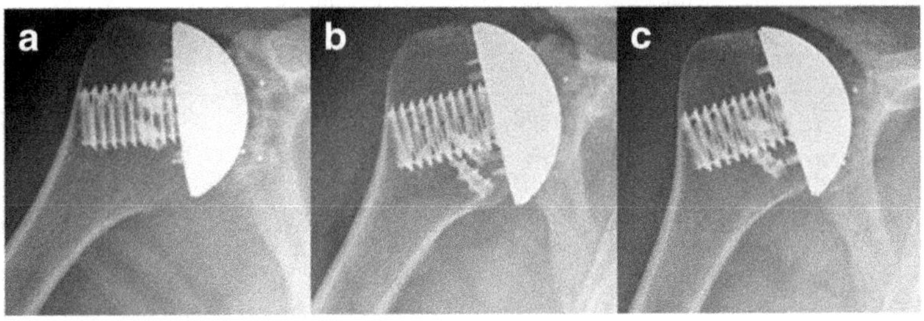

Fig. 4 Anteroposterior radiographs of a forty-year-old man made immediately after total shoulder arthroplasty (**a**), at the short-term showing partial osteolysis at the inferior trunion bone interface (**b**), and at the mid-term follow-up showing stable partial inferior osteolysis and minor superior radiolucency (**c**)

information regarding the classification protocol [15]. Nevertheless, the presence of osteolysis did not affect clinical outcome or revision rates. Comparable to Habermeyer's findings [15], internal stress shielding occurred in half of the implants in one or more zones with the majority around the greater tuberosity. Again, no influence on clinical outcome could be seen in either study.

The majority of abnormal radiological findings occurred either in the superior part of the trunion or in the inferior implant bone interface near the calcar, often leading to partial osteolysis similar to the already known phenomenon described by Raiss [14]. Radiolucencies in the superior and inferior parts of the trunion could be explained with the results of finite element analyses (FEA) [20]. FEA suggested that superposition of force and moment induced stresses in weak inferior cortical bone support is leading to higher migration values within the inferior trunion-bone interface and is therefore resulting in a shift of the centre of rotation. The bone adaptation and resorption around the implant is mostly dependent on the stability of the hollow screw and is caused by axial bending stiffness similar to the concept explained by Nagels et al. [21]. Since such radiological findings were not reflected in the clinical outcome, an arbitrary definition of an implant at risk had to be established. Thus, we assumed that if an implant showed the presence of osteolysis in two or more zones, the humeral head component might become unstable.

Currently, few different stemless shoulder implant systems are on the market with sporadic report of short-term outcome. A major strengths of the Eclipse prosthesis is that it is the only implant with a different fixation mechanism not relying on impaction implantation and therefore avoiding a potential risk of metaphyseal fracture or implant migration [19].

Revision surgeries followed an already well-known pattern. In hemiarthroplasties the majority of revisions were due to secondary glenoid erosion (20.5%), which was similar to other studies [22]. Secondary cuff failure was the main cause for revision (15.2%) in total shoulder arthroplasty. The higher revision rate due to secondary rotator cuff ruptures in the present trial compared to rates (< 8%) reported by Sperling et al. [23] could be explained with the relatively high mean age in the TSA-group. Other than that, reasons for revision were

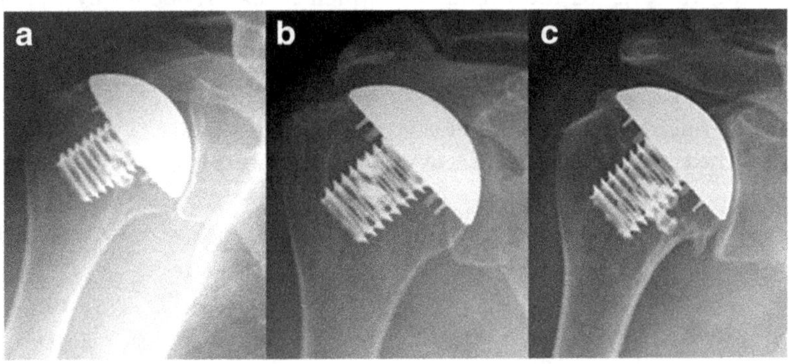

Fig. 3 Anteroposterior radiographs of a seventy-two-year-old woman made immediately after hemi shoulder arthroplasty (**a**), at the short-term follow-up showing no radiolucency or osteolysis (**b**), and at the mid-term follow-up showing osteophyte formation superior around the humeral head implant and inferior (**c**)

Table 4 Radiological Outcome with Stemless Humeral Head Replacement at Final Follow-Up

	HSA (*n* = 27)	HSA REV (*n* = 13)	TSA (*n* = 26)	TSA REV (*n* = 7)	TOTAL (*n* = 73)
Group 1 no RL/OL or minor RL in one or more zones	18	9 (4 s OA + 4 s RCT + 1 undefined pain)	16	3 (1 s RCT + 1 HH Fx + 1 undefined pain)	46
No radiolucency	16	7	12	3	38
Zone 1 (minor RL)	1	2	1	0	4
Zone 5 (minor RL)	1	0	2	0	3
Zone 1 (minor RL) + Zone 5 (minor RL)	0	0	1	0	1
Group 2 major RL or partial OL in one or more zones	1	2 (2 s OA)	2	0	5
Zone 1 (major RL)	1	1	2	0	4
Zone 1 (partial OL) + Zone 5 (partial OL)	0	1	0	0	1
Group 3 complete OL in one or more zones	8	2 (2 s OA)	8	4 (4 s RCT)	22
Zone 1 (major OL)	0	0	1	0	1
Zone 5 (major OL)	4	1	5	1	11
Zone 1(minorRL) + Zone 5 (majorOL)	2	0	0	0	2
Zone 1(majorOL) + Zone 5 (majorOL)	2	1	2	3	8
No internal stress shielding	13	9 (5 s OA + 3 s RCT + 1 undefined pain)	14	6 (5 s RCT + 1 HH Fx)	42
Internal stress shielding in one zone (1, 2, or 4)	8	2 (2 s OA)	5	0	15
Internal stress shielding in two zones (12, 23, 24, or 34)	5	2 (1 s OA + 1 s RCT)	6	1 (1 undefined pain)	14
Internal stress shielding in three zones (125 or 234)	1	0	1	0	2

Abbreviation: *HH Fx* Humeral Head Fracture, *HSA* Hemi Shoulder Arthroplasty, *OL* osteolysis, *sec OA* secondary Osteoarthritis, *REV* revision surgery, *RL* radiolucent line, *sec RCT* secondary Rotator Cuff Tear, *TSA* Total Shoulder Arthroplasty

traumatic surgical neck of humerus fracture, undefined pain for neglected long head of biceps tendon, and symptomatic mes acromion. However, no revision surgery was indicated due to humeral component loosening or polyethylene glenoid component loosening in this patient cohort.

Fortunately, but not surprisingly, revision surgery with such a stemless implant compared to stemmed prostheses were fairly easy as the removal of the humeral component does not require any special manoeuvres (e.g. osteotomy) and leaves a rather anatomic situation with the whole metaphysis in place.

Last but not least, shorter operating times, another strength of stemless humeral head surgery, with HSA as well as with TSA in comparison with a stemmed anatomic shoulder arthroplasty system could be observed. This fact is not surprising, but worth mentioning since 20 min less on operating time is a benefit for the patient regarding reduced anaesthesia time and blood loss, not to mention the advantage in time management and therefore cost effectiveness. As the humeral component implantation is a rather easy procedure, which is also reflected by the significant shorter operating time compared to stemmed shoulder arthroplasty, the learning curve for this surgical technique is quite steep.

Although results of this mid-term trial are promising, long-term outcome regarding implant stability

Table 5 Clinical mid-term outcome of 53 stemless humeral head replacements compared to radiological findings

Radiological findings	N	Constant score (%)	*p*-value
No or minor radiological findings	37	78.9 (SD, 15.7; range, 30.5–101.2)	0.891
Major radiological findings	16	78.3 (SD, 15.8; range, 49.4–97.5)	
No internal stress shielding	28	80.4 (SD, 15.6; range, 49.4–101.2)	0.411
Internal stress shielding in one or more zones	25	76.8 (SD, 15.7; range, 30.5–98.8)	

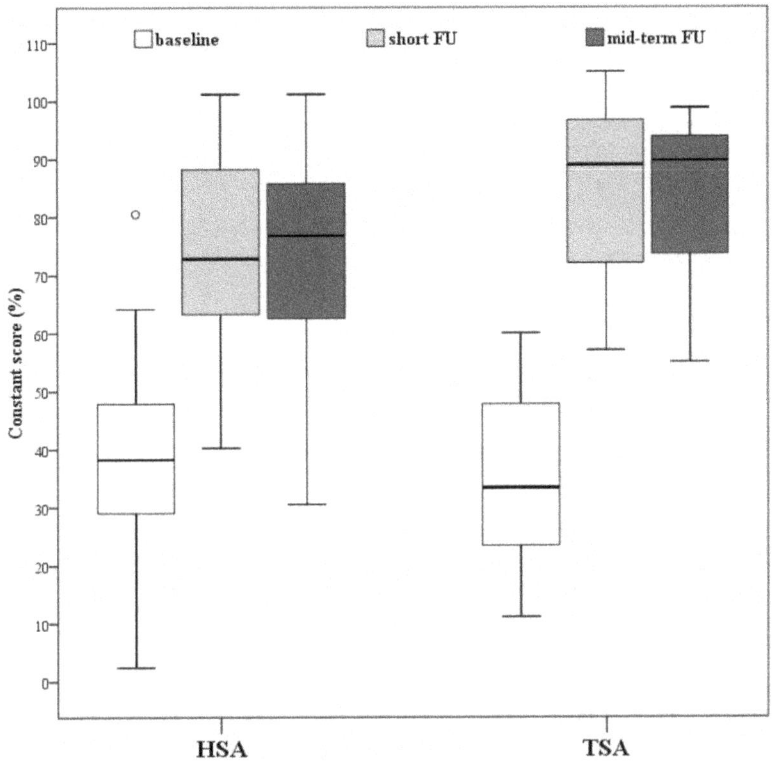

Fig. 5 Clinical outcome between hemi- (HSA; $n = 27$) and total shoulder arthroplasty (TSA; $n = 26$) at baseline (HSA: 38.8 ± 17.0% vs. TSA: 36.6 ± 13.9%, $p = 0.594$), at short (HSA: 74.0 ± 16.5% vs. TSA: 83.9 ± 14.4%, $p = 0.024$) and mid-term follow-up (HSA: 73.5 ± 17.3% vs. TSA: 84.2 ± 11.6%, $p = 0.011$)

needs to be reported. Another limitation is that in-depth subjective assessments (e.g. American Shoulder and Elbow Surgeons or quality of life scores) are missing. Furthermore, assessment of bone mineral density in the humeral head prior to implantation would have been desirable as bone mineral density might influence implant ingrowth and the possible appearance of osteolysis [24]. Unfortunately, our institution does not offer the possibility to assess bone mineral density in the shoulder. However, we believe that the present results outweigh these limitations by the thorough radiographic analysis demonstrating that radiological findings do not influence clinical outcome. We speculate that in the future a humeral head replacement with a shaft may only be indicated under rare circumstances, while the majority of patients, at least according to our results, can be successfully treated with a stemless humeral head replacement.

Conclusion

Promising clinical mid-term results with or without minor radiographic findings suggest that the concept of this stemless humeral head prosthesis might be an expedient alternative to existing shoulder replacements. Anatomical cutting of the humeral head and hollow screw fixation allow a familiar access to the glenoid combined with a shaft independent, less complex bone-sparing surgery along with shorter operating times and favourable revision situation.

Abbreviations

FEA: Finite element analyses; HSA: Hemi shoulder arthroplasties; TSA: Total shoulder arthroplasties (TSA)

Acknowledgments

The authors acknowledge the contribution of Dr. Sylvia Salem to this study.

Funding

No funding was received for this study.

Authors' contributions

WA and PRH made substantial contributions to conception and design; GB, LP, and BK collected data; PRH and BL performed analysis and interpretation of data; PRH, GB, LP, BL, BK, and WA have been involved in drafting the manuscript as well as revising it critically for important intellectual content. The final manuscript has been read and approved by all authors.

Consent for publication
Not applicable.

Competing interests
The first (PRH) and senior author (WA) are consultants for Arthrex, Inc. However, the authors have not received any financial payments or other benefits related to the subject of this article. The other authors do not have any conflict of interest.

References

1. Bohsali KI, Bois AJ, Wirth MA. Complications of shoulder arthroplasty. J Bone Joint Surg Am. 2017;99(3):256–69.
2. Singh JA, Sperling JW, Cofield RH. Revision surgery following total shoulder arthroplasty: analysis of 2588 shoulders over three decades (1976 to 2008). J Bone Joint Surg Br. 2011;93(11):1513–7.
3. Sajadi KR, Kwon YW, Zuckerman JD. Revision shoulder arthroplasty: an analysis of indications and outcomes. J Shoulder Elb Surg. 2010;19(2):308–13.
4. Chin PY, Sperling JW, Cofield RH, Schleck C. Complications of total shoulder arthroplasty: are they fewer or different? J Shoulder Elb Surg. 2006;15(1):19–22.
5. Farng E, Zingmond D, Krenek L, Soohoo NF. Factors predicting complication rates after primary shoulder arthroplasty. J Shoulder Elb Surg. 2011;20(4):557–63.
6. Iacobellis C, Berizzi A, Biz C, Camporese A. Treatment of proximal humeral fractures with reverse shoulder arthroplasty in elderly patients. Musculoskelet Surg. 2015;99(1):39–44.
7. Brunner U, Kohler S. Shoulder arthroplasty for treatment of the sequelae of proximal humerus fractures. Orthopade. 2007;36(11):1037–49.
8. Kontakis G, Tosounidis T, Galanakis I, Megas P. Prosthetic replacement for proximal humeral fractures. Injury. 2008;39(12):1345–58.
9. Levy O, SEA C. Cementless surface replacement arthroplasty of the shoulder. 5- to 10-year results with the Copeland mark-2 prosthesis. J Bone Joint Surg Br. 2001;83(2):213–21.
10. Pape G, Raiss P, Aldinger PR, Loew M. Comparison of short-term results after CUP prosthesis with cemented glenoid components and total shoulder arthroplasty: a matched-pair analysis. Z Orthop Unfall. 2010;148(6):674–9.
11. Constant CR, Murley AH. A clinical method of functional assessment of the shoulder. Clin Orthop Relat Res. 1987;(214):160-164.
12. Yian EH, Ramappa AJ, Arneberg O, Gerber C. The constant score in normal shoulders. J Shoulder Elb Surg. 2005;14(2):128–33.
13. Cil A, Veillette CJ, Sanchez-Sotelo J, Sperling JW, Schleck C, Cofield RH. Revision of the humeral component for aseptic loosening in arthroplasty of the shoulder. J Bone Joint Surg Br. 2009;91(1):75–81.
14. Raiss P, Edwards TB, Deutsch A, Shah A, Bruckner T, Loew M, Boileau P, Walch G. Radiographic changes around humeral components in shoulder arthroplasty. J Bone Joint Surg Am. 2014;96(7):e54.
15. Habermeyer P, Lichtenberg S, Tauber M, Magosch P. Midterm results of stemless shoulder arthroplasty: a prospective study. J Shoulder Elb Surg. 2015;24(9):1463–72.
16. Gartsman GM, Roddey TS, Hammerman SM. Shoulder arthroplasty with or without resurfacing of the glenoid in patients who have osteoarthritis. J Bone Joint Surg Am. 2000;82(1):26–34.
17. Sperling JW, Cofield RH, Rowland CM. Minimum fifteen-year follow-up of Neer hemiarthroplasty and total shoulder arthroplasty in patients aged fifty years or younger. J Shoulder Elb Surg. 2004;13(6):604–13.
18. Churchill RS, Chuinard C, Wiater JM, Friedman R, Freehill M, Jacobson S, Spencer E Jr, Holloway GB, Wittstein J, Lassiter T, et al. Clinical and radiographic outcomes of the Simpliciti Canal-sparing shoulder arthroplasty system: a prospective two-year multicenter study. J Bone Joint Surg Am. 2016;98(7):552–60.
19. Huguet D, DeClercq G, Rio B, Teissier J, Zipoli B, Group T. Results of a new stemless shoulder prosthesis: radiologic proof of maintained fixation and stability after a minimum of three years' follow-up. J Shoulder Elb Surg. 2010;19(6):847–52.
20. Magosch P, Habermeyer P, Bachmaier S, Metcalfe N. Biomechanics of metaphyseal fixed humeral head replacement. Obere Extremität. 2012; 7(1):11–6.
21. Nagels J, Stokdijk M, Rozing PM. Stress shielding and bone resorption in shoulder arthroplasty. J Shoulder Elb Surg. 2003;12(1):35–9.
22. Gonzalez JF, Alami GB, Baque F, Walch G, Boileau P. Complications of unconstrained shoulder prostheses. J Shoulder Elb Surg. 2011;20(4):666–82.
23. Sperling JW, Hawkins RJ, Walch G, Mahoney AP, Zuckerman JD. Complications in total shoulder arthroplasty. Instr Course Lect. 2013;62:135–41.
24. Russell LA. Osteoporosis and orthopedic surgery: effect of bone health on total joint arthroplasty outcome. Curr Rheumatol Rep. 2013;15(11):371.

4

Developing a risk prediction model for the functional outcome after hip arthroscopy

Patrick Stephan[1], Maarten A. Röling[2], Nina M. C. Mathijssen[2], Gerjon Hannink[1*] and Rolf M. Bloem[2]

Abstract

Background: Hip arthroscopic treatment is not equally beneficial for every patient undergoing this procedure. Therefore, the purpose of this study was to develop a clinical prediction model for functional outcome after surgery based on preoperative factors.

Methods: Prospective data was collected on a cohort of 205 patients having undergone hip arthroscopy between 2011 and 2015. Demographic and clinical variables and patient reported outcome (PRO) scores were collected, and considered as potential predictors. Successful outcome was defined as either a Hip Outcome Score (HOS)-ADL score of over 80% or improvement of 23%, defined by the minimal clinical important difference, 1 year after surgery. The prediction model was developed using backward logistic regression. Regression coefficients were converted into an easy to use prediction rule.

Results: The analysis included 203 patients, of which 74% had a successful outcome. Female gender (OR: 0.37 (95% CI 0.17–0.83); $p = 0.02$), pincer impingement (OR: 0.47 (95% CI 0.21–1.09); $p = 0.08$), labral tear (OR: 0.46 (95% CI 0.20–1.06); $p = 0.07$), HOS-ADL score (IQR OR: 2.01 (95% CI 0.99–4.08); $p = 0.05$), WHOQOL physical (IQR OR: 0.43 (95% CI 0.22–0.87); $p = 0.02$) and WHOQOL psychological (IQR OR: 2.40 (95% CI 1.38–4.18); p = < 0.01) were factors in the final prediction model of successful functional outcome 1 year after hip arthroscopy. The model's discriminating accuracy turned out to be fair, as 71% (95% CI: 64–80%) of the patients were classified correctly.

Conclusions: The developed prediction model can predict the functional outcome of patients that are considered for a hip arthroscopic intervention, containing six easy accessible preoperative risk factors. The model can be further improved trough external validation and/or adding additional potential predictors.

Keywords: Hip arthroscopy, Risk prediction, Clinical prediction rule, Functional outcome, Hip outcome score, Preoperative decision-making

Background

Arthroscopic intervention in the hip joint has evolved as a successful therapeutic procedure over the last decades for treating various causes of hip complaints. As diagnostic skills and surgical techniques continue to improve in managing these hip disorders, the indications for hip arthroscopy are also expanding [1, 2]. Hip arthroscopy is primarily used in the treatment of femoroacetabular impingement (FAI) caused by cam and/or pincer morphology, labral tears, focal articular cartilage injuries or the removal of loose bodies in the joint [3]. Treatment of these conditions can lead to pain relief, improvement of hip function [2] and might delay the onset of osteoarthritis and the progression to total hip arthroplasty (THA) [4, 5].

Despite that an arthroscopic treatment for FAI in general is successful, not all patients equally benefit from this procedure [6]. As with any operative procedure, multiple studies emphasize the importance of proper patient selection in achieving favorable results [7–12]. Unsuccessful treatment, e.g. insufficient reduction of complaints, requiring revision surgery or even short term progression to total hip arthroplasty caused by progressive osteoarthritis, has been associated with different preoperative factors. Progressive osteoarthritis has

* Correspondence: gerjon.hannink@radboudumc.nl
[1]Orthopaedic Research Laboratory, Radboud University Medical Center, Nijmegen, The Netherlands
Full list of author information is available at the end of the article

proven to have a negative effect on outcome results of patients treated for FAI [7–13]. A high Tönnis classification (grade ≥2) and a reduced joint space (< 2 mm) have been described as exclusion criteria for hip arthroscopy [7]. Literature suggests that age, gender, BMI, duration of symptoms, preoperative outcome scores, preoperative alpha-angle and hip dysplasia could be predictive for the outcome after hip arthroscopic surgery [7–11, 13–17].

A clinical prediction model would be a great asset in making it easier to predict the outcome of individual patients that are considered for a hip arthroscopic intervention, and could be used to guide doctors and patients in shared decision making regarding treatment and expectations [18, 19]. Therefore, the purpose of this study was to develop a clinical prediction model that can be used to predict the functional outcome 1 year after hip arthroscopy.

Methods

Study population

This study is a retrospective analysis of routinely collected data on all patients who underwent a hip arthroscopic intervention in our hospital between April 2011 and March 2015. All data were collected prospectively. Two hundred five consecutive patients underwent a hip arthroscopic intervention and surgery was performed by an experienced single orthopedic surgeon (RMB). Inclusion criteria for hip arthroscopy were a cam and/or a pincer deformity or a suspicion of a labral tear. The diagnosis was made based on clinical examination with a combination of complaints (hip/groin pain or functional disability), physical examination (FADIR and FABER tests as described by Phillippon et al. [20]) and the presence of radiographic findings that correlate with FAI hip pathology. Patients with severe signs of hip osteoarthritis (Tönnis grade 3) were not offered hip arthroscopy and were therefore excluded from the study. Also, patients unwilling to participate were excluded. All included patients were asked to fill out patient reported outcome (PRO) questionnaires preoperative and at postoperative follow up at 3 months and 1 year. Patient assessment did not differ from normal clinical practice.

The questionnaires used to assess improvement in patient outcome were the Visual Analogue Scale (VAS) for pain, modified Harris Hip Score (mHHS), Hip Outcome Score (HOS)-ADL and HOS-Sport and the physical and psychological domains of the WHOQOL. The mHHS, HOS-ADL and HOS-Sport were used to asses hip related improvement in patient outcome, which are scored percentage based on 8, 17 and 9 questions respectively. The WHOQOL-BREF [21] score was used to measure the general (non hip related) quality of life (QOL). The WHOQOL score is a generic measure designed for use in a wide spectrum of psychological and physical disorders. It is a multidimensional measure for subjective assessment of QOL. The WHOQOL-BREF has a good to excellent validity and reliability [22]. High scores indicate a good QOL. Patients in the study were scored on both the physical and psychological domains. The study protocol was assessed by the regional Medical Ethical Committee (Medisch Ethische Toetsings Commissie Zuidwest Holland (METCZH); no. METCZWH 12–083). Ethical approval was waived by the METCZH on basis of the Dutch Medical Research Involving Human Subjects Act (WMO). However, all the patients who were included gave their written informed consent. Our study was reported according to the TRIPOD guidelines [23].

Surgical technique

Patients were operated in supine position under general anesthesia. A traction table was used for subluxation of the hip joint. Fluoroscopy guided, two to three portals were inserted into the hip joint in order to adequately visualize the acetabulum, acetabular labrum, cartilage, transverse ligament and the anterior, superior and posterior aspects of the femoral head. The central and peripheral compartments were inspected for abnormalities (as described by Bond 2009) [24]. Labral tears, focal chondropathy, loose bodies, cam- and/or pincer morphologies were identified and treated accordingly: tears were repaired if possible, otherwise debrided, cam/pincer morphologies resected, loose bodies extracted and focal chondropathy > grade II were treated with microfracture.

Outcome measure

To be able to predict the risk of a successful outcome it was required to define a cutoff in the HOS-ADL, which is used as the main outcome score. To do this the Minimal Clinically Important Difference (MCID) for the HOS-ADL was used. The MCID is a common tool used to determine the smallest change in a treatment outcome that a patient would identify as important. In a recent study Chahal et al. reported an MCID of 23 for the HOS-ADL [25]. Also patients scoring above 80% in HOS-ADL score were classified as having an successful outcome [14].

Ultimately, a successful outcome was defined as either a 23% improvement in HOS-ADL from preoperative to 1 year postoperative, or a HOS-ADL score of over 80% at 1 year postoperative.

Potential predictive factors

Based on literature [7–17], the following potential predictors were considered: age, gender, years of complaints, BMI, operation indication (cam, pincer, labral tear), preoperative radiographic findings (Tönnis classification, alpha angle) and PRO scores (VAS for pain, mHHS, HOS-ADL, HOS-Sport, WHOQOL physical and psychological domains). The predictors were either continuous (age, years of complaints, BMI, alpha angle, and all outcome scores), dichotomous (gender) or categorical (indication, Tönnis classification) and used as such.

Statistical analysis

Descriptive statistics were used to summarize the data. For 12 of the 21 variables, data were missing ranging between 1% to 18% (Table 1). These missing data were imputed using multiple imputation by chained equations procedure (predictive mean matching) [26, 27]. Missing data were assumed to be missing at random (MAR), five imputed datasets were created.

Logistic regression was used to evaluate the association between each prognostic factor and outcome. Potential prognostic variables were entered into a logistic regression model, taking into account the multiple imputed datasets. The univariable odds ratios of the variables were calculated using univariable logistic regression analyses to evaluate their individual contribution. Multivariable logistic regression with a backward stepwise selection procedure was used to achieve the most informative and parsimonious combination of predictors. Akaike's information criterion ($p < 0.157$) was used as a selection criterion [28, 29]. The probability of having an successful functional outcome can be calculated by using the following formula: $P_{\text{successful outcome}} = e^{(\beta_0+\beta_1*x_1+\beta_2*x_2+\ \dots\ +\beta_n*x_n)} / 1 + e^{(\beta_0+\beta_1*x_1+\beta_2*x_2+\ \dots\ +\beta_n*x_n)}$.

In this formula, $P_{\text{successful outcome}}$ is the probability of having a successful functional outcome, β_0 represents the constant and β_1, β_2 and β_n are the regression coefficients of the predictors x_1, x_2, and x_n, respectively, after having been pooled.

The model performance was assessed on calibration with the Hosmer-Lemeshow goodness-of-fit test and a calibration plot to estimate its reliability [29, 30]. The model's ability to discriminate between patients with successful or unsuccessful outcomes was estimated as the area under the curve (AUC) of the receiver operating characteristic (ROC) curve of the model [31]. Prediction models derived with multivariable regression analyses are known for over fitting, which results in too extreme predictions when applied in new cases. Therefore, the model was validated internally using bootstrapping techniques. Five hundred samples were drawn with replacement from the development sample. Bootstrapping techniques provide information on the performance of the model in comparable datasets and generate a shrinkage factor to adjust the regression coefficients [31, 32]. After this adjustment, the model performance was reevaluated. A nomogram was created to easily calculate the risk of a successful outcome after hip arthroscopy for a given patient.

All statistical analyses were performed using SPSS version 22 (IBM, New Jersey, US) and R version 3.3.1 (R Foundation, Vienna, Austria) with package 'rms' [33].

Results

Our database yielded 205 patients, 203 were eligible for statistical analysis. Two patients were excluded: one because of a different indication (free body), and the other because at the start of surgery it was not possible to reach the joint space as the capsule was too tight. The latter patient was afterwards referred for a Ganz osteotomy. Out of the 203 participating patients 74% had a successful outcome 1 year after hip arthroscopy according to our composite outcome. Temporal changes (pre-operative, 3 months and 1 year) in HOS-ADL scores are shown in Fig. 1. Additional information on the two components of our composite outcome (i.e. > 23 points improvement in preoperative HOS-ADL at 1 year postoperative, or an HOS-ADL > 80 at 1 year postoperative) is presented in Table 1.

Of the 203 eligible patients 114 (56%) were female. The patients had a mean age of 40 years (SD±11), a mean BMI of 26 (SD±4), and the mean time of complaints prior to surgery was 4 years (SD±4). The indications for surgery were cam morphology (121 (60%)), pincer morphology (46 (22%)) (both causing FAI) and labral tear (138 (67%)). Patients had a mean alpha angle of 65° (SD±14). Table 1 presents the demographic and clinical characteristics of the study population.

Gender, cam, preoperative PRO scores of the HOS-ADL and WHOQOL psychological showed to be significantly ($p < 0.05$) associated with outcome in univariable analysis (Table 2).

After backward selection, the following variables remained in the multivariable model: gender, pincer, labral tear, HOS-ADL, WHOQOL physical, and WHOQOL psychological (Table 2). The reduced model's AUC of the ROC curve was 0.72 (95% CI: 0.65–0.80) and the Hosmer-Lemeshow goodness-of-fit test was not statistically significant, indicating that the model fits the data well.

Through bootstrapping the maximum absolute difference in predicted and calibrated probabilities (E_{max}) and a shrinkage factor were determined, 0.15 and 0.61, respectively. After multiplying the regression coefficients with the shrinkage factor the models performance was reevaluated. The mean probability of having a successful functional outcome was 67% (SD±12%). Female patients in our population had a lower chance on a successful outcome 1 year after hip arthroplasty

Table 1 Demographic and clinical characteristics of study participants

Characteristic	Total sample ($n = 203$)		Patients with successful outcome[a] ($n = 133$)		Patients with unsuccessful outcome[a] ($n = 46$)		Patients with missing outcome ($n = 24$)	
	Value	Missing	Value	Missing	Value	Missing	Value	Missing
Gender (female)	114 (56%)	–	64 (48%)	–	33 (72%)	–	17 (71%)	–
Age (yrs)	40 (11, 15–67)	–	40 (11, 17–67)	–	40 (10, 18–55)	–	39 (13, 15–64)	–
BMI (kg/m^2)	26 (4, 18–42)	–	25 (4, 18–35)	–	26 (5, 20–42)	–	27 (6, 20–40)	–
Duration of complaints (yrs)	4 (4, 1–30)	–	4 (4, 1–25)	–	3 (2, 1–10)	–	5 (6, 1–30)	–
Tönnis classification	193	10 (5%)	128	5 (4%)	45	1 (2%)	20	4 (17%)
Grade 0	142 (74%)	–	94 (73%)	–	35 (78%)	–	13 (65%)	–
Grade 1	46 (23%)	–	32 (25%)	–	9 (20%)	–	5 (25%)	–
Grade 2	5 (3%)	–	2 (2%)	–	1 (2%)	–	2 (10%)	–
Alpha angle (°)	64 (14, 39–99)	–	66 (14, 39–99)	–	62 (13, 39–91)	–	62 (14, 43–89)	–
Cam	120 (59%)	–	87 (65%)	–	20 (44%)	–	13 (54%)	–
Pincer	45 (22%)	–	26 (20%)	–	12 (26%)	–	7 (29%)	–
Labral tear	138 (68%)	–	87 (65%)	–	37 (80%)	–	14 (58%)	–
Preoperative PRO scores								
VAS pain, mean	6 (2, 1–10)	–	6 (2, 1–10)	–	6 (2, 2–9)	–	7 (1,3–9)	–
mHHS, mean (SD, range)	55 (12, 22–90)	–	57 (12, 26–90)	–	53 (11, 23–80)	–	50 (14, 22–72)	–
HOS-ADL, mean (SD, range)	58 (20, 7–96)	2 (1%)	60 (20, 7–96)	–	53 (18, 14–84)	–	55 (22, 15–91)	2 (8%)
HOS-Sport, mean (SD, range)	40 (22, 0–94)	11 (5%)	42 (23, 0–94)	3 (2%)	38 (19, 3–78)	3 (7%)	34 (22, 0–72)	5 (21%)
WHOQOL physical, mean (SD, range)	49 (16, 7–86)	30 (15%)	50 (16, 7–86)	17 (13%)	48 (14, 21–82)	6 (13%)	45 (19, 7–75)	7 (29%)
WHOQOL psychological, mean (SD, range)	71 (15, 13–100)	29 (14%)	72 (15, 13–100)	16 (12%)	67 (16, 25–95)	6 (13%)	69 (16, 38–96)	7 (29%)
PRO scores at 3 months postoperative								
VAS pain	3 (2, 0–9)	12 (6%)	2 (2, 0–9)	6 (5%)	4 (3, 0–8)	1 (2%)	2 (2, 0–6)	5 (21%)
mHHS	73 (15, 17–91)	12 (6%)	77 (12, 41–91)	5 (4%)	63 (18, 17–91)	1 (2%)	69 (15, 41–87)	6 (25%)
HOS-ADL	76 (20, 27–100)	118 (58%)	81 (15, 38–100)	77 (58%)	64 (23, 28–100)	27 (59%)	73 (25, 27–100)	14 (58%)
HOS-Sport	62 (27, 6–100)	129 (64%)	65 (24, 6–100)	83 (62%)	51 (32, 6–100)	29 (63%)	63 (26, 33–97)	17 (71%)
WHOQOL physical								
WHOQOL psychological								

Table 1 Demographic and clinical characteristics of study participants *(Continued)*

Characteristic	Total sample ($n = 203$)		Patients with successful outcome[a] ($n = 133$)		Patients with unsuccessful outcome[a] ($n = 46$)		Patients with missing outcome ($n = 24$)	
	Value	Missing	Value	Missing	Value	Missing	Value	Missing
PRO scores at 1 year postoperative								
VAS pain	3 (3, 0–9)	20 (10%)	1 (2, 0–9)	–	5 (2, 0–9)	–	6 (4, 1–9)	20 (83%)
mHHS	77 (16, 27–91)	25 (12%)	84 (9, 47–91)	1 (1%)	57 (15, 27–91)	3 (7%)	60 (31, 29–91)	21 (88%)
HOS-ADL	81 (21, 14–100)	24 (12%)	91 (9, 56–100)	–	51 (17, 14–78)	–	–	24 (100%)
HOS-Sport	71 (26, 11–100)	36 (18%)	83 (16, 28–100)	7 (5%)	36 (18, 11–81)	6 (13%)	38 (38, 38–38)	23 (96%)
WHOQOL physical	70 (20, 7–100)	26 (13%)	77 (15, 7–100)	3 (2%)	48 (17, 14–79)	1 (2%)	50 (25, 32–68)	22 (92%)
WHOQOL psychological	76 (14, 29–100)	26 (13%)	79 (13, 29–100)	3 (2%)	68 (13, 38–92)	1 (2%)	52 (9, 46–58)	22 (92%)
Components of composite outcome								
Increase in HOS-ADL > 23	85 (47%)	24 (12%)	85 (64%)	–	0 (0%)	–	–	24 (100%)
Postoperative HOS-ADL > 80	120 (67%)	24 (12%)	120 (90%)	–	0 (0%)	–	–	24 (100%)

[a]Successful outcome is defined as an HOSADL > 80 or HOSADL increase > 23 1 year postoperative
Unless otherwise indicated values between parentheses are (sd, range)

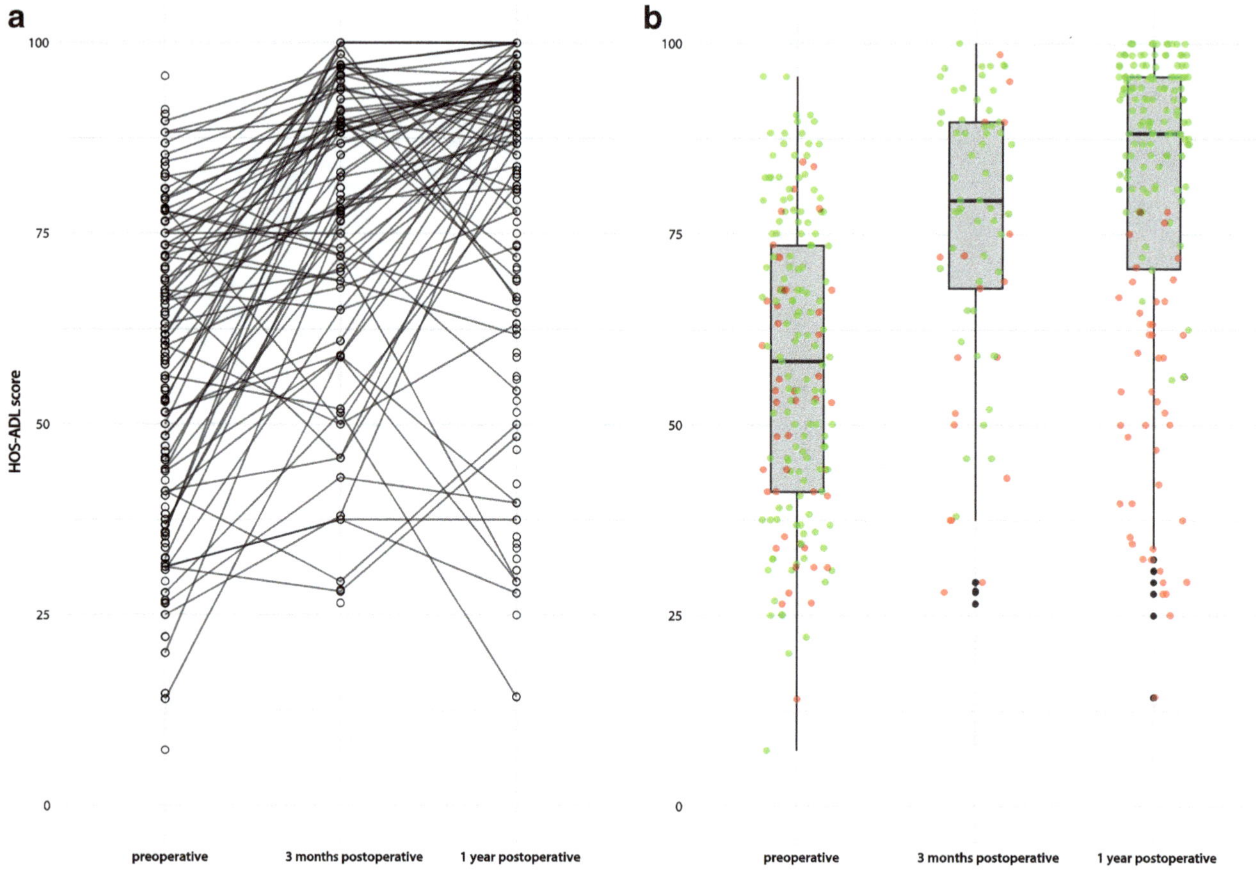

Fig. 1 **a** Graphical representation of temporal changes in HOS-ADL scores for each patient. Please note that due to missing values for some patients scores at certain time points are not available and connecting lines not drawn. **b** Boxplots showing distribution of preoperative HOS-ADL scores and scores at 3 months and 1 year postoperative. Green dots represent patients with successful outcome after hip arthroscopy at 1 year follow-up. Red dot represent patient without successfull outcome

compared to men (OR: 0.37 (95% CI 0.17–0.83); $p = 0.02$). Patients with indications pincer morphology (OR: 0.47 (95% CI 0.21–1.09); $p = 0.08$) or labral tear (OR: 0.46 (95% CI 0.20–1.06); $p = 0.07$) had a lower chance on a successful outcome. Patients with a higher preoperative HOS-ADL had a higher chance on a successful outcome (IQR OR: 2.01 (95% CI 0.99–4.08); $p = 0.05$). A lower score on the WHOQOL physical domain (IQR OR: 0.43 (95% CI 0.22–0.87); $p = 0.02$) and a higher psychological score (IQR OR: 2.40 (95% CI 1.38–4.18); $p = < 0.01$) gave a higher chance on a successful outcome. The final model's discrimination yielded an AUC of the ROC curve of 0.71 (95% CI: 0.64–0.80). The model's calibration was visualized with a calibration plot (Fig. 2). The Hosmer-Lemeshow goodness-of-fit test was not significant ($p = 0.48$), indicating that the model fits the data well.

The risk of a successful functional outcome after hip arthroscopy for a given patient can be calculated as follows:

$$P_{\text{successful outcome}} = e^{(\text{lp})}/1 + e^{(\text{lp})},$$

where

$$\begin{aligned} \text{lp} = -0.19 &+ (-0.97 * \text{female}) + (-0.74 * \text{pincer}) \\ &+ (-0.77 * \text{labral tear}) \\ &+ (0.02 * \text{HOS-ADL score}) \\ &+ (-0.04 * \text{WHOQOL physical score}) \\ &+ (0.05 * \text{WHOQOL psychological score}) \end{aligned}$$

The nomogram created as a tool to easily calculate the risk of a successful outcome after hip arthroscopy for a given patient is shown in Fig. 3.

Discussion

Arthroscopic procedures for FAI caused by cam/pincer morphologies or labral tears, can significantly resolve complaints and impairment in patients. However, not all patients equally benefit from this procedure. Careful

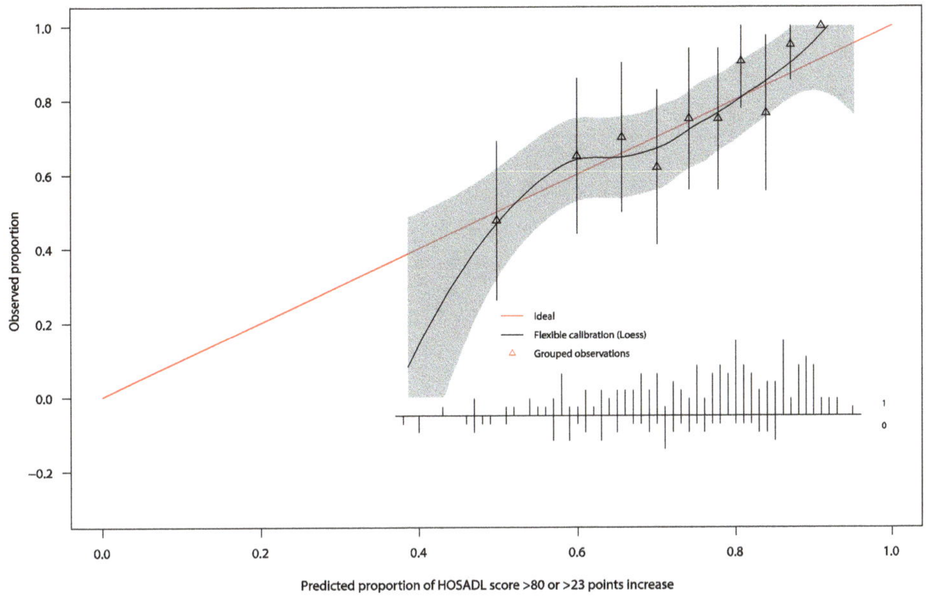

Fig. 2 Calibration plot. Distribution of predicted probabilities shown separately for patients with and without a successful outcome after hip arthroscopy. Triangles indicate observed proportions of successful outcome after hip arthroscopy, by tenths of predicted probability

patient selection is of great importance for success of this procedure. In this study a clinical prediction model was developed using logistic regression for functional outcome 1 year after hip arthroscopy, containing six easy accessible preoperative risk factors: gender, indication: pincer and labral tear, and the preoperative PRO scores: HOS-ADL and WHOQOL physical and psychological domains. Based on this model, a nomogram was created that can be used to easily calculate the risk of a successful outcome after hip arthroscopy for a given patient.

Table 2 Logistic regression analysis of predictor variables for successful outcome 1 year after hip arthroscopy

Predictors		Univariable analysis		Multivariable analysis		
		Odds ratio (95% CI)	*P* value	Odds ratio (95% CI)	Regression coefficient	*P* value
Constant					−0.19	
Gender	female vs male	0.38 (0.19–0.76)	0.01	0.37 (0.17–0.83)	−0.97	0.02
Age (IQR 31–48)		1.07 (0.67–1.72)	0.77	–	–	–
BMI (IQR 23–28)		0.75 (0.48–1.16)	0.20	–	–	–
Years of complaints (IQR 2–4)		0.95 (0.81–1.13)	0.59	–	–	–
Tönnis classification	grade ≥ 1 vs grade 0	1.30 (0.36–4.66)	0.69	–	–	–
Alpha angle (IQR 52–75)		1.66 (0.97–2.83)	0.06	–	–	–
CAM	yes vs no	2.38 (1.25–4.55)	0.01	–	–	–
Pincer	yes vs no	0.58 (0.28–1.21)	0.15	0.47 (0.21–1.09)	−0.74	0.08
Labral tear	yes vs no	0.55 (0.27–1.15)	0.11	0.46 (0.20–1.06)	−0.77	0.07
Preoperative VASpain (IQR 5–8)		0.91 (0.50–1.63)	0.75	–	–	–
Preoperative mHHS (IQR 48–64)		1.44 (0.95–2.18)	0.09	–	–	–
Preoperative HOS-ADL (IQR 41–74)		1.84 (1.08–3.15)	0.02	2.01 (0.99–4.08)	0.02	0.05
Preoperative HOS-Sport (IQR 48–64)		1.38 (0.83–2.29)	0.21	–	–	–
Preoperative WHOQOL physical (IQR 48–64)		1.35 (0.88–2.06)	0.16	0.43 (0.22–0.87)	−0.04	0.02
Preoperative WHOQOL psychological (IQR 60–79)		1.69 (1.12–2.57)	0.01	2.40 (1.38–4.18)	0.05	0.002

IQR interquartile range. Odds ratios for continuous predictors are presented as IQR odds ratios

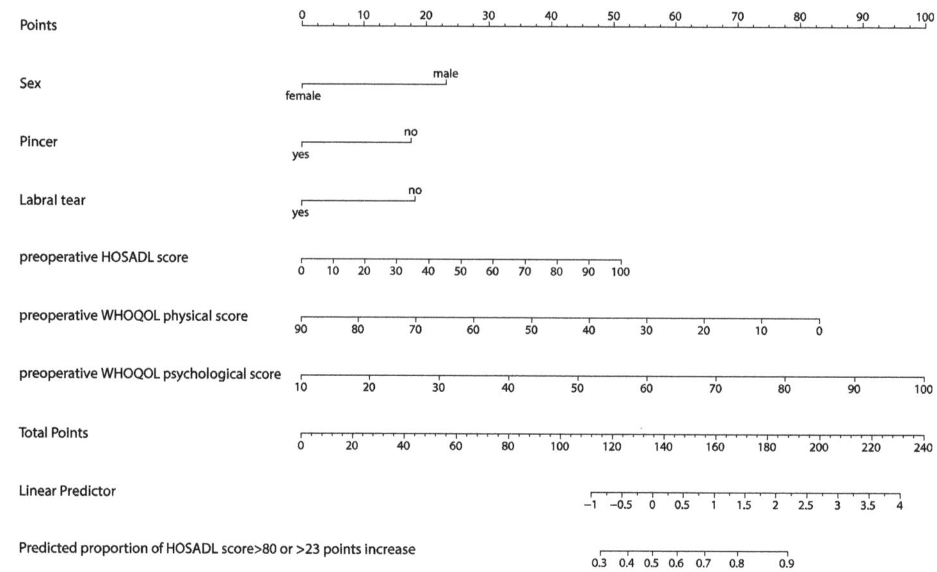

Fig. 3 Nomogram for prediction of a successful outcome after hip arthroscopy in a given patient. To calculate the probability of a successful outcome, first obtain the value for each predictor by drawing a vertical line straight upward from that predictor to the points' axis, then sum the points obtained for each predictor, and locate this sum on the total points' axis of the nomogram, where the probability of a successful outcome after hip arthroscopy can be located by drawing a vertical line downward

The discriminating accuracy of this model as assessed by the AUC of the ROC curve turned out to be fair, 71% (95% CI: 64–80%) of the patients were classified correctly. The model has a relatively high predictive probability (67%) for successful outcome after hip arthroscopy, as most patients in the cohort had a successful outcome after surgery. The developed model is a first step to predict the course of functional outcome of patients that are considered for a hip arthroscopic intervention, as its accuracy can still be improved through external validation to examine the generalizability for other hip arthroscopic populations [30]. However, the model can be used as a guidance tool to optimize preoperative decision-making.

Female gender was identified as a predictor in the final model. Findings out of previous studies on gender as a predictor showed to be inconsistent [34, 35]. The study of McCarthy et al. [34] identified predictors for long term survivorship after hip arthroscopy and analyzed that gender had no predictive value. The study of Frank et al. [35] compared clinical outcomes (HOS and mHHS) before and after hip arthroscopy and pointed out that gender was predictive for both HOS-Sport and mHHS. Women presenting with hip pain have different hip morphology compared to men (smaller alpha angles, increased acetabular version, and increased femoral anteversion), and speculations are made that this difference is caused by a greater component of soft-tissue laxity and difference in muscle mass, as it results in less protective dynamic stabilization of the painful hip joint [36]. Also hip dysplasia is known to have a higher occurrence in women and can lead to inferior results and higher failure rates after arthroscopic treatment of FAI [16].

Our model identified pincer morphologies and labral tear indications as predictors that have a negative effect on a successful outcome. Multiple studies demonstrate that cam and pincer morphologies and labral tears induced FAI, in the absence of significant degenerative changes, are appropriate indications for arthroscopic hip surgery resulting in improvements in functional outcome [37, 38]. In our population patients with these indications had a lower chance to get the desired improvement in functional outcome. Therefore, more cautious consideration is advised compared to patients with cam impingement.

The other predictors in our model were based on preoperative PRO scores. Preoperative HOS-ADL showed to be a predictor in the prediction model. That a preoperative outcome score can have predictive value in predicting postoperative outcome seems logical, but there is still limited evidence on this subject, as only Philippon et al. [11] identified the preoperative mHHS as predictor for postoperative outcome. The physical and psychological domains of quality of life, based on the WHOQOL-BREF, were also identified as predictors in the final model. There have been no studies known by the authors to use this quality of life score as a predictor for functional outcome. Yet, there are studies that describe a strong correlation between psychological factors and post-operative outcome in other fields of orthopedic surgery (including total joint arthroplasty, anterior cruciate ligament reconstruction, and spine surgery for degenerative disease) [39]. Several intervention strategies exist to address these psychological factors when they appear to contribute suboptimal postoperative rehabilitation or recovery [39].

Previous studies show there is evidence that demographic factors such as age, BMI and duration of symptoms can be predictors of outcome after hip arthroscopy, but are inconsistent [7, 9–11, 13–15, 34, 35]. Our model does not show this predictive relationship either. However, some of the risk factors (the cam type FAI (IQR OR: 2.38 (95% CI 1.25–4.55); $p = 0.01$) and preoperative alpha angle (IQR OR: 1.66 (95% CI 0.97–2.83); $p = 0.06$)) that did not make it into the final predictive model, showed to have a correlation with successful outcome in univariable analysis.

In addition to assisting clinicians in patient selection for hip arthroscopic interventions, the model can be used for consulting patients on their expectations of successful surgery. A study examining satisfaction in total knee arthroplasty patients found that preoperative expectations affect satisfaction [19]. As patients with a lower risk score have a lower chance on a successful outcome, patients and clinicians should adjust their expectations accordingly.

Some potential limitations of our study have to be discussed. We had to define improved functional outcome after hip arthroscopy (composite of HOS-ADL score above 80 or increase of 23 points). Despite the limitations related to the use of composite outcomes, the impossibility for patients with preoperative HOS-ADL scores of > 80 points to increase 20 points or more necessitated the use of a composite outcome (as these patients otherwise would have been considered unsuccessful irrespective of their score at 1 year postoperative). The HOS-ADL was chosen as the main outcome score because it is a validated, self-administered score and is designed for younger patients with hip pathology without relevant arthritic degeneration [40–42]. The cutoff value for improved outcome was based on the MCID of 23 determined in a recent study done by Chahal et al. [25] Other studies show different MCID values, e.g. Martin et al. [43] found an MCID of 9 (which we considered to be too low to be of clinical importance). Repeating the analysis with a cutoff based on this MCID (HOS-ADL score above 80 or increase of 9 points) resulted in a very similar model, yielding the same predictive factors as our current prediction model. Furthermore, in order to use this prediction model, the suggested PROs have to be used.

There are also limitations in our follow-up duration, population size and missing values in the outcome scores. Our study has a relatively short follow-up time (1 year) and a small study group size (205), although it is larger than presented by most previous authors. Models developed from datasets with too few outcome events relative to the number of candidate predictors are likely to yield biased estimates of regression coefficients. They lead to unstable prediction models that are overfit to the development sample and perform poorly on new data. It has been suggested that an EPV of 10 or more is needed to avoid the problem of overfitting [44–46]. To make sure that the model would not overfit the data, the number of variables included in the model was kept within the limit of 10 events per predictive variable. Another limitation is the influence of pre-, peri- and postoperative factors on functional outcome. All patients had a standardized preoperative selection process, based on known indications, contraindications and the surgeon's clinical expertise. Outcome can also be affected by factors as perioperative findings or treatment, complications during surgery or injuries after surgery. Examples are, e.g. unexpected chondral damage based on the Outerbridge classification [7, 10, 11, 13, 34], labral repair versus debridement [11], and residual FAI after surgery [47]. These factors are not in the prediction model but still influence the outcome of hip arthroscopic interventions.

Finally, this study included a relatively diverse range of preoperative risk factors, as the addition of preoperative PRO scores as potential risk factors, which is unique in this research field. However, not all possible preoperative risk factors were included in the study. For example, risk factors based on physical examination [48] or radiographic measurements (CT/MRI) [9, 49] can still be added to the model, as every predictor adds to a more accurate identification of patients at risk for an successful outcome.

Conclusion

This study identified six easy accessible preoperative risk factors that can be used to predict functional outcome 1 year after a hip arthroscopic intervention, i.e. gender (female), indication (pincer and labral tear), HOS-ADL (low), WHOQOL physical (high) and WHOQOL psychological (low) score. The proposed clinical prediction model is a first step to predict the functional outcome of patients that are considered for a hip arthroscopic intervention, as it can still be improved through external validation and/or adding additional potential predictors.

Abbreviations

95% CI: 95% Confidence interval; ADL: Activities of daily living; AUC: Area under the curve; BMI: Body mass index; CT: Computed tomography; EPV: Events per variable; FAI: Femoroacetabular impingement; HOS: Hip outcome score; IQR: Inter-quartile range; MAR: Missing at random; MCID: Minimal clinically important difference; mHHS: Modified Harris Hip score; MRI: Magnetic resonance imaging; OR: Odds ratio; PRO: Patient reported outcome; ROC: Receiver operating characteristic; THA: Total hip arthroplasty; TRIPOD: Transparent reporting of a multivariable prediction model for individual prognosis or diagnosis; VAS: Visual analogue scale; WHOQOL-BREF: World Health Organization's quality of life assessment (abbreviated version)

Acknowledgements
We would like to show our gratitude to the patients who made this study possible.

Funding
No funding was received.

Authors' contributions
All authors (PS, MAR, NMCM, GH, RMB) designed the study and interpreted data. PS and GH made the statistical analyses. PS, MAR, NMCM, and GH wrote the first version of the manuscript. All authors critically revised different versions of the manuscript, and all authors read and approve the final version of the manuscript. GH is the corresponding author.

Consent for publication
Not applicable

Competing interests
The authors declare that they have no competing interest.

Author details
[1]Orthopaedic Research Laboratory, Radboud University Medical Center, Nijmegen, The Netherlands. [2]Department of Orthopaedics, Reinier de Graaf Groep, Delft, The Netherlands.

References

1. McCarthy J, Mc MS. Arthroscopy of the hip: factors affecting outcome. Orthop Clin North Am. 2013;44:489–98.
2. Stevens MS, Legay DA, Glazebrook MA, Amirault D. The evidence for hip arthroscopy: grading the current indications. Arthroscopy. 2010;26:1370–83.
3. Leunig M, Beaule PE, Ganz R. The concept of femoroacetabular impingement: current status and future perspectives. Clin Orthop Relat Res. 2009;467:616–22.
4. Kemp JL, Makdissi M, Schache AG, Pritchard MG, Pollard TC, Crossley KM. Hip chondropathy at arthroscopy: prevalence and relationship to labral pathology, femoroacetabular impingement and patient-reported outcomes. Br J Sports Med. 2014;48:1102–7.
5. Meermans G, Konan S, Haddad FS, Witt JD. Prevalence of acetabular cartilage lesions and labral tears in femoroacetabular impingement. Acta Orthop Belg. 2010;76:181–8.
6. Nwachukwu BU, Rebolledo BJ, McCormick F, Rosas S, Harris JD, Kelly BT. Arthroscopic versus open treatment of Femoroacetabular impingement: a systematic review of medium- to long-term outcomes. Am J Sports Med. 2016;44:1062–8.
7. Domb BG, Gui C, Lodhia P. How much arthritis is too much for hip arthroscopy: a systematic review. Arthroscopy. 2015;31:520–9.
8. Horisberger M, Brunner A, Herzog RF. Arthroscopic treatment of femoral acetabular impingement in patients with preoperative generalized degenerative changes. Arthroscopy. 2010;26:623–9.
9. Larson CM, Giveans MR, Taylor M. Does arthroscopic FAI correction improve function with radiographic arthritis? Clin Orthop Relat Res. 2011;469:1667–76.
10. McCormick F, Nwachukwu BU, Alpaugh K, Martin SD. Predictors of hip arthroscopy outcomes for labral tears at minimum 2-year follow-up: the influence of age and arthritis. Arthroscopy. 2012;28:1359–64.
11. Philippon MJ, Briggs KK, Yen YM, Kuppersmith DA. Outcomes following hip arthroscopy for femoroacetabular impingement with associated chondrolabral dysfunction: minimum two-year follow-up. J Bone Joint Surg Br. 2009;91:16–23.
12. Skendzel JG, Philippon MJ, Briggs KK, Goljan P. The effect of joint space on midterm outcomes after arthroscopic hip surgery for femoroacetabular impingement. Am J Sports Med. 2014;42:1127–33.
13. Kemp JL, MacDonald D, Collins NJ, Hatton AL, Crossley KM. Hip arthroscopy in the setting of hip osteoarthritis: systematic review of outcomes and progression to hip arthroplasty. Clin Orthop Relat Res. 2015;473:1055–73.
14. Nabavi A, Olwill CM, Harris IA. Preoperative predictors of outcome in the arthroscopic treatment of femoroacetabular impingement. Hip Int. 2015;25:402–5.
15. Bech NH, Kodde IF, Dusseldorp F, Druyts PA, Jansen SP, Haverkamp D. Hip arthroscopy in obese, a successful combination? J Hip Preserv Surg. 2016;3:37–42.
16. Larson CM, Ross JR, Stone RM, Samuelson KM, Schelling EF, Giveans MR, et al. Arthroscopic Management of Dysplastic hip Deformities: predictors of success and failures with comparison to an arthroscopic FAI cohort. Am J Sports Med. 2016;44:447–53.
17. Board TN. Predictive factors of success in hip impingement surgery. Hip Int. 2015;25:393.
18. Moons KG, Royston P, Vergouwe Y, Grobbee DE, Altman DG. Prognosis and prognostic research: what, why, and how? BMJ. 2009;338:b375.
19. Noble PC, Conditt MA, Cook KF, Mathis KB. The John Insall award: patient expectations affect satisfaction with total knee arthroplasty. Clin Orthop Relat Res. 2006;452:35–43.
20. Philippon MJ, Maxwell RB, Johnston TL, Schenker M, Briggs KK. Clinical presentation of femoroacetabular impingement. Knee Surg Sports Traumatol Arthrosc. 2007;15:1041–7.
21. Development of the World Health Organization WHOQOL-BREF quality of life assessment. The WHOQOL group. Psychol Med. 1998;28:551–8.
22. Skevington SM, Lotfy M, O'Connell KA. The World Health Organization's WHOQOL-BREF quality of life assessment: psychometric properties and results of the international field trial. A report from the WHOQOL group. Qual Life Res. 2004;13:299–310.
23. Collins GS, Reitsma JB, Altman DG, Moons KG. Transparent reporting of a multivariable prediction model for individual prognosis or diagnosis (TRIPOD): the TRIPOD statement. BMJ. 2015;350:g7594.
24. Bond JL, Knutson ZA, Ebert A, Guanche CA. The 23-point arthroscopic examination of the hip: basic setup, portal placement, and surgical technique. Arthroscopy. 2009;25:416–29.
25. Chahal J, Van Thiel GS, Mather RC, Lee S, Salata MJ, Nho SJ. The minimal clinical important difference (MCID) and patient acceptable symptomatic state (PASS) for the modified Harris hip score and hip outcome score among patients undergoing surgical treatment for femoroacetabular impingement. Orthopaedic Journal of Sports Medicine. 2014;2: 2325967114S00105.
26. White IR, Royston P, Wood AM. Multiple imputation using chained equations: issues and guidance for practice. Stats in Med. 2011;30:377–99.
27. van Buuren S. Flexible imputation of missing data. Boca Raton, FL: CRC Press; 2012.
28. Wood AM, White IR, Royston P. How should variable selection be performed with multiply imputed data? Stat Med. 2008;27:3227–46.
29. Royston P, Moons KG, Altman DG, Vergouwe Y. Prognosis and prognostic research: developing a prognostic model. BMJ. 2009;338:b604.
30. Altman DG, Vergouwe Y, Royston P, Moons KG. Prognosis and prognostic research: validating a prognostic model. BMJ. 2009;338:b605.
31. Harrell FE Jr, Lee KL, Mark DB. Multivariable prognostic models: issues in developing models, evaluating assumptions and adequacy, and measuring and reducing errors. Stat Med. 1996;15:361–87.
32. Steyerberg EW, Vergouwe Y. Towards better clinical prediction models: seven steps for development and an ABCD for validation. Eur Heart J. 2014; 35:1925–31.
33. Harrell Jr FE. rms: Regression Modeling Strategies. R package version 4.5–0. 2016. https://CRAN.R-project.org/package=rms
34. McCarthy JC, Jarrett BT, Ojeifo O, Lee JA, Bragdon CR. What factors influence long-term survivorship after hip arthroscopy? Clin Orthop Relat Res. 2011; 469:362–71.
35. Frank RM, Lee S, Bush-Joseph CA, Salata MJ, Mather RC 3rd, Nho SJ. Outcomes for hip arthroscopy according to sex and age: a comparative matched-group analysis. J Bone Joint Surg Am. 2016;98:797–804.
36. Hetsroni I, Dela Torre K, Duke G, Lyman S, Kelly BT. Sex differences of hip morphology in young adults with hip pain and labral tears. Arthroscopy. 2013;29:54–63.
37. Khan M, Habib A, de Sa D, Larson CM, Kelly BT, Bhandari M, et al. Arthroscopy up to date: hip Femoroacetabular impingement. Arthroscopy. 2016;32:177–89.
38. Amar E, Wong IH, Coady CM, Glazebrook MA. Despite its current widespread use, evidence to support the indications for hip arthroscopy

lags behind: a review of current literature. Journal of ISAKOS: Joint Disorders & Orthopaedic Sports Medicine. 2016;1:87–92.
39. Flanigan DC, Everhart JS, Glassman AH. Psychological factors affecting rehabilitation and outcomes following elective Orthopaedic surgery. J Am Acad Orthop Surg. 2015;23:563–70.
40. Tijssen M, van Cingel R, van Melick N, de Visser E. Patient-reported outcome questionnaires for hip arthroscopy: a systematic review of the psychometric evidence. BMC Musculoskelet Disord. 2011;12:117.
41. Kemp JL, Collins NJ, Roos EM, Crossley KM. Psychometric properties of patient-reported outcome measures for hip arthroscopic surgery. Am J Sports Med. 2013;41:2065–73.
42. Levy DM, Kuhns BD, Chahal J, Philippon MJ, Kelly BT, Nho SJ. Hip arthroscopy outcomes with respect to patient acceptable symptomatic state (PASS) and minimal clinically important difference (MCID). Arthroscopy. 2016;32:1877–86.
43. Martin RL, Philippon MJ. Evidence of reliability and responsiveness for the hip outcome score. Arthroscopy. 2008;24:676–82.
44. Peduzzi P, Concato J, Feinstein AR, Holford TR. Importance of events per independent variable in proportional hazards regression analysis. II. Accuracy and precision of regression estimates. J Clin Epidemiol. 1995;48: 1503–10.
45. Concato J, Peduzzi P, Holford TR, Feinstein AR. Importance of events per independent variable in proportional hazards analysis. I. Background, goals, and general strategy. J Clin Epidemiol. 1995;48:1495–501.
46. Peduzzi P, Concato J, Kemper E, Holford TR, Feinstein AR. A simulation study of the number of events per variable in logistic regression analysis. J Clin Epidemiol. 1996;49:1373–9.
47. Bogunovic L, Gottlieb M, Pashos G, Baca G, Clohisy JC. Why do hip arthroscopy procedures fail? Clin Orthop Relat Res. 2013;471:2523–9.
48. Tijssen M, van Cingel RE, de Visser E, Holmich P, Nijhuis-van der Sanden MW. Hip joint pathology: relationship between patient history, physical tests, and arthroscopy findings in clinical practice. Scand J Med Sci Sports. 2017;27:342–50.
49. Krych AJ, King AH, Berardelli RL, Sousa PL, Levy BA. Is subchondral acetabular edema or cystic change on MRI a contraindication for hip arthroscopy in patients with Femoroacetabular impingement? Am J Sports Med. 2016;44:454–9.

5

A controlled before-after study to evaluate the effect of a clinician led policy to reduce knee arthroscopy in NSW

H. Y. Chen[1*], I. A. Harris[2], K. Sutherland[1] and J-F. Levesque[1,3,4]

Abstract

Background: Clinical evidence shows knee arthroscopy has little benefit for degenerative conditions and considerable variation in the incidence of knee arthroscopy in Australia has been identified. This study aimed to evaluate a clinician-led evidence-based policy which was implemented in one local health district in New South Wales (NSW) in 2012 to reduce the use of knee arthroscopy for patients aged 50 years or over.

Methods: Trends in rates and volume of knee arthroscopy for patients 50 years or over in NSW between 2004 and 2015 by district were examined. Changes at four hospitals that adopted the policy were assessed by a quasi-experimental before and after study design with control groups, using the generalised estimating equations (GEE) Poisson model. Each case hospital was matched with four control hospitals in terms of the volume of knee arthroscopy surgeries performed in the five years prior to the intervention.

Results: Between 2004 and 2015, the number of knee arthroscopies in NSW initially increased and then decreased after 2011, with considerable variation across districts. While an overall reducing trend in NSW was observed between 2011 and 2015 (39%), a 58% reduction (95% CI: 55–62%) was found in the intervention district, including the private sector, being the greatest reduction found in all districts. The GEE Poisson results show that, compared with control hospitals, the number of knee arthroscopy was significantly reduced by 56% (95% CI: 11%–79%) at four hospitals that adopted the policy during the follow-up period ($p = 0.02$).

Conclusions: Clinicians in one local health district initiated a policy to restrict knee arthroscopy for patients aged 50 years or over, which may explain the greater reduction seen in that district compared to all others, despite an overall decrease noted in the state. A significant reduction found at intervened hospitals proved the effect of the policy, suggesting that the implementation of a simple clinical governance process may help reduce inappropriate surgery.

Keywords: Performance and evaluation, Quality and safety, Hospitals, Clinical guidelines

Background

Clinical variation has been extensively documented across a wide range of specialties in many healthcare systems. J. Alison Glover was a pioneer in publishing a seminal study on tonsillectomy rates in 1938 [1] and around forty years later, Wennberg and Gittelsohn conducted work that culminated in the highly influential Dartmouth Atlas of Clinical Variation [2]. Some of their early work highlighted the role of clinical leadership in discontinuing procedures or low value care. *"The drop, we subsequently learned, occurred because of conscious change in treatment policy among local physicians .... Upon learning of the high rate in their area, two physicians... undertook an active review process that led to the rapid decline of their use of the procedure"* [2].

The Dartmouth Atlas catalysed efforts to explore clinical variation across many healthcare systems and focused attention on identifying treatments and procedures that are overused or provided to patients despite insufficient evidence about their efficacy and effectiveness [3–5].

Knee arthroscopy is a commonly performed orthopaedic surgical procedure, with approximately one

* Correspondence: tom.chen@health.nsw.gov.au
[1]Bureau of Health Information, Level 11, 67 Albert Avenue, Chatswood, NSW 2067, Australia
Full list of author information is available at the end of the article

million performed annually in the USA [6] and over 70,000 annually in Australia [7]. Significant geographic variation has been demonstrated in the rates of knee arthroscopy internationally [8] and within Australia [3]. This may represent variation in surgeon preferences or 'supply-sensitive care' –variation that arises not in response to evidence but due to availability of resources such as doctors or hospital beds [9].

Around 55% of knee arthroscopies in New South Wales (NSW), Australia, are performed for people aged 50 years or over, in whom degenerative changes such as osteoarthritis and meniscal tears are common [10–12]. The correlation between knee symptoms (e.g. pain, stiffness and mechanical symptoms) and the presence of meniscus tears and degenerative changes is weak. Population studies have shown that knee symptoms are not more likely in patients with meniscal tears, and that most patients with meniscus tears do not have knee pain [10, 11].

The evidence on knee arthroscopy for degenerative conditions has been accumulating for many years [13–16] and has been recently summarised in three systematic reviews [17–19] and a combined systematic review and practice guideline [20], yet observational studies using administrative data have shown that the rates of knee arthroscopy are not falling significantly, particularly for patients with degenerative conditions [21, 22]. One systematic review concluded that this surgery had no clinically important benefit in middle aged or older populations, regardless of their osteoarthritis status and found that knee arthroscopy surgery was associated with risk of harm [18]. A recent review pointed out that compared with conservative management strategies, patients who undergo knee arthroscopy do not have important benefits in pain or function over the long term [19]. Current guidelines make "a strong recommendation against the use of arthroscopy in nearly all patients with degenerative knee disease" and conclude that "further research is unlikely to alter this recommendation" [20].

In 2011, the orthopaedic department head covering two public hospitals in South Western Sydney Local Health District (SWSLHD, one of 16 districts in NSW) suggested a policy change in response to increasing evidence against the use of arthroscopy in degenerative knees, particularly affecting the middle aged and older people [13, 16]. As of 2012, the policy change restricted knee arthroscopy to patients aged less than 50 years unless approved by the department head. For patients aged 50 or over, cases presenting for knee arthroscopy were reviewed by admissions staff and forwarded to the department head. The department head reviewed but did not refuse any procedures that were submitted for surgery. The intervention involved education of the surgeons and the insertion of an extra step in the process, but not refusal to perform the surgery. This method was chosen due mainly to its simplicity and because of experience of previous success using this method to reduce the use of bone morphogenetic protein intra-operatively. The decline in case numbers was due to a lower number of patients recommended for surgery, not due to cancellation of those cases. Patients already on the waiting list for knee arthroscopy at the time of the intervention were not removed from the list. The maximum wait for surgery in NSW is 12 months.

A third public hospital adopted the policy in late 2012, and, in 2013, the orthopaedic surgeons at a fourth hospital agreed to participate. The other (fifth) orthopaedic department did not participate in the policy based on their perception of the effectiveness of the procedure in degenerative knees. While four of the five public hospitals performing knee arthroscopy in SWSLHD participated, no private hospitals were involved in the policy, although the department members involved also worked in private hospitals.

This paper describes changes in the rate and volumes of knee arthroscopy following this natural experiment. It reports trends in the volume and rate of knee arthroscopies in the state of NSW, grouped by Local Health District (LHD). The impact of policy was assessed by comparing the reductions in knee arthroscopy in SWSLHD with those in other districts and also the reductions in the four public hospitals that adopted the policy versus matched control hospitals.

Methods

Data

We used the Admitted Patient Data Collection including records for admitted patients from both public and private hospitals in NSW (population 7.6 million at the end of 2015), between January 1, 2004 and September 30, 2016 [23]. There are more than 220 public hospitals and health services in NSW which provide free health care to Australian citizens and permanent residents. People with private health insurance can choose to go to private hospitals ($n = 190+$). While public hospitals cover a full range of services, the majority of elective surgeries occurred in private hospitals [24]. Private hospital data after June 30, 2015 were incomplete when the analyses was conducted. The complete data in 2015 are now included in Additional file 1: Table S3, along with the overall reduction in arthroscopies between the 12 months to December 31, 2011 and the 12 months to June 30, 2017 (most recent data available). Procedure codes for knee arthroscopy are provided in Additional file 1: Table S1. Procedures associated with ligament reconstruction were excluded. Admitted patients with a knee arthroscopy procedure code in the principal or any secondary procedures between 2004 and 2016 were identified. The number of knee arthroscopies by public/private sector, and by the location of surgery (local: patients received surgery at public hospitals at their residential LHD/outflow: patients received surgery in other LHD's public hospitals) are presented in Additional file 1: Table S2 with estimated mid-year population for the same age group. As the policy only focus on aged 50 years or over, this study only presented and discussed the results for this age group.

Intervention

A policy was introduced in participating hospitals that involved a clinical governance process requiring department head approval for knee arthroscopy surgery for patients aged 50 years or older. The evidence was presented at a department meeting in 2011 prior to the initial decision by the first two hospitals. No further surgeon education was performed. Additionally, a letter was written to all primary care providers (general practitioners) in the LHD explaining the evidence against knee arthroscopy in this group and against unnecessary investigations (MRI).

Ethical consideration

According to the policy activities that constitute research at the NSW Ministry of Health, this work met criteria for operational improvement activities exempt from ethics review.

Analysis

Rates of knee arthroscopy in people aged 50 and over were estimated for each calendar year (i.e., the number of knee arthroscopy performed for residents aged 50 or over in SWSLHD divided by the number of SWSLHD residents aged 50 or over). Results for NSW and districts include patients aged 50 years and over, taking into account patient flows between districts (inflow: patients lived in other LHDs received surgery in this LHD's public hospitals; outflow: patients lived in this LHD received surgery in other LHD's public hospitals). The reduction in knee arthroscopy in both public and private hospitals between 2011 and 2015 for each district was assessed in order to capture any reduction since the first implementation in 2011 (Additional file 1: Table S3 includes an update of the complete data in 2015 and the reduction up to June 30, 2017).

Reductions in knee arthroscopy at four SWSLHD 'intervention' hospitals were further examined by a controlled before and after study design using a GEE Poisson model. Due to a possible lag in uptake of the recommendation and the fact that waiting lists were not altered, we chose 1st January of the year following the intervention to be the cut-off between pre- and post-implementation. Therefore, the post intervention period for three hospitals started on January 1, 2013 and the last one started at January 1, 2014. Earlier time points (January 1, 2012 and July 1, 2012) were used in sensitivity analyses. Trends in the number of arthroscopies before and after the policy change were compared with other matched control hospitals (one intervention hospital matched with four controls). All hospitals included in this part of the analysis are acute public hospitals. Control and intervention hospitals were also matched for the total number of knee arthroscopies between January 1, 2008 and December 31, 2012 (the fourth hospital was matched based on January 1, 2009 and December 31, 2013). All arthroscopies performed by September 30, 2016 were included in the follow-up analyses. The GEE Poisson model was used to examine arthroscopy volumes after the policy change, taking into account different follow-up times at each intervention hospital. Analyses are based on five years of data preceding the policy change and 45 months of follow-up data for three hospitals and 33 months for the remaining hospital. Due to a small number of intervention hospitals ($n = 4$), model-based standard errors were used to assess the significance of the findings. In the GEE analysis, the regression coefficient (β) represents the log-scale of the outcome variable so that the reduction rate at intervened hospitals is given by $1\text{-}e^{\beta}$. A negative value for β indicates that the rates for knee arthroscopy decreased following intervention, and vice versa for a positive value for β. This is also known as difference in difference regression which is often used to estimate the effect of a specific intervention or treatment by comparing the changes in outcomes over time between the intervention group and the control group. The analyses were performed using SAS software, version 9.4 (Cary, NC) [25].

Results

Between 2004 and 2016, there were more than 10,000 knee arthroscopies performed on people aged 50 years or over in NSW each year of the study period (Data is provided in Additional file 1: Table S2).

Examining the knee arthroscopy volumes in the intervention district, by the amount of arthroscopies provided by public hospitals within the district (Supply) and the total arthroscopies performed on the district residents, regardless of where they received surgery (Demand), there was a clear drop after 2011 (Fig. 1a and b). The reduction in arthroscopies performed on SWSLHD residents was not only seen in public hospitals but also the surgeries performed in the private sector, including residents treated in private hospitals at other LHDs (Fig. 1b). A 40% or greater decrease in rates of knee arthroscopy in public sector was observed in five of 15 districts over the study period (Fig. 2a). In the period 2011–15, the largest decrease (from 1.4 to 0.5 per 1000 population) was found in the intervention district (SWSLHD). A similar drop in private sector was observed in SWSLHD between 2011 and 2014, from 3.6 to 2.3 per 1000 population, which was also the largest reduction among all districts in NSW (Fig. 2b). In view of the overall decrease noted, we

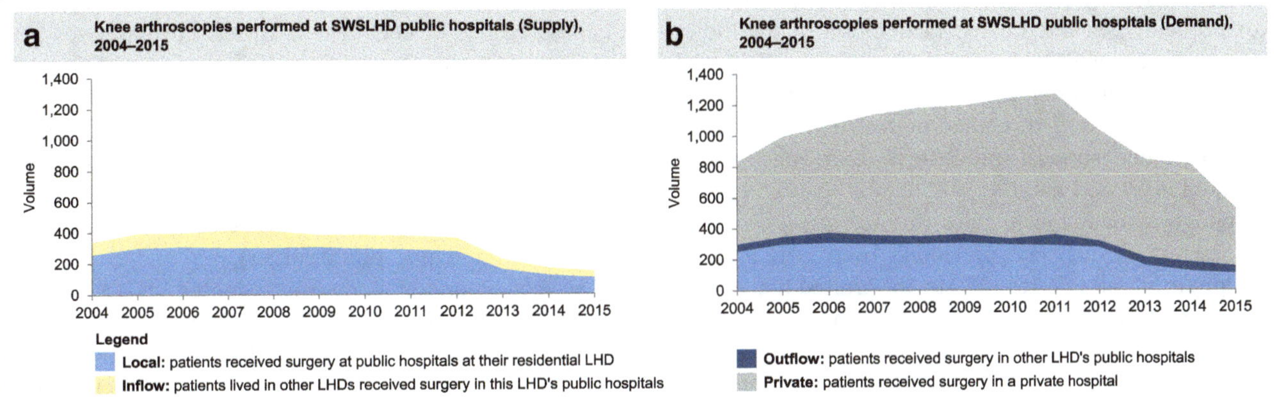

Fig. 1 Knee arthroscopy (**a**) supply and (**b**) demand, for age 50+ years in SWSLHD between 2004 and 2015

calculated the overall (state-wide) decrease in the rate of knee arthroscopy in people aged 50 years or older using the most recent data available (Additional file 1: Table S3). This showed a decrease from a peak of 5.4 per 1000 people in 2011 to 2.8 per 1000 people in the 12 months up to June 30, 2017, a decline of 48% over 4.5 years.

Table 1 presents the reduction from 2011 to 2015 for NSW overall and by district. Between 2011 and 2015, the number of knee arthroscopies in NSW reduced by 39% (95% CI: 38–40%). Considering arthroscopies in both public and private hospitals by district, a clear reduction in arthroscopies (range from 7% to 58%) was shown for all districts except for Far West (number of arthroscopy in Far West LHD increased from 31 to 41 over the same period). The reduction in SWSLHD was the highest among all districts (58%, 95% CI: 55–62%) (Table 1).

Table 2 summarised the number of knee arthroscopy before and after the policy implementation at both intervention and control hospitals. For example, in the first intervention hospital, there were 102 and 53 knee arthroscopies performed before and after the intervention, respectively. The corresponding figures in control hospitals were, in average, 104 and 87. It was clear that the number of knee arthroscopy reduced after the intervention at both intervention and control hospitals, despite the reduction scale at intervention hospitals seemed to be greater than that at control hospitals. Tables 3 present the estimation of reductions in knee arthroscopies in four hospitals where the policy was implemented. The number of knee arthroscopy at four intervention hospitals reduced by 56% (95% CI: 11%–79%, $p = 0.02$). Sensitivity analyses adjusting cut off dates resulted in similar findings.

Discussion

Our results provide empirical evidence of practice change in response to an evidence-based policy in SWSLHD. The rate of knee arthroscopy in patients aged 50 years or over in SWSLHD decreased by almost 60% between 2011 and 2015 following the policy change. Despite an overall reduction over time seen at state level, the reduction was significantly larger in the intervention LHD. The results of difference in difference regression also found intervention hospitals had statistically significant more reductions than control hospitals. It is worthwhile to mention the fact that the intervention in the intervention hospital was not a complex intervention requiring heavy investments. It was

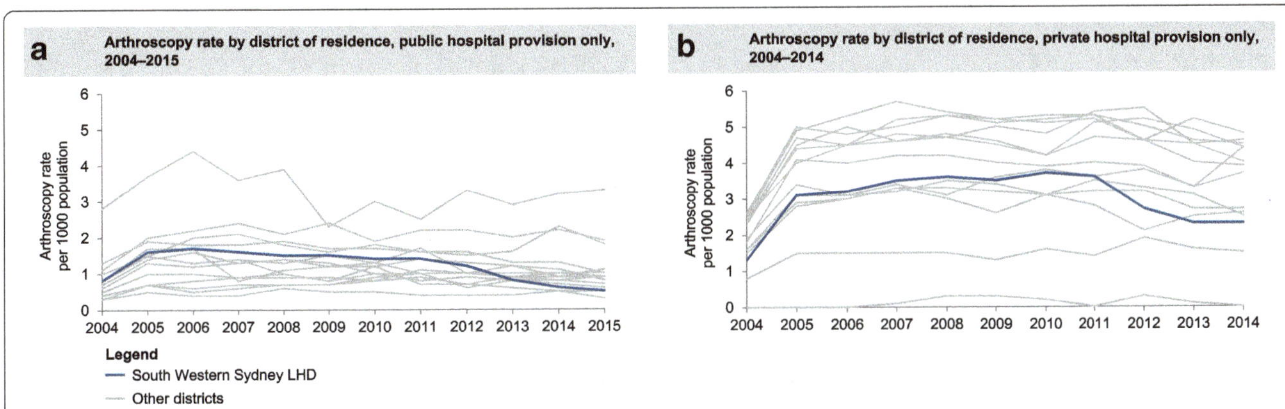

Fig. 2 Knee arthroscopy demand rates for age 50+ by districts, (**a**) public and (**b**) private, between 2004 and 2015

a simple clinical governance and education process that most probably generated a reconsideration of the indication for arthroscopies and referral to surgeons. This study provide empirical evidence to show a very simple process worked, and therefore, this could be scaled and potentially tried for other surgical procedures that may not be warranted in all patients.

Although a reduction in rates of knee arthroscopy has been warranted, there has previously been little evidence of a significant fall in rates [26]. In the United States, both increase and decrease in the knee arthroscopies were found [6, 27] and the trends are not consistent with a recent study showing the annual rate of knee arthroscopy dropped between 1998 and 2002 but increased between 2006 and 2010 [28]. Studies from UK and Canada showed a reduction from 1993 to 2004 [29]. Furthermore, Mattila et al. [30] reported recent reductions in knee arthroscopy rates in Sweden and Finland, which could be attributed to well-established scientific evidence against knee arthroscopy for osteoarthritis. A recent study found there was a reducing trend in meniscus surgeries in the Netherlands following a nationwide guideline and the incidence seemed to increase in the last year of the study period [31].

Due to evidence showing that there was great variation between hospitals in patients with knee osteoarthritis receiving knee arthroscopy in Australia [32], and evidence against the effectiveness of knee arthroscopy, some clinicians at SWSLHD initiated a policy in 2011 to restrict knee arthroscopy for patients 50 years and over, regardless of the presence of knee osteoarthritis. Further steps have been taken in this district to reduce the rates of inappropriate knee arthroscopy by educating primary care providers, in order to reduce referrals and unnecessary investigations (MRI scans) for people with knee pain. Our initial findings demonstrated that clinician led policy change, based on high quality evidence is associated with a reduction in inappropriate surgery.

The policy under study was adopted by four public hospitals in SWSLHD in 2011–2013; however a drop in volumes was also observed over the study period in the other hospitals in the district as well as in other districts and in NSW overall. The fall in knee arthroscopy rates after 2011 observed in various districts suggests some practice change in response to the evidence. However, it was not possible to determine the extent to which the reduction observed in the intervention district was a result of the policy change. The interpretation of rate reduction observed should be cautious as rates were estimated based on "demand" rather than "supply" (no fixed denominator). The reduction in rate based on "demand" reflects the change in need for knee arthroscopy for residents in this particular LHD. This is because "demand" includes "outflow" as it measures surgery on patients living within an LHD, regardless of where they have surgery. Supply data reflects the number of surgeries performed in this LHD, regardless of where the patient lives. By using demand

Table 1 Reductions in numbers of knee arthroscopies for age 50+ between 2011 and 2015 by district, public and private hospitals, NSW

NSW district	Arthroscopy surgeries, 12 months to December 31, 2011	Arthroscopy surgeries, 12 months to December 31, 2015[b]	Reduction	Reduction percentage (%)	95% CI	
Central Coast	792	430	362	46%	42%	49%
Far West	31	41	−10	−32%	−14%	−50%
Hunter New England	2021	1554	467	23%	21%	25%
Illawarra Shoalhaven	497	370	127	26%	22%	29%
Mid North Coast	735	516	219	30%	26%	33%
Murrumbidgee	438	383	55	13%	9%	16%
Nepean Blue Mountains	601	354	247	41%	37%	45%
Northern NSW	476	409	67	14%	11%	17%
Northern Sydney	2012	905	1107	55%	53%	57%
South Eastern Sydney	2133	1187	946	44%	42%	46%
South Western Sydney	899	374	525	58%	55%	62%
Southern NSW	133	124	9	7%	2%	11%
Sydney	659	325	334	51%	47%	55%
Western NSW	390	254	136	35%	30%	40%
Western Sydney	841	541	300	36%	32%	39%
NSW overall	12,703	7786	4917	39%	38%	40%

[a]Figures included knee arthroscopies in both public and private hospitals; St Vincent district data is not presented due to confidentiality issue
[b]Due to incomplete private hospital data after July 1, 2015 at the time of this analysis, the number of knee arthroscopy in private hospitals during 2015 is underestimated

Table 2 The number of knee arthroscopy pre- and post- intervention at intervention and control hospitals (public only)

Policy		Intervention 1	Control 1	Intervention 2	Control 2	Intervention 3	Control 3	Intervention 4	Control 4	All interventions ($n = 4$)	All control ($n = 16$)
Before[a]	Sum	102	415	595	2080	410	1539	142	612	1249	4646
	Average	102	104	595	520	410	385	142	153	312	290
After	Sum	53	349	138	1181	133	1040	40	371	364	2941
	Average	53	87	138	295	133	260	40	93	91	184
	Follow up Period (months)	45	45	45	45	45	45	33	33	39	39

[a]Both Intervention and control hospitals have 5 year pre intervention data; the number of knee arthroscopy are rounded

(and including outflow), we have addressed the criticism that the reduction in rates of surgery was due to patients seeking treatment outside the LHD.

A controlled before and after study design was used to assess the cause-effect of the policy implementation at the four intervention hospitals (within the intervention district). Four control hospitals from other LHDs were matched with each intervention hospitals in terms of hospital type (public), acute hospital and total volume of knee arthroscopies performed in the 5 years before the policy implementation.

The results showed that compared with hospitals without the policy, intervention hospitals reduced the number of knee arthroscopy by 56%. This reduction figure echoes the observation comparing the number of knee arthroscopy supplied by LHDs, which found that district of the intervention had the greatest reduction (58%) among all districts. Despite a small sample size, the reductions found comparing with control hospitals were statistically significant, suggesting the success of the policy. The reduction translates to 26 less cases performed per year in each hospital between 2012 and 2015 (95% CI: 22–30). Over the study period, we did not observe significant change in knee replacement rate for SWSLHD residents in the same age group (data not shown). The longer trend of knee replacement may need to be re-examined to ensure the reduction in knee arthroscopies does not lead to an increase in knee replacement surgery. This study is strengthened by using administrative datasets covering the whole state, which allowed comprehensive coverage and allowed measurement of district inflow and outflow and diversion to private hospitals. It also allowed measurement of the lead-in period prior to the policy change. The quasi-experimental design with control group enabled to examine the effect of the policy despite the overall reduction in arthroscopies in NSW.

Evidence on behavioural interventions that reduce inappropriate practice can be found [33–35] but not specifically for knee arthroscopy. From the review of interventions that reduce inappropriate transfusion, the results from the pre- and post-intervention, including education, retrospective audit, prospective audit along with a new request form, patient-specific decision support or new transfusion algorithm, have shown some reductions in inappropriate transfusion [34]. Different definitions of inappropriateness may make comparison difficult, but Wilson et al. concluded that there is evidence to support the possibility of behavioural interventions to change inappropriate practice among health care providers [34].

It is not possible to determine the relative contribution of the administrative intervention (department head approval) and the letter sent to general practitioners in the district.

A limitation of the study is that it did not measure 'leakage' (or patient flows) across state borders. This mainly affects the few districts that are adjacent to other states. Due to incomplete private hospital data in 2015, the overall reduction might be overestimated, but this should not influence the comparison between LHDs. Additional file 1: Table S3, with the complete data in 2015 and the overall reduction in arthroscopies between the 12 months to December 31, 2011 and the 12 months to June 30, 2017, consolidates our findings. While a reduction in private sector arthroscopies was observed in SWSLHD between 2012 and 2014, we could not properly assess the significance of reductions in the private sector as we have limited information to differentiate which private hospitals were influenced by the policy. Similarly, some clinicians at 'intervention' hospitals may work at private hospitals at other LHDs. Due to the control groups not being selected

Table 3 Model estimations of reduction in knee arthroscopy in intervention hospitals (vs. control hospitals[a], public only)

	Point estimates	95% CI		*p*-value	Incidence rate ratio
Intervention	0.08	−0.23	0.38	0.630	
Time	−0.13	−0.40	0.13	0.323	
Intervention [a] Time	−0.82	−1.52	−0.12	0.022	0.44 (0.21–0.89)

[a]Control hospitals were matched by volume of knee arthroscopy, and one intervention matches with four controls

randomly, selection bias may also exist [36]. We have not adjusted for the number of orthopaedic surgeons in each department or the surgical volume of the department but these variables may not be associated with the timing or extent of practice change. In addition, the sample size maybe too small to limit the ability to generalise the findings to all hospitals in NSW or other countries. Nevertheless, the results from comparison between districts and to external controls showing similar reductions support the effect of the policy on reducing the knee arthroscopies despite the overall reduction in NSW.

Conclusion

This is the first study in Australia to report a decrease in knee arthroscopy as a result of clinician-led policy change, which involved a simple clinical governance process and education letter. This study shows a significant reduction in the rate of knee arthroscopic surgery in patients aged 50 years and over after local implementation of the policy, despite an overall reduction in NSW since 2011. While evidence in this study generally supports the effect of the policy in reducing knee arthroscopies in the four hospitals and potentially in the whole district, a future assessment with more participating hospitals with sufficient follow-up period of data is recommended to verify the causal effect of the policy.

Abbreviations

GEE: Generalised estimating equations; LHD: Local Health District; NSW: New South Wales; SWSLHD: South Western Sydney Local Health District

Acknowledgements

We thank the NSW Ministry of Health for access to population health data and the NSW Centre for Health Record Linkage for linking the data sets. We also thank Dr. Renee Carter for initial statistical guidance.

Authors' contributions

HYC had main responsibility for study design, data analyses and writing of manuscript. IAH, KS and JFL all contributed to study design and writing of manuscript. All authors have read and approved the manuscript.

in according to the policy activities that constitute research at the NSW Ministry of Health [37].

Competing interests

The authors declare that they have no competing interests.

Author details

[1]Bureau of Health Information, Level 11, 67 Albert Avenue, Chatswood, NSW 2067, Australia. [2]Whitlam Orthopaedic Research Centre, Ingham Institute for Applied Medical Research, South Western Sydney Clinical School, University of NSW, High St, Kensington, NSW 2052, Australia. [3]Centre for Primary Health Care and Equity, University of NSW, Sydney, NSW, Australia. [4]Agency for Clinical Innovation, Level 4, 67 Albert Avenue, Chatswood, NSW 2067, Australia.

References

1. Glover JA. The incidence of tonsillectomy in school children. Indian J Pediatr. 1938;5(4):252–8.
2. Wennberg J. Commentary: a debt of gratitude to. J Alison Glover Int J Epidemiol. 2008;37(1):26–9.
3. Australian Commission on Safety and Quality in Health Care. Australian Atlas of Healthcare Variation. Sydney: ACSQHC; 2015. p. 27.
4. Public Health England. The NHS Atlas of Variation in Healthcare: Reducing unwarranted variation to increase value and improve quality. London: Public Health England; 2015.
5. Health Quality and Safety Commission New Zealand: Atlas of Healthcare Variation. http://www.hqsc.govt.nz/our-programmes/health-quality-evaluation/projects/atlas-of-healthcare-variation. Accessed 8 Mar 2016.
6. Kim S, Bosque J, Meehan JP, Jamali A, Marder R. Increase in outpatient knee arthroscopy in the United States: a comparison of National Surveys of ambulatory surgery, 1996 and 2006. J Bone Joint Surg Am. 2011;93(11):994–1000.
7. Australian Commission on Safety and Quality in Health Care. Australian Institute of Health and Welfare: Exploring Healthcare Variation in Australia: Analyses Resulting from an OECD Study. Sydney: ACSQHC; 2014. p. 27.
8. OECD: Geographic Variations in Health Care: What Do We Know and What Can Be Done to Improve Health System Performance? In. Edited by Studies OHP: OECD Publishing; 2014.
9. Hiscock H, Perera P, McLean K, Roberts G. Variation in paediatric clinical practice: an evidence check review brokered by the sax institute for NSW kids and families. In. Sydney: The Sax Institute; 2014.
10. Englund M, Guermazi A, Gale D, Hunter DJ, Aliabadi P, Clancy M, et al. Incidental meniscal findings on knee MRI in middle-aged and elderly persons. N Engl J Med. 2008;359(11):1108–15.
11. Guermazi A, Niu J, Hayashi D, Roemer FW, Englund M, Neogi T, et al. Prevalence of abnormalities in knees detected by MRI in adults without knee osteoarthritis: population based observational study (Framingham osteoarthritis study). BMJ. 2012;345:e5339.
12. March LM, Bagga H. Epidemiology of osteoarthritis in Australia. MJA. 2004; 180(5 Suppl):S6–10.
13. Moseley JB, O'Malley K, Petersen NJ, Menke TJ, Brody BA, Kuykendall DH, et al. A controlled trial of arthroscopic surgery for osteoarthritis of the knee. N Engl J Med. 2002;347(2):81–8.
14. Sihvonen R, Paavola M, Malmivaara A, Itälä A, Joukainen A, Nurmi H, et al. Arthroscopic partial meniscectomy versus sham surgery for a degenerative meniscal tear. N Engl J Med. 2013;369(26):2515–24.
15. Sihvonen R, Englund M, Turkiewicz A, Järvinen TL. Mechanical symptoms and arthroscopic partial meniscectomy in patients with degenerative meniscus tear: a secondary analysis of a randomized trial. Ann Intern Med. 2016;164(7):449–55.
16. Kirkley A, Birmingham TB, Litchfield RB, Giffin JR, Willits KR, Wong CJ, et al. A randomized trial of arthroscopic surgery for osteoarthritis of the knee. N Engl J Med. 2008;359(11):1097–107.
17. Khan M, Evaniew N, Bedi A, Ayeni OR, Bhandari M. Arthroscopic surgery for degenerative tears of the meniscus: a systematic review and meta-analysis. CMAJ. 2014;186(14):1057–64.
18. Thorlund JB, Juhl CB, Roos EM, Lohmander LS. Arthroscopic surgery for degenerative knee: systematic review and meta-analysis of benefits and harms. BMJ. 2015;350:h2747.
19. Brignardello-Petersen R, Guyatt GH, Buchbinder R, Poolman RW, Schandelmaier S, Chang Y, et al. Knee arthroscopy versus conservative management in patients with degenerative knee disease: a systematic review. 2017;7(5):e016114.
20. Siemieniuk RAC, Harris IA, Agoritsas T, Poolman RW, Brignardello-Petersen R, Van de Velde S, et al. Arthroscopic surgery for degenerative knee arthritis and meniscal tears: a clinical practice guideline. BMJ. 2017;357:j1982.
21. Bohensky MA, Sundararajan V, Andrianopoulos N, de Steiger RN, Bucknill A, Kondogiannis CM, et al. Trends in elective knee arthroscopies in a population-based cohort, 2000-2009. MJA. 2012;197(7):399.
22. Harris IA, Madan NS, Naylor JM, Chong S, Mittal R, Jalaludin BB. Trends in knee arthroscopy and subsequent arthroplasty in an Australian population: a retrospective cohort study. BMC Musculoskelet Disord. 2013;14(1):1.
23. NSW Ministry of Health: Secure analytics for population health research and intelligence (SAPHaRI): Admitted Patient, Emergency Department Attendance and Deaths Register. 2016.
24. Australian Institute of Health and Welfare. Admitted patient care 2015–16: Australian hospital statistics. In: Health services series. Canberra: AIHW; 2017.
25. SAS Institute Inc. SAS/STAT® software. Cary, NC: SAS Institute Inc; 2013.

26. Jarvinen TL, Sihvonen R, Englund M. Arthroscopy for degenerative knee–a difficult habit to break? Acta Orthop. 2014;85(3):215–7.
27. Potts A, Harrast JJ, Harner CD, Miniaci A, Jones MH. Practice patterns for arthroscopy of osteoarthritis of the knee in the United States. Am J Sports Med. 2012;40(6):1247–51.
28. Adelani MA, Harris AH, Bowe TR, Giori NJ. Arthroscopy for knee osteoarthritis has not decreased after a clinical trial. Clin Orthop Relat Res. 2016;474(2):489–94.
29. Hawker G, Guan J, Judge A, Dieppe P. Knee arthroscopy in England and Ontario: patterns of use, changes over time, and relationship to total knee replacement. J Bone Joint Surg Am. 2008;90(11):2337–45.
30. Mattila VM, Sihvonen R, Paloneva J, Fellander-Tsai L. Changes in rates of arthroscopy due to degenerative knee disease and traumatic meniscal tears in Finland and Sweden. Acta Orthop. 2016;87(1):5–11.
31. Rongen JJ, van Tienen TG, Buma P, Hannink G. Meniscus surgery is still widely performed in the treatment of degenerative meniscus tears in the Netherlands. Knee Surg Sports Traumatol Arthrosc. 2017; https://doi.org/10.1007/s00167-017-4473-2.
32. Duckett SJ, Breadon P, Romanes D. Identifying and acting on potentially inappropriate care. MJA. 2015;203(4):183.
33. Loeb M, Hunt D, O'Halloran K, Carusone SC, Dafoe N, Walter SD. Stop Orders to Reduce Inappropriate Urinary Catheterization in Hospitalized Patients: A Randomized Controlled Trial. 2008;23(6):816–20.
34. Wilson K, MacDougall L, Fergusson D, Graham I, Tinmouth A, Hébert PC. The effectiveness of interventions to reduce physician's levels of inappropriate transfusion: what can be learned from a systematic review of the literature. 2002;42(9):1224–9.
35. Cossette B, Bergeron J, Ricard G, Éthier JF, Joly-Mischlich T, Levine M, et al. Knowledge translation strategy to reduce the use of potentially inappropriate medications in hospitalized elderly adults. 2016;64(12):2487–94.
36. Harris AD, McGregor JC, Perencevich EN, Furuno JP, Zhu J, Peterson DE, et al. The use and interpretation of quasi-experimental studies in medical informatics. J Am Med Inform Assoc. 2006;13(1):16–23.
37. Office for Health and Medical Research: Human Research Ethics Committees - Quality Improvement & Ethical Review: A Practice Guide for NSW. Edited by NSW Ministry of Health; 2007.

6

Tourniquet use in arthroscopic anterior cruciate ligament reconstruction

Liang-Tseng Kuo[1,2,3], Pei-An Yu[1], Chi-Lung Chen[1], Wei-Hsiu Hsu[1,4*†] and Ching-Chi Chi[2,4,5*†]

Abstract

Background: To assess the effects of tourniquet use in arthroscopic anterior cruciate ligament (ACL) reconstruction surgery.

Methods: We conducted a systematic review and meta-analysis of randomised controlled trials (RCTs) that compared surgical outcomes following tourniquet use against non-tourniquet use during ACL reconstruction surgery. We searched the Cochrane Central Register of Controlled Trials, MEDLINE, and EMBASE for relevant RCTs. We used the Cochrane Collaboration's tool to assess the risk of bias of included RCTs, and performed a random-effects meta-analysis in calculating the pooled risk estimates. The primary outcomes was postoperative pain measured by visual analogue scale, verbal rating scale, or required morphine dose. The secondary outcomes were blood loss in drainage, operative time, muscle strength, and calf and thigh girth.

Results: We included 5 RCTs with 226 participants (116 in the tourniquet group and 110 in the non-tourniquet group). Postoperative pain and morphine doses were not significantly different between the two groups. Compared to the non-tourniquet group, the tourniquet group had a significantly increased blood loss in the drain (mean difference: 94.40 ml; 95% CI 3.65–185.14; P = 0.04). No significant differences in the operative time and muscle strength were found between the two groups. Tourniquet use was associated with a greater decrease in thigh girth but not in calf girth.

Conclusions: The current evidence shows that compared to tourniquet use, ACL reconstruction surgery without tourniquet does not appear to have any major disadvantages and does not prolong operation time. There might be less drain blood loss associated with tourniquet use, though drains are no longer routinely used in ACL reconstruction surgery.

Keywords: Knee, Anterior cruciate ligament, Tourniquet, Arthroscopy, Systematic review, Meta-analysis

* Correspondence: 7572@cgmh.org.tw; chingchi@cgmh.org.tw; chingchichi@gmail.com
[†]Equal contributors
[1]Department of Orthopedic Surgery, Division of Sports Medicine, Chang Gung Memorial Hospital, 6, Sec West, Chia-Pu Rd, Puzih, Chiayi 61363, Taiwan
[2]Centre for Evidence-Based Medicine, Chang Gung Memorial Hospital, Chiayi, Taiwan
Full list of author information is available at the end of the article

Background

Whether a tourniquet should be used in arthroscopic anterior cruciate ligament (ACL) reconstruction surgery is unclear. The advantages of tourniquet use include less intra-articular blood loss, improved visualization, and hence potential shortening of operative time [1–5]. However, there are reports of adverse effects of tourniquet use. The disadvantages include increased postoperative pain, neuropathies, muscle weakness, and atrophy [6–8]. Rare complications like rhabdomyolysis and a high incidence of thromboembolic events have also been reported [9–11].

There are studies in favour of and against the use of tourniquet. Tsarouhas et al. [4] reported that tourniquet use did not affect postoperative pain and return to light work and jogging. Hoogeslag et al. [12] proposed that tourniquet use improved visibility in arthroscopic knee surgery. The meta-analyses and reviews of Smith and Hing [13] claimed that tourniquet use during arthroscopic ACL reconstruction improved surgical visualization but were contradicted by Zhang et al. [11], who found that it did not reduce blood loss or improve surgical visualisation. Wu et al. [5] published a systematic review on this issue, which reported no significant benefit in operative time using a tourniquet. However, due to heterogeneity over outcomes and limited data provided with a small number of participants (mainly based on two trials), only one outcome could be noted by meta-analysis, thus the value of tourniquet use remains largely unclear.

A recent randomised controlled trial (RCT) on tourniquet use has been published in 2014 [14]. Adding this new trial to systematic review make participant number larger and more synthesis of outcomes possible. To clarify the pros and cons of tourniquet use during ACL reconstruction, we performed a systematic review and meta-analysis of RCTs that evaluated the effects of tourniquet use on surgical outcomes including postoperative pain, muscle strength, blood loss, and operative time as well as thigh and calf girth. Our hypothesis was that the use of tourniquet would provide little benefits in ACL reconstruction surgery.

Methods

Data source and search strategy

We searched comprehensively for all RCTs that compared surgical outcomes following tourniquet use against non-tourniquet use during ACL reconstruction surgery. We searched the Cochrane Central Register of Controlled Trials, MEDLINE, and EMBASE for relevant RCTs from inception to February 20, 2017. The search terms were "(tourniquet OR tourniquets OR tourniquets [Mesh Terms]) AND (anterior cruciate ligament [MeSH Terms] OR (anterior AND cruciate AND ligament) OR anterior cruciate ligament)" without restrictions for language or gender. We also searched the U.S. National Institutes of Health trials register (https://clinicaltrials.gov). In addition, we contacted specialists in this field for any ongoing trial or relevant unpublished data on this topic.

Trials were included if they met the following criteria: (1) designed as a RCT; (2) compared surgical outcomes after using and not using a tourniquet during ACL reconstruction surgery. There were no restrictions on the graft type. Two authors (author A and author B) independently checked the citations identified from the searches against the inclusion criteria. The reference lists of included trials were also checked to identify relevant RCTs.

Data extraction and quality assessment

Two authors (LTK and PAY) independently extracted the following data from the included trials using a standardized data extraction form: first author, year of publication, study design (patient selection and concealment), sample size, participant characteristics (e.g. age, sex, etc.), use of tourniquet (tourniquet pressure and time), and outcome data (subjective outcome: pain score; objective outcomes: operative time (min), blood loss through intra-articular drain (ml), morphine dose (mg), thigh girth (cm), calf girth (cm), and isokinetic quadriceps and hamstring strength). A third author (CCC) arbitrated when the two authors disagreed.

The same two authors independently used the Cochrane Collaboration's tool to assess the risk of bias of included RCTs [15, 16]. A third author resolved differences of opinion. We assessed the following seven domains related to biased estimates of intervention effects: random sequence generation, allocation concealment, blinding of patient and personnel, blinding of outcome assessment, incomplete outcome data, selective reporting, and other biases [16]. For each domain, high risk of bias, low risk of bias, or unclear risk of bias was judged according to the quality of each RCT [15].

The primary outcome was the postoperative pain level on day one, which was judged using a patient-reported visual analogue scale (VAS), a verbal rating scale (VRS), or the required morphine dose. Secondary outcomes included operative time, blood loss in the drain, isokinetic quadriceps strength, and thigh and calf girth.

Statistical analysis

Quantitative analysis was undertaken for pain intensity represented with postoperative morphine consumption dose within 24 h after surgery, operative time, blood loss, and Data were reported as mean difference (MD) or standardized mean difference (SMD) with a 95% CI for continuous data. The χ^2 and I^2 statistics were used to examine statistical heterogeneity: significance was set at $P < 0.10$. I^2 values of 0–24.9%, 25–49.9%, 50–74%, and 75–100% were considered none, low, moderate, and high heterogeneity, respectively [17, 18]. We also estimated the between-study variance using tau-square (τ^2) statistic [16]. We used a random-effects model meta-analysis for all outcomes because we expected clinical heterogeneity across the included RCTs [19]. When analysing continuous data, if the standard deviation was not reported, we estimated the mean and variance from the reported median, range, and sample size [20]. When the standard deviation and range were not available, the variance was estimated from the *P* value in the *t* test. When only graphs were available without raw data for analysis, a software was used to extract the details [21]. A forest plot was applied for summary of results. The Review Manager 5.3 (The Nordic Cochrane Centre, The Cochrane Collaboration, 2014) was used for meta-analysis.

Results

The PRISMA study flow diagram is shown in Fig. 1 [22]. We found 179 published RCTs after searching the MEDLINE, EMBASE, and CENTRAL databases. Three additional records were identified from the bibliography of included RCTs. After we had removed 80 duplicates and excluded 97 studies because they had irrelevant topics or a non-randomised design, we included 5 RCTs for this meta-analysis: Arciero et al. [1], Hooper et al. [3], Nakayama et al. [23], Nicholas et al. [24], and Reda et al. [14]. No ongoing trials were identified after consulting specialists and searching the trial register.

Study characteristics

The included RCTs were published between 1996 and 2015 (Table 1). The sample sizes ranged from 29 to 58, with a total of 226 participants (116 in the tourniquet group and 110 in the non-tourniquet group). All the included studies reported how they used tourniquets. The tourniquet pressure ranged from 269 to 350 mmHg and the mean tourniquet time ranged from 69 to 86 min. For the non-tourniquet groups, diluted epinephrine was added to the irrigation solution in Nakayama et al. [23],

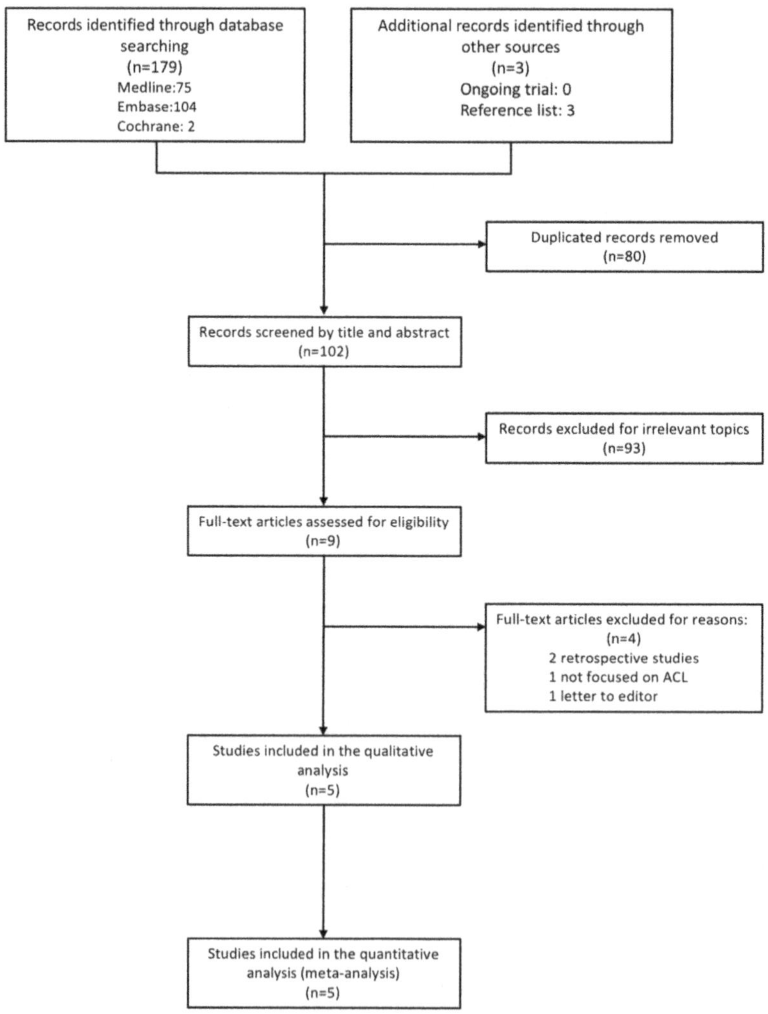

Fig. 1 PRISMA flow diagram of the study

Table 1 Characteristics of included studies

First Author	Place/Year	Type of		Sample size	Gender ratio (M/F)		Mean age[d]		Epinephrine use in NT group	Tourniquet Setting		Follow-up time[f]
		Autograft	Anaesthesia	n (T/NT)	T	NT	T	NT		Pressure[d]	Duration[e]	
Arciero [1]	Canada/1996	BPTB	NR	40 (20/20)	13/7	17/3	24.8	26.7	NR	269	87 (64–105)	12
Hooper [3]	Canada/1999	Hamstring	GA	29 (14/15)	5/9	10/9	35.3	35.7	NR	300	NR	NR
Nakayama [23]	Japan/2013	Hamstring	GA[a]	51 (28/23)	11/17	16/7	26.0	22.0	1:3,000,000	300	NR	3
Nicholas [24]	USA/2001	BPTB	GA/EA[b]	48 (25/23)	13/12	16/7	33.0	32.0	1:100,000	300	85 ± 7.0	6
Reda [14]	Egypt/2015	Hamstring	SA	58 (29/29)	25/4	17/3	26.0	22.0	1:250,000	269	87 (64–105)	6

T tourniquet, NT non-tourniquet, M male, F female, BPTB bone-patella-tendon-bone, GA general anaesthesia, EA epidural anaesthesia, SA spinal anaesthesia, NR not reported

[a]An additional femoral nerve block using 20 ml of 0.25% bupivacaine was done for all participants

[b]GA = 38; EA = 16, [c]Mean age in years, [d]Pressure in mmHg, [e]Duration in minutes, [f]Follow-up in months

	Random sequence generation (selection bias)	Allocation concealment (selection bias)	Blinding of participants and personnel (performance bias)	Blinding of outcome assessment (detection bias)	Incomplete outcome data (attrition bias)	Selective reporting (reporting bias)	Other bias
Arciero 1996	?	?	?	+	+	+	+
Hooper 1999	+	+	+	+	+	+	+
Nakayama 2013	+	?	-	-	+	+	-
Nicholas 2001	+	+	-	+	+	+	-
Reda 2015	+	?	?	+	?	+	-

Fig. 2 Risk of bias summary: authors' judgments about each risk of bias item for each included study. The "–" sign means low risk of bias, the "+" sign means high risk of bias, and the "?" sign means unclear risk of bias

Nicholas et al. [24], and Reda et al. [14]. ACL reconstruction was achieved with bone-patella-tendon-bone (BPTB) autografts in Arciero et al. [1] and Nicholas et al. [24]. Hamstring autografts were used in the remaining three. The types of anaesthesia used were different across trials and included: general (GA), epidural (EA), spinal anaesthesia (SA) (Table 1).

Double blinding was used only in Hooper et al. [3]. Blinding of participants and researchers (performance bias) in all trials was generally unclear or at a high risk, except in Hooper et al. [3]. Blinding of outcome assessment (detection bias) was generally at a low risk, except in Nakayama et al. [23]. All the included trials were at an unclear or a high risk of bias when appraised using the Cochrane Collaboration's tool for assessing the risk of bias in RCTs [17, 18] (Fig. 2).

Postoperative pain

Pain score

Only three studies with 138 patients reported postoperative patient-reported pain score [3, 14, 23]. Hooper et al. provided data on the VRS for pain within 6 h after surgery [3], and Reda et al. reported pain VAS (from 0 to 10) at 4, 10, 16 and 22 h following surgery [14], while Nakayama et al. reported pain VAS of the Japan Society of Pain Clinicians (from 0 to 5) 1 day following surgery [23]. The random-effects meta-analysis showed no significant differences between the two group in the patient-reported pain score at either 6 h (SMD = 1.94, 95% CI = −1.17 to 5.05, P = 0.22) or 22 h after surgery (SMD = 0.13, 95% CI = −−0.24 to 0.51, P = 0.49) (Figs. 3 and 4). The power for this outcome was 0.14.

Required postoperative morphine dose

Hooper et al. [3] and Reda et al. [14] with a total 87 participants reported the required postoperative morphine doses within 24 h after surgery. A random-effects meta-analysis showed no significant difference in the mean dose

Study or Subgroup	Touniquet Mean	SD	Total	Non-Tourniquet Mean	SD	Total	Weight	Std. Mean Difference IV, Random, 95% CI
1.6.1 Visual analogue scale (0–10)								
Reda 2015	8.5	1.1	29	4.9	0.9	29	49.8%	3.53 [2.69, 4.38]
Subtotal (95% CI)			**29**			**29**	**49.8%**	**3.53 [2.69, 4.38]**
Heterogeneity: Not applicable								
Test for overall effect: Z = 8.23 (P < 0.00001)								
1.6.2 Verbal pain scale (0–10)								
Hooper 1999	0.75	0.813131	14	0.45	0.813131	15	50.2%	0.36 [−0.38, 1.09]
Subtotal (95% CI)			**14**			**15**	**50.2%**	**0.36 [−0.38, 1.09]**
Heterogeneity: Not applicable								
Test for overall effect: Z = 0.96 (P = 0.34)								
Total (95% CI)			**43**			**44**	**100.0%**	**1.94 [−1.17, 5.05]**

Heterogeneity: Tau² = 4.88; Chi² = 31.01, df = 1 (P < 0.00001); I² = 97%
Test for overall effect: Z = 1.22 (P = 0.22)
Test for subgroup differences: Chi² = 31.01, df = 1 (P < 0.00001), I² = 96.8%

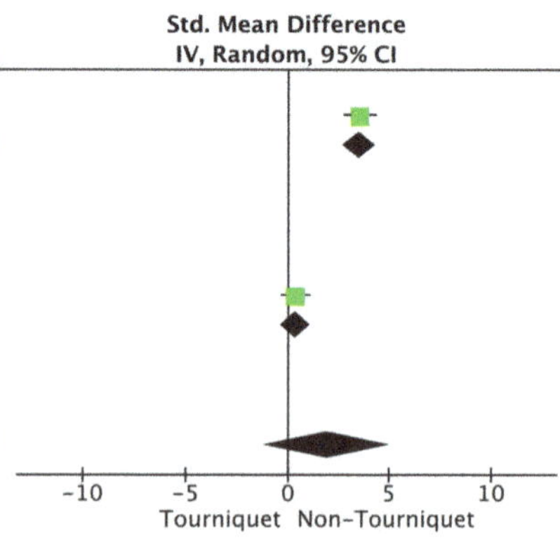

Fig. 3 Forest plot of patient-reported pain score for tourniquet group versus non-tourniquet group. There was no significant difference in patient-reported pain score 6 h after surgery between the tourniquet and non-tourniquet groups

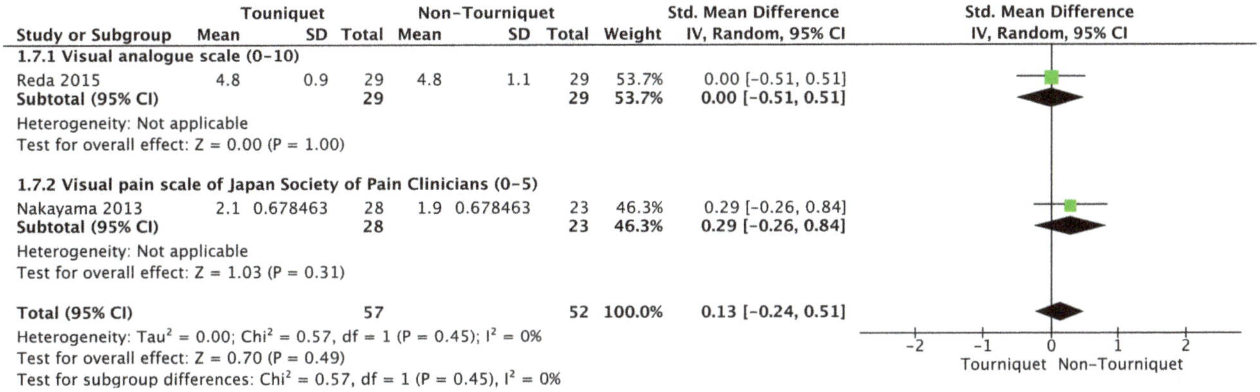

Fig. 4 Forest plot of patient-reported pain score for tourniquet group versus non-tourniquet group. There was no significant difference in patient-reported pain score 22 h after surgery between the tourniquet and non-tourniquet groups

between the two group (MD = 2.25 mg, 95% CI = −3.52 to 8.02, $P = 0.44$) (Fig. 5). The power for this outcome was 0.27. Statistical heterogeneity across the included RCTs was found ($\tau^2 = 12.96, \chi^2 = 3.29, P = 0.07, I^2 = 70\%$).

Operative time

Only Hooper et al. [3], Nakayama et al. [23], and Reda et al. [14] with a total of 138 participants reported operative time. The tourniquet group appeared to have a slightly shorter operative time, but a meta-analysis using the random-effects model found no significant differences between the two groups (MD = 1.52 min when using a tourniquet, 95% CI = −7.20 to 4.16, $P = 0.60$) (Fig. 6). The power for this outcome was 0.37.

There was no significant heterogeneity across the RCTs ($\tau^2 = 10.15, \chi^2 = 3.21, P = 0.20, I^2 = 38\%$).

Blood loss in the drain

Nakayama et al. [23] and Reda et al. [14] with a total of 109 participants reported blood loss in surgical drains during the first 24 h after surgery. There was significant heterogeneity across the trials ($\tau^2 = 4116.68, \chi^2 = 25.12, P < 0.00001, I^2 = 96\%$). Nakayama et al. [23] reported significantly more blood loss in the drain in the tourniquet group than in the non-tourniquet group (133.6 ± 6.4 ml vs. 85.3 ± 47.3 ml, $P = 0.02$). Reda et al. [14] also reported significantly more blood loss in the tourniquet group (327.6 ± 57.2 ml vs. 186.7 ± 47.1 ml, $P = 0.001$). Pooling the two trials together using a random-effects meta-analysis found more blood loss in the surgical drain in the tourniquet group than in the non-tourniquet group (MD = 94.40 ml, 95% CI = 3.65 to 185.14, $P = 0.04$) (Fig. 7).

Muscle strength

Except for Hooper et al. [3], four included RCTs with a total of 197 participants reported postsurgical muscle strength. Nakayama et al. [23] and Reda et al. [14] reported that the isokinetic quadriceps and hamstring strengths were not significantly different between the two groups either before or after surgery. There were insufficient data available for meta-analysis.

Only Arciero et al. [1] and Nicholas et al. [24] reported detailed data on isokinetic muscle strength. A random-effects meta-analysis found no significant differences in isokinetic quadriceps strength measured at 60°/S at 6 months after surgery between the tourniquet and non-tourniquet groups (MD = 0.01 more than for a normal limb site compared with non-tourniquet patients, 95% CI = −0.07–0.09, $P = 0.82$) (Fig. 8). The power for this outcome was 0.47. There was no significant heterogeneity across the trials ($\tau^2 = 0.00, \chi^2 = 1.03, P = 0.31, I^2 = 3\%$).

Thigh and calf girth

Three studies with a total of 157 participants evaluated postsurgical thigh and calf girth. Nakayama et al. [23]

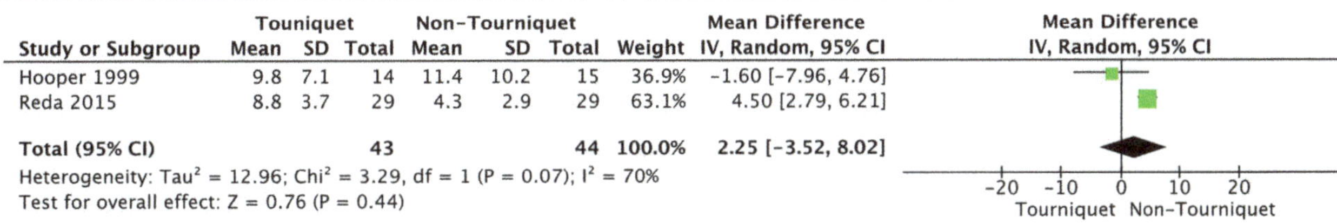

Fig. 5 Forest plot of postoperative morphine consumption for tourniquet group versus non-tourniquet group. There was no significant difference in required postoperative morphine doses between the tourniquet and non-tourniquet groups

Study or Subgroup	Touniquet Mean	SD	Total	Non-Tourniquet Mean	SD	Total	Weight	Mean Difference IV, Random, 95% CI
Hooper 1999	60.8	9.6	14	65.3	15.5	15	25.6%	-4.50 [-13.82, 4.82]
Nakayama 2013	115	18	20	122	17	20	20.6%	-7.00 [-17.85, 3.85]
Reda 2015	64	8.7	29	62	9.1	29	53.8%	2.00 [-2.58, 6.58]
Total (95% CI)			**63**			**64**	**100.0%**	**-1.52 [-7.20, 4.16]**

Heterogeneity: $Tau^2 = 10.15$; $Chi^2 = 3.21$, df = 2 (P = 0.20); $I^2 = 38\%$
Test for overall effect: Z = 0.52 (P = 0.60)

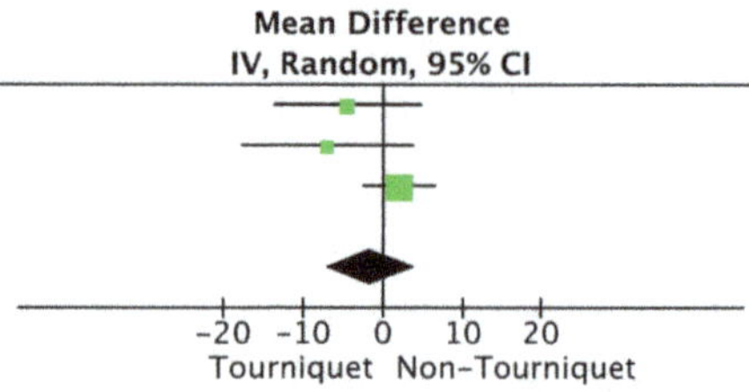

Fig. 6 Forest plot of operation time for tourniquet group versus non-tourniquet group. There was no significant difference in postoperative operation time between the tourniquet and non-tourniquet groups

measured thigh girth at the level of the proximal pole of the patella, and found no significant side-to-side difference between the two groups. Nicholas et al. [24] and Reda et al. [14] both measured the thigh girth at the same level (1/3 the distance between the patella and the anterior superior iliac spine above the superior pole of the patella). Nicholas et al. [24] compared the thigh girth difference between healthy and non-healthy limb, and reported a greater decrease in thigh girth 3 weeks following surgery in the tourniquet group than that in the non-tourniquet group (mean decrease: 2.5 cm vs. 1.1 cm, $P < 0.05$). Reda et al. [14] also found that thigh girth in the tourniquet group decreased more than that in the non-tourniquet group 2 weeks after surgery (mean thigh girth 33.4 ± 1.9 cm vs. 35.6 ± 3 cm, respectively, $P = 0.001$). The available data were insufficient for meta-analysis.

Nicholas et al. [24] and Reda et al. [14] measured the calf girth at the same level (1/3 the distance from the lateral joint line to the lateral malleolus). The postsurgical decrease in calf girth was significantly different between the tourniquet and non-tourniquet groups in Reda et al. [14] (mean calf girth 30.9 ± 1.8 cm vs. 33.1 ± 3 cm, respectively, $P = 0.001$), but not significantly different in Nicholas et al. [24] (mean decrease: 1.1 cm versus 1.0 cm $P = 0.78$). There were insufficient data available for meta-analysis.

Discussion

Our major finding was that tourniquet use during arthroscopic ACL reconstruction surgery significantly increased postoperative blood loss in the drain. There were no significant differences in postoperative pain, the required postoperative morphine dose, operative time, or quadriceps muscle strength at 6 months after surgery. That is, comparing to tourniquet use, ACL reconstruction surgery without tourniquet did not have major disadvantages and complications, and there might be less blood loss in the drain.

There are still debates on whether tourniquet use increases the intensity of postoperative pain and hence the amounts of analgesics administered. Some studies supported this notion [14, 25] but others did not [3, 23]. The findings of our study do not support the effect of tourniquet in worsening postoperative pain, no matter from the view of patient-reported pain score 6 h or 16 h after surgery or from the view of morphine doses within 24 h after surgery. Thus, tourniquet use appears not associated with increased postoperative pain.

The type of anaesthesia administered, especially regional anaesthesia (EA, SA and nerve block), did affect the levels of postoperative pain, but the effects on the tourniquet and non-tourniquet groups were comparable in most of the included RCTs [1, 3, 14, 23]. And the result of meta-analysis of morphine consumption was reported with mean difference between T and NT group, which also minimize the potential bias by type of anaesthesia. Only Nicholas et al. used a mixed type of anaesthesia, but no pain measurements were reported [24]. Two RCTs that reported morphine consumption used hamstring autografts but different types of anaesthesia (GA and SA) [3, 14]; however, it is sensible to combine these two studies because the effect of SA did not exceed 4–6 h after surgery.

Tourniquet use in arthroscopic surgery decreases intra-articular bleeding and increases surgical visualization, which

Study or Subgroup	Touniquet Mean	SD	Total	Non-Tourniquet Mean	SD	Total	Weight	Mean Difference IV, Random, 95% CI
Nakayama 2013	133.6	6.4	14	85.3	47.3	15	50.2%	48.30 [24.13, 72.47]
Reda 2015	327.6	57.2	29	186.7	47.1	29	49.8%	140.90 [113.93, 167.87]
Total (95% CI)			**43**			**44**	**100.0%**	**94.40 [3.65, 185.14]**

Heterogeneity: $Tau^2 = 4116.68$; $Chi^2 = 25.12$, df = 1 (P < 0.00001); $I^2 = 96\%$
Test for overall effect: Z = 2.04 (P = 0.04)

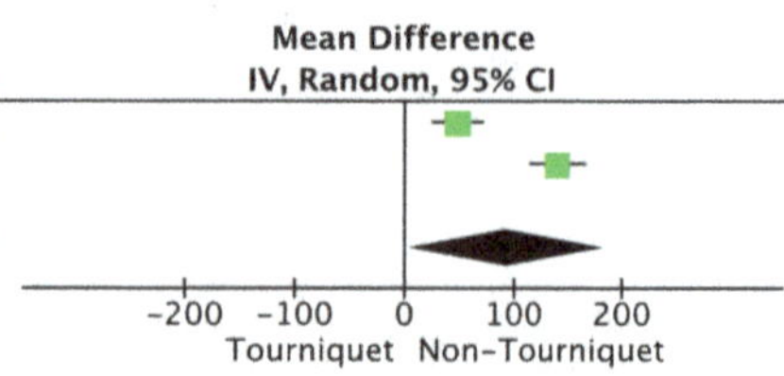

Fig. 7 Forest plot of blood loss in surgical drain for tourniquet group versus non-tourniquet group. The tourniquet group had 94.4 ml more blood loss in the surgical drain than did the non-tourniquet group

Study or Subgroup	Touniquet Mean	SD	Total	Non-Tourniquet Mean	SD	Total	Weight	Mean Difference IV, Random, 95% CI
Arciero 1996	0.71	0.178	20	0.66	0.178	20	49.0%	0.05 [-0.06, 0.16]
Nicholas 2001	0.32	0.191	25	0.35	0.191	23	51.0%	-0.03 [-0.14, 0.08]
Total (95% CI)			**45**			**43**	**100.0%**	**0.01 [-0.07, 0.09]**

Heterogeneity: $Tau^2 = 0.00$; $Chi^2 = 1.03$, df = 1 (P = 0.31); $I^2 = 3\%$
Test for overall effect: Z = 0.23 (P = 0.82)

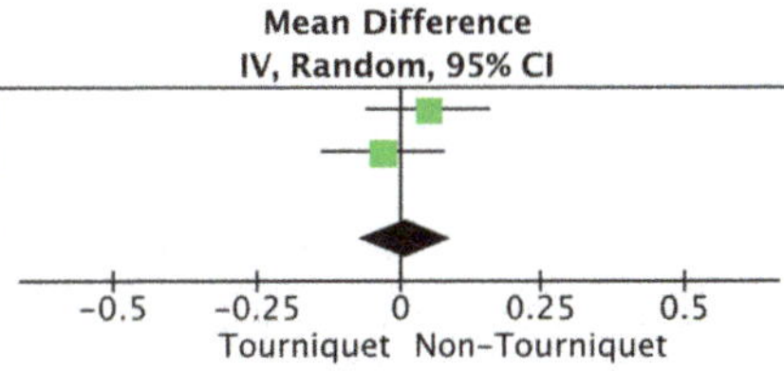

Fig. 8 Forest plot of isokinetic quadriceps strength (60°/S) at 6 months after surgery for tourniquet group and non-tourniquet group. There was no significant difference in isokinetic quadriceps strength at 60°/S at 6 months after surgery between the tourniquet and non-tourniquet groups

potentially shortens operative time [26]. Reda et al. [14] and Hooper et al. [3] evaluated arthroscopic visualization during surgery. Only Hooper et al. [3] reported poorer arthroscopic visibility in the non-tourniquet group. However, satisfactory visualisation is possible by increasing the flow of irrigation fluid or adding epinephrine to the irrigation solution without having to inflate the tourniquet. The operative time did not significantly differ between the two groups. Also, in a recent systematic review that compared using and not using a tourniquet in arthroscopic ACL reconstruction, the operative times were not significantly different [5]. Our meta-analysis showed similar results, i.e. tourniquet use did not shorten the operative time.

We found that tourniquet use in arthroscopic ACL reconstruction surgery might increase blood loss in the drain by about 100 ml, which might cause discomfort during postoperative rehabilitation exercises. That is, a drain is necessary to prevent a large haemarthrosis and other potential complications when using a tourniquet in arthroscopic ACL reconstruction surgery. However, the association between tourniquet use and blood loss in the drain may not be applicable since the drain is not used in most ACL reconstruction surgery nowadays. Meanwhile, the three studies that reported blood loss in the drain had a major flaw [14, 23, 24]. The diluted epinephrine was added to irrigation solution in the non-tourniquet group but not in the tourniquet group. That is, tourniquet use was actually compared with not using a tourniquet plus using epinephrine solution. In other words, ACL reconstruction surgery without tourniquet, but instead using irrigation with epinephrine, is an alternative to tourniquet use in ACL reconstruction surgery.

Furthermore, compared to drainage volume, the haemoglobin level or calculated total blood loss is the preferable way to assess the intraoperative blood loss instead. However, except for Nakayama's trial [23], no other trials employed the two outcomes in assessing intraoperative blood loss. Further study evaluating effect of tourniquet on intraoperative blood loss should report these two outcomes instead to make this issue clearer.

Muscle weakness and atrophy are other concerns related to tourniquet use. Some studies [14, 27–29] showed that using a tourniquet was associated with prolonged muscle weakness and delayed functional recovery. Although Reda et al. [14] reported a significant decrease in the thigh and calf girth, there were no significant differences in quadriceps muscle strength at 6 months after surgery between using and not using a tourniquet. Our study confirmed that tourniquet use was not associated with quadriceps muscle weakness.

None of the studies reported serious complications associated with tourniquet use, e.g. nerve palsy, vascular damage, and thromboembolic events. This might be attributable to the relatively small sample size in each RCT, all of which lacked adequate power to detect these rare complications (i.e. Type II error). The question of whether tourniquet use for arthroscopic ACL reconstruction is safe remains unanswered based on the current available evidence.

Strengths and limitations

This meta-analysis has some strengths: (1) it is the most updated systematic review and meta-analysis of RCTs to explore the effects of tourniquet use in arthroscopic ACL reconstruction; (2) we comprehensively searched the three largest and most comprehensive databases for relevant RCTs; (3) all included RCTs were assessed using the Cochrane Collaboration's tool for the risk of bias; (4) for all but one outcome included in the meta-analyses, no heterogeneity was observed between the two groups.

Our meta-analysis also has some limitations: First, our study only included one additional study than previous systematic review by Wu et al. [5]. However, our study provides more information via meta-analysis including patient-reported pain score, morphine dose, blood loss, and isokinetic quadriceps strength than previous systematic review. Second, the included studies in this review did not have sufficient data for all outcomes available for meta-analysis. The pain score level was one of the primary outcomes of interest. However due to variation of measures and lack of data in some studies, we could not perform a meta-analysis and could not compare the data between studies. Third, due to relatively low methodological quality, small sample size, and clinical heterogeneity of clinical setting and outcome assessment across included studies, it should be very cautious while applying these results to clinical practice. Larger-scale high-quality RCTs might be warranted to clarify this issue.

Conclusions

The current evidence shows that compared to using tourniquet, ACL reconstruction surgery without tourniquet, but using irrigation with epinephrine instead, does not appear to have any major disadvantages and does not prolong operation time. There might also be less drain blood loss; though drains are no longer routinely used in ACL reconstruction surgery.

Abbreviations

ACL: anterior cruciate ligament; EA: epidural anaesthesia; GA: general anaesthesia; MD: mean difference; RCT: randomised controlled trial; SA: spinal anaesthesia; VAS: visual analogue scale; VRS: verbal rating scale

Acknowledgements

Not applicable.

Conflict of interest

The authors declare that they have no conflict of interest.

Funding

No funding was obtained for this study.

Authors' contributions

LTK was responsible for the study concept and design and drafting of the manuscript. LTK and PAY were responsible for the trials selection and appraisal of methodological quality. LTK and CLC participated in acquisition, analysis, and interpretation of data. CCC provided consultation of statistics and methodology. WHH and CCC were in charge of the study concept and design, supervised the study and critically revised the manuscript for important intellectual content. All authors read and approve the final manuscript.

Consent for publication

Not applicable.

Competing interests

The authors declare that they have no competing interests.

Author details

[1]Department of Orthopedic Surgery, Division of Sports Medicine, Chang Gung Memorial Hospital, 6, Sec West, Chia-Pu Rd, Puzih, Chiayi 61363, Taiwan. [2]Centre for Evidence-Based Medicine, Chang Gung Memorial Hospital, Chiayi, Taiwan. [3]Chang Gung University of Science and Technology, Chiayi, Taiwan. [4]College of Medicine, Chang Gung University, Taoyuan, Taiwan. [5]Department of Dermatology, Chang Gung Memorial Hospital, Linkou, 5, Fuxing St, Guishan Dist, Taoyuan 33305, Taiwan.

References

1. Arciero RA, Scoville CR, Hayda RA, Snyder RJ. The effect of tourniquet use in anterior cruciate ligament reconstruction. A prospective, randomized study. Am J Sports Med. 1996;24:758–64.
2. Daniel DM, Lumkong G, Stone ML, Pedowitz RA. Effects of tourniquet use in anterior cruciate ligament reconstruction. Arthroscopy. 1995;11:307–11.
3. Hooper J, Rosaeg OP, Krepski B, Johnson DH. Tourniquet inflation during arthroscopic knee ligament surgery does not increase postoperative pain. Can J Anaesth. 1999;46:925–9.
4. Tsarouhas A, Hantes ME, Tsougias G, Dailiana Z, Malizos KN. Tourniquet use does not affect rehabilitation, return to activities, and muscle damage after arthroscopic meniscectomy: a prospective randomized clinical study. Arthroscopy. 2012;28:1812–8.
5. Wu H, Chen LX, Li YL, Wu Q, Wu QL. Tourniquet used in anterior cruciate ligament reconstruction: a system review. Eur J Orthop Surg Traumatol. 2014;24:999–1003.
6. Delee JC. Complications of arthroscopy and arthroscopic surgery: results of a national survey. Committee on complications of Arthroscopy Association of North America. Arthroscopy. 1985;1:214–20.
7. Johnson DS, Stewart H, Hirst P, Harper NJ. Is tourniquet use necessary for knee arthroscopy? Arthroscopy. 2000;16:648–51.
8. Thorblad J, Ekstrand J, Hamberg P, Gillquist J. Muscle rehabilitation after arthroscopic meniscectomy with or without tourniquet control. A preliminary randomized study. Am J Sports Med. 1985;13:133–5.
9. Lee YG, Park W, Kim SH, Yun SP, Jeong H, Kim HJ, Yang DH. A case of rhabdomyolysis associated with use of a pneumatic tourniquet during arthroscopic knee surgery. Korean J Intern Med. 2010;25:105–9.
10. Small NC. Complications in arthroscopic surgery performed by experienced arthroscopists. Arthroscopy. 1998;4:215–21.
11. Zhang Y, Li L, Wang J, Li ZH, Shi ZJ. Do patients benefit from tourniquet in arthroscopic surgeries of the knee? Knee Surg Sports Traumatol Arthrosc. 2013;21:1125–30.
12. Hoogeslag RA, Brouwer RW, van Raay JJ. The value of tourniquet use for visibility during arthroscopy of the knee: a double-blind, randomized controlled trial. Arthroscopy. 2010;26(Suppl 9):S67–72.
13. Smith TO, Hing CB. A meta-analysis of tourniquet assisted arthroscopic knee surgery. Knee. 2009;16:317–21.
14. Reda W, ElGuindy AM, Zahry G, Faggal MS, Karim MA. Anterior cruciate ligament reconstruction; is a tourniquet necessary? A randomized controlled trial. Knee Surg Sports Traumatol Arthrosc. 2016;24:2948–52.
15. Higgins JP, Altman DG, Gøtzsche PC, Jüni P, Moher D, Oxman AD, Savovic J, Schulz KF, Weeks L, Sterne JA. Cochrane bias methods group. Cochrane Statistical Methods Group The Cochrane Collaboration's tool for assessing risk of bias in randomised trials BMJ. 2011;343:d5928.
16. Higgins JP, Green S. Cochrane Handbook for Systematic Reviews of Interventions Version 5.1.0. The Cochrane Collaboration; 2011. http://handbook-5-1.cochrane.org. Accessed 15 Feb 2017.
17. Higgins JP, Thompson SG. Quantifying heterogeneity in a meta-analysis. Stat Med. 2002;21:1539–58.
18. Higgins JP, Thompson SG, Deeks JJ, Altman DG. Measuring inconsistency in meta-analyses. BMJ. 2003;327:557–60.
19. DerSimonian R, Laird N. Meta-analysis in clinical trials. Control Clin Trials. 1986;7:177–88.
20. Hozo SP, Djulbegovic B, Hozo I. Estimating the mean and variance from the median, range, and the size of a sample. BMC Med Res Methodol. 2005;5:13.
21. Mitchell M, Muftakhidinov B, Winchen T, et al. Engauge Digitizer Software. Webpage: http://markummitchell.github.io/engauge-digitizer. Accessed 11 May 2017.
22. Moher D, Liberati A, Tetzlaff J, Altman DG; PRISMA Group. Preferred reporting items for systematic reviews and meta-analyses: the PRISMA statement. PLoS Med. 2009; 6(7):e1000097. Doi: https://doi.org/10.1371/journal.pmed.1000097
23. Nakayama H, Yoshiya S. The effect of tourniquet use on operative performance and early postoperative results of anatomic double-bundle anterior cruciate ligament reconstruction. J Orthop Sci. 2013; 18:586–91.
24. Nicholas SJ, Tyler TF, McHugh MP, Gleim GW. The effect on leg strength of tourniquet use during anterior cruciate ligament reconstruction: a prospective randomized study. Arthroscopy. 2001;17:603–7.
25. Brookes B, Jamil W, Khunda A, Ryan W. Post-operative pain and length of hospital stay in patients undergoing knee arthroscopy: does tourniquet use make a difference? Bone Jt J Orthop Proc Suppl. 2013;95-B:4.
26. Gutin B, Warren R, Wickiewicz T, O'Brien S, Altchek D, Kroll M. Does tourniquet use during anterior cruciate ligament surgery interfere with postsurgical recovery of function? A review of the literature. Arthroscopy. 1991;7:52–6.

7

Update on the risks of complications after knee arthroscopy

Katarina Friberger Pajalic[1], Aleksandra Turkiewicz[1] and Martin Englund[1,2*]

Abstract

Background: Knee arthroscopy is one of the most common surgical procedures worldwide and the number of arthroscopies has substantially increased in the last 30 years. Thus, our aim was to provide updated estimates on the risk of complications and compare it with the background risk in the general population.

Methods: We identified patients aged 15–84 years with knee arthroscopy in the years 2005–2016 in southern Sweden. We calculated the risk of pyogenic arthritis, venous thromboembolism, and other typical complications within 30 days. As a reference cohort we included the regional population in the corresponding age interval. We estimated the relative and absolute risks of complications compared to the reference cohort using logistic regression adjusted for age, sex, and level of education. We also estimated the proportion of complications in the population explained by knee arthroscopy (population attributable fraction).

Results: We identified 18,735 knee arthroscopy patients (mean age 39 years) and 1,171,084 reference subjects (mean age 46 years). The absolute risk of one or more complications was 1.1% after knee arthroscopy and 0.16% in references. The odds ratio of *any* complication after knee arthroscopy vs. the reference cohort was 9.4 (95% confidence interval [CI] 8.1, 10.9) with an absolute risk difference of 1.4% (1.1, 1.6%). The relative risk (95% CI) for pyogenic arthritis was 115 (75, 174), venous thromboembolism 6.8 (5.1, 9.1), and other complications 7.7 (6.3, 9.5). The population attributable fraction for pyogenic arthritis was 5%.

Conclusions: The absolute risks of complications associated with knee arthroscopy remain small at about 1%. Still, 5% of all pyogenic knee arthritis cases in adults are attributable to knee arthroscopy, thus risks with knee arthroscopy should be carefully considered in the choice of treatment.

Keywords: Knee arthroscopy, Complications, Pyogenic arthritis, Venous thromboembolism, Epidemiology

Background

Knee arthroscopy is one of the most common surgical procedures worldwide [1] and the number of arthroscopies has substantially increased in the last 30 years [2]. The patients are often younger or middle-aged physically active individuals. Annually, there are about one million such procedures performed in the United States and in Sweden (population 9.5 million) the corresponding number is about 35,000 [2, 3]. The most common procedures are meniscectomy, meniscal repair, and cruciate ligament reconstruction [2, 4, 5].

Knee arthroscopy is widely acknowledged to be a safe procedure [4, 6]. Still, there are also known serious complications such as joint infection, deep vein thrombosis, pulmonary embolism, and there are even deaths reported [5, 7, 8]. For more complex arthroscopic procedures that involve ligament reconstruction, the risk of complication has been reported to be the highest followed by meniscal repair, chondroplasty, and meniscectomy [5, 7]. However, there is a substantial variation in the reported absolute risks for complications – pyogenic arthritis between 0.08% [4] and 0.42% [9], deep vein thrombosis between 0.12% [5] and 41% [10], and pulmonary embolism between 0.03% [11] and 0.11% [7].

Because knee arthroscopy has become high volume surgery, and the procedure is also more and more frequently performed in older patients, it is of importance

* Correspondence: martin.englund@med.lu.se
[1]Department of Clinical Sciences Lund, Orthopaedics, Clinical Epidemiology Unit, Faculty of Medicine, Lund University, Remissgatan 4, 221 85 Lund, Sweden
[2]Clinical Epidemiology Research & Training Unit, Boston University School of Medicine, Boston, MA, USA

to gain updated information on safety of the procedure. Further, there are as of yet *no* studies comparing the risks of complications to the underlying risks for these events in the background population. Such comparisons are needed to get a better understanding of the share of complications attributable to the arthroscopy. Hence, the two main purposes of our study were to: 1) determine updated risks for a number of pre-specified complications within 30 days after knee arthroscopy in absolute terms as well in relative terms compared to the background population, and 2) to estimate the proportion of the total number of complications in the society explained by knee arthroscopies.

Methods

Data sources

The Skåne Healthcare Register (SHR)

In Skåne region, the most southern part of Sweden, information about all healthcare visits (primary and secondary outpatient care and hospitalizations) is collected in the Skåne Healthcare Register (SHR). Doctors register the diagnostic codes according to the International Classification of Diseases (ICD)-10 system. Codes for surgical procedures are registered according to the classification of healthcare procedures [12]. In addition, information about the type and level of the health care and the date of the visit is included.

The Swedish population register

The Swedish population register contains information about deaths, gender, and residential address for all residents. This register is continuously updated by the Swedish Tax Agency.

Study cohorts and exposure

For both patients having had knee arthroscopy and the reference population we used the same principal inclusion criteria: we required all persons to be *i*) aged 15 to 84 years and *ii*) to be residents in the Skåne region at the time of the index visit.

In our *exposed* cohort, the exposure of interest was a knee arthroscopy (index visit), defined by the surgical codes in the SHR between February 1st 2005 and November 30th 2016. In brief, the selected surgical knee procedures included exploration of the joint, resection of the meniscus, meniscus repair, ligament reconstruction, and synovectomy (Table 1). We included each person only *once*, at the time of their *first* knee arthroscopy during the inclusion period.

In our *unexposed* cohort, i.e., background population *not* having knee arthroscopy, we included all persons in the Skåne region with at least one healthcare visit in outpatient care or day surgery (excl. Cases of knee arthroscopy) between the February 1st 2005 and November 30th 2016. We randomly selected an index date from a calendar year with at least one healthcare visit (Fig. 1).

Table 1 The different knee arthroscopic procedures included in the study

Code[a]	Knee arthroscopic procedure
NGA01	Exploration of soft tissue of knee or lower leg; arthroscopic
NGA11	Exploration of knee joint; arthroscopic
NGA21	Biopsy of soft tissue of knee or lower leg; arthroscopic
NGA31	Biopsy of bone of knee or lower leg; arthroscopic
NGD01	Total excision of meniscus; arthroscopic
NGD11	Partial excision of meniscus; arthroscopic
NGD21	Reinsertion of meniscus; arthroscopic
NGD91	Other operation on meniscus; arthroscopic
NGE01	Incision or suture of joint capsule of knee; arthroscopic
NGE11	Transcision or excision of ligament of knee; arthroscopic
NGE21	Suture or replantation of ligament of knee; arthroscopic
NGE31	Transposition of ligament of knee; arthroscopic
NGE41	Reconstruction of ligament of knee without foreign object; arthroscopic
NGE51	Reconstruction of ligament of knee with foreign object; arthroscopic
NGE91	Other surgery on capsule or ligament of knee; arthroscopic
NGF01	Total synovectomy of knee; arthroscopic
NGF11	Partial synovectomy of knee; arthroscopic
NGF21	Fixation of fragment of surface of knee; arthroscopic
NGF31	Partial excision of joint cartilage of knee; arthroscopic
NGF91	Other operation on synovia or joint surface of knee; arthroscopic
NGH31	Freeing of adhesions of knee joint; arthroscopic
NGH51	Excision of intraarticular exostosis or osteophyte of knee; arthroscopic
NGH71	Surgery for habitual dislocation of knee joint; arthroscopic
NGH91	Other operation of knee joint; arthroscopic

[a]Surgical codes according to "Klassifikation av. vårdåtgärder" (KVÅ) [in Swedish]

We did not include hospitalizations (i.e. stays at hospital overnight) because all the diagnostic codes are registered once, at the time of discharge. Thus, the true temporal order of diagnoses is unknown, e.g., if pyogenic arthritis developed due to other reasons and was the *indication* to perform the arthroscopic lavage there would have been a risk for reverse causality and thus inflated estimates of risk. Of all knee arthroscopies 6.5% were

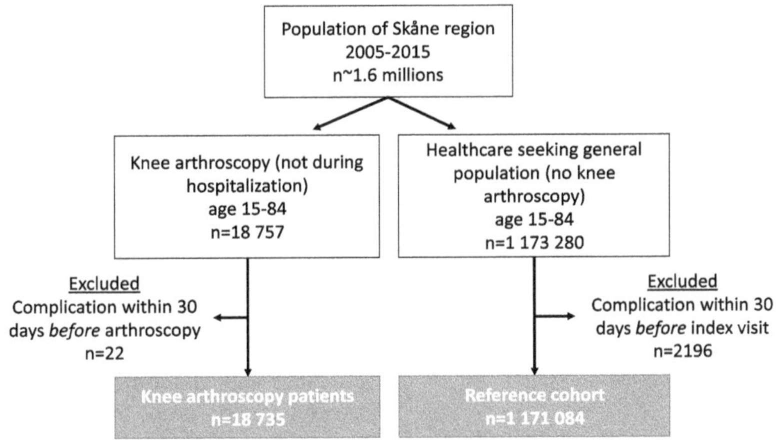

Fig. 1 Flow chart of the study cohorts

made during hospitalisations and were thus *not* included in the present study.

Outcome

The outcome was having at least *one* of our pre-specified complications diagnosed in specialist care within 30 days *after* the index visit (Table 2).

The main diagnoses of interest were pyogenic arthritis (ICD-10 code M00), venous thrombotic event (VTE, including thrombophlebitis, ICD-10 code I80 and pulmonary embolism, ICD-10 code I26), complications of procedures (ICD-10 code T81), local infections (ICD-10 code L08), sepsis (ICD-10 code A41) and mistakes done during the surgery (ICD-10 codes Y60, 61, 69 and 71). Primarily, the outcome was having *any* of the aforementioned complications. Additionally, we performed analyses with the specific complication of pyogenic arthritis, VTE, and other complications, respectively.

Data analysis strategy

To avoid the risk of bias due to reverse causality we only included complications registered from day 1 to day 30 *after* the index visit. The number of complications registered on day 0 was only 15 in the arthroscopy patients and 84 in the reference cohort. In addition, we *excluded* all subjects (both in the arthroscopy group and the reference group) who had *any* of the aforementioned complications up to 30 days *before* the index visit.

We also evaluated the risk for complications after cruciate ligament reconstructions (code NGE41 group within the KVÅ system, Table 1) as compared to the other arthroscopies. Additionally, we estimated the risk of complications after arthroscopy compared to the background population, after excluding cruciate ligament reconstruction from the arthroscopy group. The rationale with these two latter analyses was that cruciate ligament reconstructions have been reported to have a higher risk for complications due to e.g. the drilling of bone tunnels and the typically long duration of the procedure [5, 7].

For the purpose of a sensitivity analysis we created an alternative reference group only containing patients who had consulted for a knee problem but having *no* knee arthroscopy. We used the same study period and age criterion as detailed above. However, we sampled reference subjects, who all have had at least one clinic visit to a physician, with at least one primary diagnostic code for a knee problem which may have represented an indication for knee arthroscopy, but the patient did *not* have knee surgery. The included diagnostic codes were: Meniscus tear, old (M23.2), Chronic instability of knee (M23.5), Unilateral primary osteoarthritis of knee (M17.1), Traumatic tear of meniscus (S83.2), Sprain and strain involving cruciate ligament of knee (S83.5), Other post-traumatic gonarthrosis (M17.3), Tear of articular cartilage of knee, current (S83.3), Other secondary gonarthrosis (M17.5), Injury to multiple structures of knee (S83.7), Patellofemoral disorders (M22.2), Dislocation of patella (S83.0), Other internal derangements of knee (M23.8), and Recurrent dislocation of patella (M22.0). In this sensitivity analysis we also only included arthroscopies with one the above diagnoses registered as main diagnosis. In the analysis, the date of the healthcare visit (reference subjects) or arthroscopy was the index visit. A reference subject was excluded if he/she had any knee surgery (KVÅ code starting with "NG") within 30 days *before* the index visit as well as a knee surgery other than knee arthroscopy 0 to 30 days *after* the index visit.

Statistical analysis

We present descriptive data for the study sample as means and standard deviations (SD) for the continuous variables and as counts and percentages for categorical variables. We estimated the odds ratios (ORs) and risk differences using a logistic regression model. We present both crude

Table 2 ICD-10 codes for the complications included in the study

ICD-10 code	Complication (Adverse event, outcome). Specialist in and out-patient care	Complication group
I80	Phlebitis and thrombophlebitis	VTE
I26	Pulmonary embolism	
M00[a]	Pyogenic arthritis	Pyogenic arthritis
A41	Other sepsis	Other
L08	Other local infections of skin and subcutaneous tissue	
T81	Complications of procedures, not elsewhere classified	
T81.0	Bleeding and hematoma as complication due to surgical and medical procedures, not elsewhere classified	
T81.1	Post procedural shock	
T81.2	Accidental puncture or damage during surgical and medical procedure, not elsewhere classified	
T81.3	Disruption of wound, not elsewhere classified	
T81.4	Infection following a procedure	
T81.5	Complications of foreign body accidentally left in body following procedure	
T81.6	Acute reaction to foreign substance accidentally left during a procedure	
T81.7	Vascular complications following a procedure, not elsewhere classified	
T81.8	Other complications of procedures, not elsewhere classified	
T81.9	Unspecified complication of procedure	
Y60	Unintentional cut, puncture, perforation or haemorrhage during surgical and medical care	
Y61	Foreign object accidentally left in body during surgical and medical care	
Y69	Unspecified misadventure during surgical and medical care	
Y79	Orthopaedic devices associated with adverse incidents	
Death[b]		

[a]M00 in joints other than the knee were not included
[b]Data on death date were retrieved from the Population Register

results (i.e. from an unadjusted model) and results from a model that was adjusted for 3 pre-specified confounders, i.e., characteristics that we considered to be associated with both knee surgery and the risk of complications [13, 14]. These were age (included as continuous variable), sex (male or female), and level of education with four categories (primary school, high school, higher education < 3 years, and higher education ≥3 years). *Individual-level* data on level of education were retrieved from Statistics Sweden (provider of official statistics in Sweden) by register cross-linking. Please note, due to low prevalence of the outcome the ORs can be interpreted as risk ratios [15]. The risk difference was calculated from the adjusted logistic regression model as the difference of the mean probabilities predicted by the model, as implemented in the command *adjrr* in Stata [16]. The population attributable fraction was estimated from the adjusted risk ratios and the prevalence of exposure among cases (i.e. those with outcome) as prevalence_among_cases*((risk_ratio-1)/risk_ratio). All estimates are presented with its 95% confidence intervals (95% CI).

Results

Demographics

Out of our 1,171,084 included subjects, 18,735 (1.6%) had undergone knee arthroscopy. Mean age for the knee arthroscopy cohort and the reference cohort was 39.4 years (SD 15.4) and 45.5 years (SD 20.3), respectively (Table 3).

Indications for knee arthroscopy and type of procedures

The four most common diagnoses registered as the primary diagnosis for the knee arthroscopy were: meniscus tear, old (ICD-10 M23.2, 35%), chronic instability of knee (M23.5, 19%), unilateral primary osteoarthritis of knee (M17.1, 11%) and traumatic tear of meniscus (S83.2, 6%).

The three most frequent arthroscopic procedures were partial excision of meniscus (44%), reconstruction of ligament of knee with/without foreign object (17%) and exploration of knee joint (diagnostic arthroscopy) (16%).

Risk of complications

We found that the risk for any of our pre-specified complications in the knee arthroscopy cohort was 1.1% (210 persons) and in the reference cohort 0.16% (1818 persons) during the follow-up period of 30 days. The most common complications were: complications of procedures not classified elsewhere (33% of all complications), thrombophlebitis (24%) and pulmonary embolism (14%).

The crude OR of having any complication after a knee arthroscopy compared to the reference cohort was 7.3 while it was 9.4 (95% CI 8.1, 10.9) adjusted for age, gender, and level of education (Table 4). The corresponding risk difference was 1.4%. Among the adjusted ORs for the specific complications, pyogenic arthritis yielded by far the highest OR; 115 (95% CI 75, 174). The OR for VTE was 6.8 and for having other complications the OR was 7.7 (Table 4).

In our sensitivity analysis (the comparison against knee patients but *without* knee arthroscopy) the OR of any aforementioned complication (knee arthroscopy vs. the

Table 3 The description of the study cohorts

	Main analysis		Sensitivity analysis	
	Arthroscopy patients, *n* = 18,735	References (general population), *n* = 1,171,084	Arthroscopy patients, *n* = 15,528	References (knee patients), *n* = 44,804
Age, *mean (SD) years*	39.4 (15.4)	45.5 (20.3)	40.1 (15.4)	49.8 (19.5)
Women, *n (%)*	7398 (39.5)	604,583 (51.6)	5900 (38)	22,721 (51)
Level of education (years), *n (%)*				
Primary school (up to 9)	3824 (21)	282,043 (27)	3114 (21)	11,611 (27)
High school (10–12)	8984 (50)	436,465 (41)	7555 (50)	18,863 (44)
Higher education (13–14)	2419 (13)	141,418 (13)	2057 (14)	5277 (12)
Higher education (15+)	2855 (16)	204,085 (19)	2407 (16)	6803 (16)

references) was 4.9 in the adjusted model with an absolute risk difference of 1.0%. The corresponding ORs for pyogenic arthritis, VTE, and other complications were 10.3, 2.3, and 7.9, respectively (Table 4).

The population attributable fraction was 5.1% for pyogenic arthritis, 0.2% for VTE, and 0.3% for the other complications (i.e., about 5% of all pyogenic knee arthritis cases were attributable to the knee arthroscopy).

The OR for complications after *ligament reconstruction surgery* compared to *other arthroscopies* adjusted for age, sex, and level of education was 4.1 (95% CI 2.9, 5.8). The OR for complications after a knee arthroscopy *excluding* ligament reconstruction compared to the reference population was 6.6 (95% CI 5.5, 8.0) with a corresponding risk difference of 0.92% (95% CI 0.73, 1.10%).

Discussion

The absolute risk of having a complication such as pyogenic arthritis, VTE, or other surgical complications after knee arthroscopy was 1.1%. The increase in risk of these conditions as compared to the general population was about 9-fold, and compared to other patients with a knee condition (but no knee arthroscopy) about 5-fold.

There is a need for updated estimates on the risks associated with knee arthroscopy as there has been an increase in number of procedures, but the procedure is also more and more frequently performed also in middle-aged patients. Also the surgical routines may have improved which calls for a need of new estimates of risks associated with the procedure. Thus, we used comprehensive Swedish health care data over a 12-year time period to evaluate the risks for the most frequent complications during a 30-day follow-up period.

It has been previously reported that knee arthroscopy is associated with complications such as pyogenic arthritis and VTE [4, 7, 10, 17]. However, the estimated over-all risk of complications varies from 0.27 to 8.2% with the risk being higher after more complex and longer lasting arthroscopies [7]. Reigstad et al. [8] presented an over-all risk of 5%, but pain and swelling were included in this study which represented almost 50% of all complications. In our study, we focused on the more *severe* complications which explain why our estimate is lower. Sherman et al. [6] presented the over-all risk of complications after knee arthroscopy to be about 8%. In the study the authors classified complications into minor and major. Several of the *major* complications were more similar to the ones selected in our study such as infections, cardiovascular, neurological and instrument failure. Further, the relatively high over all risk could also potentially partly be explained by the study being 20 years old and that arthroscopic surgery has developed

Table 4 Odds ratios (OR) and risk differences (RD) with 95% confidence intervals (CI) for complications after knee arthroscopy compared to reference persons. Results are from a logistic regression model, crude (unadjusted) or adjusted for age, sex and education level

	Main analysis[a]			Sensitivity analysis[b]		
	Crude	Adjusted		Crude	Adjusted	
	OR (95%CI)	OR (95%CI)	RD (95%CI), %	OR (95%CI)	OR (95%CI)	RD (95%CI), %
Any complication	7.3 (6.3,8.4)	9.4 (8.1, 10.9)	1.35 (1.14, 1.56)	5.0 (3.9, 6.4)	4.9 (3.8, 6.4)	0.95 (0.76, 1.15)
Pyogenic arthritis	127 (85, 191)	115 (75, 174)	0.37 (0.27, 0.47)	13.8 (7.6, 25.1)	10.3 (5.6, 19.0)	0.30 (0.21, 0.39)
VTE[c]	4.8 (3.6, 6.4)	6.8 (5.1, 9.1)	0.37 (0.25, 0.49)	2.0 (1.4, 3.0)	2.3 (1.5, 3.5)	0.17 (0.07, 1.30)
Other	6.4 (5.2, 7.8)	7.7 (6.3, 9.5)	0.61 (0.47, 0.60)	7.8 (5.3, 11.6)	7.9 (5.2, 11.9)	0.54 (0.40, 0.68)

[a]knee arthroscopy compared to general population
[b]knee arthroscopy compared to persons consulting for knee problems
[c]venous thrombotic event

since with better equipment and better surgical routines at large. In the rest of the existing literature, which is somewhat more recent, the reported risk of complications is reported to be below 5%. In one study from Japan [4] the investigators report a very low over all risk for complications of merely 0.27% in a relatively small cohort. In larger cohort studies the risk is typically reported to be between 0.64 and 4.7% [7, 18, 19], which is more in line with our findings. The follow-up period in most studies has typically been up to some 30 days [5, 7, 9, 18, 19] with the exception of a few studies with 90 days of follow-up [8, 11, 18]. In our study, we chose 30 days of follow-up because the most common complications, such as infections and VTE, attributed to the surgery are likely to be diagnosed within that time frame.

Partial meniscectomy was the most common procedure in our study (44% of all knee arthroscopies) which is in line with existing literature [2, 5, 8, 11]. Although arthroscopic partial meniscectomy carries a smaller risk for complications as compared to more complex surgery, such as ligament reconstruction, the reported overall risk is still not negligible [7]. This is in line with our results, where even after *excluding* the ligament reconstruction from the arthroscopy group, the relative risk of a complication was still almost 7-fold as compared to the general population.

Since knee arthroscopy is the most common orthopaedic procedure this results quite many patients experiencing a complication even though the absolute risk is low. For example, our data suggests that 5% of all cases of pyogenic arthritis are caused by knee arthroscopy. Thus, indications for arthroscopic surgery need to be scrutinized as proper evidence of efficacy above non-surgical management is sometimes lacking and compliance to new guidelines still needs to be verified, e.g. for degenerative meniscal lesions and knee osteoarthritis [20, 21].

Our study is based on a large study population from an entire Swedish region without selection bias. The original data is all prospectively registered in the electronic medical records, i.e., free of any potential recall bias from both the patient and doctor. We estimated not only the absolute risk for complications after knee arthroscopy but also the relative risk compared to the background population. Still, we would like to acknowledge some important limitations: As in all register-based research, there is a risk of misclassification of procedures and diagnostic codes which may lead to biased results. However, the validity of the diagnostic codes in SHR and Swedish health care registers in general has been reported to be high [22–24]. We would like to emphasize that these registers are not just administrative data per se, as in many other countries, but diagnoses are actually set by the doctors' themselves and data is drawn directly from the patients' electronic medical records. Further, we only included complications diagnosed within specialist care, where the validity of the diagnostic codes (such as pyogenic arthritis or VTE) is expected to be higher than in primary care. We did not include the complications registered on day 0 to minimize the risk of reverse causality (pyogenic arthritis). Thus, the true absolute risks may rather have been underestimated, but is not expected to substantially influence the relative risks or the population attributable fraction. Another important limitation is a potential for bias from unmeasured confounding (e.g. smoking and body mass index) and bias by indication – i.e. the systematic differences between persons undergoing arthroscopic surgery and the underlying population. We aimed to take the latter into account in our sensitivity analysis, where only persons with a potential indication for a knee arthroscopy were included which yielded similar results, except for pyogenic arthritis where we noted a substantial attenuation of the risk estimate. Unfortunately, there is no data on body length and body weight available in the register.

Conclusions

To conclude, although the absolute risk of complication of 1.1% is small, knee arthroscopy should not be considered a completely benign intervention. In particular as it is high volume surgery at most knee surgery clinics. For example, the procedure may be responsible for 5% of cases of pyogenic arthritis of the knee. Thus, it remains important to communicate risks with the patient, and consider non-surgical treatment options when appropriate.

Abbreviations

CI: confidence interval; ICD: International Classification of Diseases; OR: odds ratio; SHR: Skåne healthcare register; VTE: venous thrombotic event

Funding

The study was supported by the Swedish Research Council, Kock Foundations, The Swedish Rheumatology Association, Österlund Foundation, the Faculty of Medicine, Lund University, Sweden, and Governmental Funding of Clinical Research within National Health Service (ALF). The funders had no role in the design of the study, data collection, analysis, interpretation of data, in writing the manuscript, or decision to publish.

Authors' contributions

KFP participated in study design, did results interpretation and drafted the first version of manuscript. AT did the study design, data acquisition, lead the statistical analyses, results interpretation, and participated in manuscript revision. ME conceived the study and participated in study design, data acquisition, results interpretation, and lead the manuscript revision. All authors have approved the final version of manuscript for submission.

Competing interests

The authors declare that they have no competing interests.

References

1. Treuting R. Minimally invasive orthopedic surgery: arthroscopy. Ochsner J. 2000;2(3):158–63.
2. Kim S, Bosque J, Meehan JP, Jamali A, Marder R. Increase in outpatient knee arthroscopy in the United States: a comparison of National Surveys of ambulatory surgery, 1996 and 2006. J Bone Joint Surg Am. 2011;93(11):994–1000.
3. Artroskopi- knä [http://www.internetmedicin.se/page.aspx?id=4299]. Accessed Oct 2016.
4. Hagino T, Ochiai S, Watanabe Y, Senga S, Wako M, Ando T, Sato E, Haro H. Complications after arthroscopic knee surgery. Arch Orthop Trauma Surg. 2014;134(11):1561–4.
5. Jameson SS, Dowen D, James P, Serrano-Pedraza I, Reed MR, Deehan DJ. The burden of arthroscopy of the knee: a contemporary analysis of data from the English NHS. J Bone Joint Surg Br. 2011;93(10):1327–33.
6. Sherman OH, Fox JM, Snyder SJ, Del Pizzo W, Friedman MJ, Ferkel RD, Lawley MJ. Arthroscopy–"no-problem surgery". An analysis of complications in two thousand six hundred and forty cases. J Bone Joint Surg Am. 1986;68(2):256–65.
7. Salzler MJ, Lin A, Miller CD, Herold S, Irrgang JJ, Harner CD. Complications after arthroscopic knee surgery. Am J Sports Med. 2014;42(2):292–6.
8. Reigstad O, Grimsgaard C. Complications in knee arthroscopy. Knee Surg Sports Traumatol Arthrosc. 2006;14(5):473–7.
9. Armstrong RW, Bolding F, Joseph R. Septic arthritis following arthroscopy: clinical syndromes and analysis of risk factors. Arthroscopy. 1992;8(2):213–23.
10. Sun Y, Chen D, Xu Z, Shi D, Dai J, Qin J, Qin J, Jiang Q. Deep venous thrombosis after knee arthroscopy: a systematic review and meta-analysis. Arthroscopy. 2014;30(3):406–12.
11. Hetsroni I, Lyman S, Do H, Mann G, Marx RG. Symptomatic pulmonary embolism after outpatient arthroscopic procedures of the knee: the incidence and risk factors in 418,323 arthroscopies. J Bone Joint Surg Br. 2011;93(1):47–51.
12. Åtgärdskoder (KVÅ) [http://www.socialstyrelsen.se/klassificeringochkoder/atgardskoderkva]. Accessed Oct 2016.
13. Wetterholm M, Turkiewicz A, Stigmar K, Hubertsson J, Englund M. The rate of joint replacement in osteoarthritis depends on the patient's socioeconomic status. Acta Orthop. 2016;87(3):245–51.
14. Rahman MM, Kopec JA, Sayre EC, Greidanus NV, Aghajanian J, Anis AH, Cibere J, Jordan JM, Badley EM. Effect of sociodemographic factors on surgical consultations and hip or knee replacements among patients with osteoarthritis in British Columbia, Canada. J Rheumatol. 2011;38(3):503–9.
15. Modern Epidemiology, 3rd edn. Edited by Rothman KJ, Greenland S, Lash TL. Philadelphia: Lippincott Williams and Wilkins; 2008. p. 60–1.
16. Norton EC, Arbor A, Miller MM, Kleinman LC. Computing adjusted risk ratios and risk differences in Stata. Stata J. 2013;13(3):492–509.
17. Allum R. Complications of arthroscopy of the knee. J Bone Joint Surg Br. 2002;84(7):937–45.
18. Bohensky MA, deSteiger R, Kondogiannis C, Sundararajan V, Andrianopoulos N, Bucknill A, McColl G, Brand CA. Adverse outcomes associated with elective knee arthroscopy: a population-based cohort study. Arthroscopy. 2013;29(4):716–25.
19. Martin CT, Pugely AJ, Gao Y, Wolf BR. Risk factors for thirty-day morbidity and mortality following knee arthroscopy: a review of 12,271 patients from the national surgical quality improvement program database. J Bone Joint Surg Am. 2013;95(14):e98 91–10.
20. Siemieniuk RAC, Harris IA, Agoritsas T, Poolman RW, Brignardello-Petersen R, Van de Velde S, Buchbinder R, Englund M, Lytvyn L, Quinlan C, et al. Arthroscopic surgery for degenerative knee arthritis and meniscal tears: a clinical practice guideline. BMJ. 2017;357:j1982.
21. Beaufils P, Becker R, Kopf S, Englund M, Verdonk R, Ollivier M, Seil R. Surgical management of degenerative meniscus lesions: the 2016 ESSKA meniscus consensus. Knee Surg Sports Traumatol Arthrosc. 2017;25(2):335–46.
22. Turkiewicz A, Petersson IF, Bjork J, Hawker G, Dahlberg LE, Lohmander LS, Englund M. Current and future impact of osteoarthritis on health care: a population-based study with projections to year 2032. Osteoarthr Cartil. 2014;22(11):1826–32.
23. Rosengren BE, Karlsson M, Petersson I, Englund M. The 21st-century landscape of adult fractures: cohort study of a complete adult regional population. J Bone Miner Res Off J Am Soc Bone Miner Res. 2015;30(3):535–42.
24. Ludvigsson JF, Andersson E, Ekbom A, Feychting M, Kim JL, Reuterwall C, Heurgren M, Olausson PO. External review and validation of the Swedish national inpatient register. BMC Public Health. 2011;11:450.

8

A comparison of zero-profile anchored spacer (ROI-C) and plate fixation in 2-level noncontiguous anterior cervical discectomy and fusion

Zongyu Zhang[1†], Yawei Li[2†] and Weimin Jiang[1*]

Abstract

Background: Anterior cervical discectomy and fusion (ACDF) is the classic surgical treatment for symptomatic cervical degenerative disc disease (CDDD). However, there is controversy over the best surgical management in patients with two noncontiguous symptomatic levels of CDDD.

Methods: From April 2011 to May 2014, 44 patients with two noncontiguous symptomatic levels of CDDD underwent skip-level ACDFs. In Group NoPlate, 23 cases underwent 2 noncontiguous levels of ACDF using zero-profile anchored spacer; and in Group Plate, 21 cases underwent 2 noncontiguous levels of ACDF using cages and plates. Operation-related paraeters for each group were recorded and compared. Japanese Orthopedic Association (JOA) scores and Neck Disability Index (NDI) scores at preoperation and postoperation were compared with at least a 2-year follow-up. Cervical lordosis was analyzed before surgery, 1 month after surgery, 3 months after surgery, and at final follow-up.

Results: Mean follow-up was 35.4 ± 6.5 (range 24–48) months. Significant improvement on the JOA, NDI scores and cervical lordosis was noted in each group ($p < 0.05$), and there were no significant difference in terms of JOA, NDI scores, cervical lordosis and fusion rate between the two groups ($P > 0.05$). The operation time in Group NoPlate was significantly shorter than in Group Plate ($p < 0.05$), and the incidence of dysphagia and adjacent segment degeneration in Group NoPlate was significantly lower than in Group Plate ($p < 0.05$).

Conclusions: ROI-C and cages with plate fixation were both effective in two-level noncontiguous ACDF, and there were no significant difference in clinical outcomes, fusion rate, and cervical lordosis. However, ROI-C was associated with shorter operative time, lower incidence of dysphagia and adjacent segment degeneration.

Keywords: Anterior cervical discectomy and fusion (ACDF), Cervical disk degenerative disease (CDDD), Two noncontiguous levels

Background

Anterior cervical discectomy and fusion (ACDF) was first reported in the 1950s [1], which then has become the classic surgical treatment for symptomatic cervical degenerative disc disease (CDDD) [2]. Many studies showed that single- and multilevel continuous ACDFs achieved good results [3–7]; however, there is controversy over the best surgical management in patients with two noncontiguous symptomatic levels of CDDD. Surgeons may choose to perform a 3-level ACDFs rather than just treat symptomatic levels for fear of significant additive stress on the intermediate intervertebral disc. However, 3-level anterior fusions are associated with increased rates of pseudarthrosis and poorer clinical outcomes than shorter constructs [8, 9].

In 2-level noncontiguous ACDF, 2 plates are often used to provide the immediate postoperative stability and improve the fusion rate. However, the procedure of implanting plates is associated with the risk of perforation

* Correspondence: jwmpaper@126.com
†Equal contributors
[1]Department of Orthopaedic Surgery, The First Affiliated Hospital of Soochow University, 899 Pinghai Road, Suzhou, China
Full list of author information is available at the end of the article

of esophagus and dysphagia. Besides, it may raise the risk of adjacent-level ossification [10, 11]. Previously, we investigated ACDF with zero-profile anchored spacer (ROI-C, LDR, Troyes, France) for the treatment of 1-level and 2-level contiguous CDDD, achieving satisfactory clinical and radiological outcomes [12]. This implant system is constructed of a polyether-ether-ketone (PEEK) cage and two integrated self-locking clips. The clips can enter the vertebral body through the endplate and provide anterior column fixation (Fig. 1). Two-level noncontiguous ACDFs with ROI-C, which only fuses the symptomatic levels without anterior plates, may therefore be the optimal treatment choice. The aim of the present study was to compare surgical parameters, clinical and radiological outcomes in patients who underwent 2-level noncontiguous ACDF with ROI-C or with cages and plates.

Methods

Patient population

From April 2011 to May 2014, a total of 44 patients underwent skip-level ACDFs.

Inclusion criteria were (1) symptomatic CDDD which was unresponsive to non-operative management; and (2) spinal cord or root compression at two noncontiguous intervertebral levels confirmed by magnetic resonance imaging (MRI). Exclusion criteria were: (1) significant instability of cervical spine; (2) developmental cervical spinal stenosis; (3) severe cervical deformity; (4) a previous history of cervical spine surgery; and (5) fracture, tumor, ossification of posterior longitudinal ligament and any serious general illness.

The 44 patients were divided into 2 groups: Group NoPlate (23 patients), who underwent fusion using ROI-C (Fig. 2); and Group Plate (21 patients), who underwent fusion using cages and plates (Medtronic, Minneapolis, American) (Fig. 3). There were no significant differences in the demographic data between the two groups ($P > 0.05$) (Table 1). This study was approved by the Institutional Ethics Committee of Soochow University.

Surgical technique

Operations were performed in supine position under general anesthesia using the standard right-sided anterior approach. The basic procedures including exposure, discectomy, and decompression were performed as described previously [1]. To achieve adequate decompression, the posterior longitudinal ligament, osteophytes, and other compressive elements should be removed after discectomy. Great care was taken to remove the cartilaginous tissue, but preserve the bony endplate to prevent cage subsidence. Cages were then implanted into the intervertebral space.

Zero-profile anchored spacers were used in Group NoPlate. In Group Plate, PEEK cages were inserted, and anterior plates were applied. In both groups, each appropriate-sized cage was packed with 0.25 mg of recombinant human bone morphogenetic protein (rhBMP-2, pharmaceutical group investment limited corporation, Hangzhou, China) and excised local osteophytes.

Patients were allowed to sit up on the first day postoperatively and walk on the second day postoperatively with a Philadelphia neck collar, which was applied for 4 weeks.

Collected data and outcome assessment

Collected data included age, gender, operated segments, intraoperative blood loss, operative time, complications, and clinical and radiologic outcomes. The complete cervical spine X-ray, computed tomography (CT), and magnetic resonance imaging (MRI) were performed preoperatively. After surgery, the cervical spine X-ray were routinely taken. Clinical and radiological evaluations were performed preoperatively (1 day before operation) and postoperatively at 2 weeks, 1 month, 3 months, and the final follow-up. Radiological outcomes were measured using the Picture Archiving and Communication System (PACS) imaging system.

The Japanese Orthopaedic Association (JOA; scored from 0 to 17, with a lower score indicating more severe symptoms) scoring system was used to evaluate the

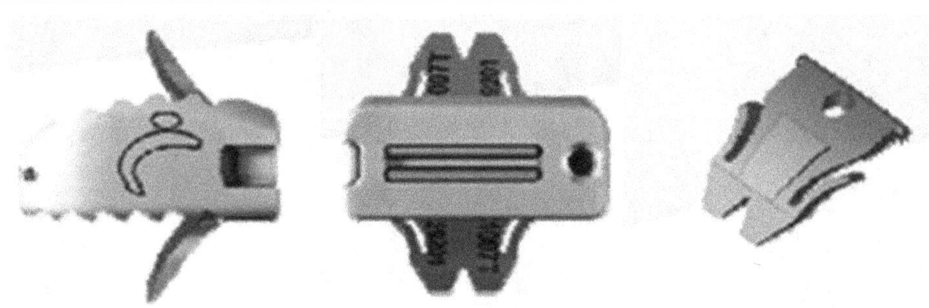

a b c

Fig. 1 Lateral (**a**) and anteroposterior (**b**) views of the zero-profile anchored spacer (ROI-C, LDR, Troyes, France); (**c**) the integrated self-locking and self-directing clip

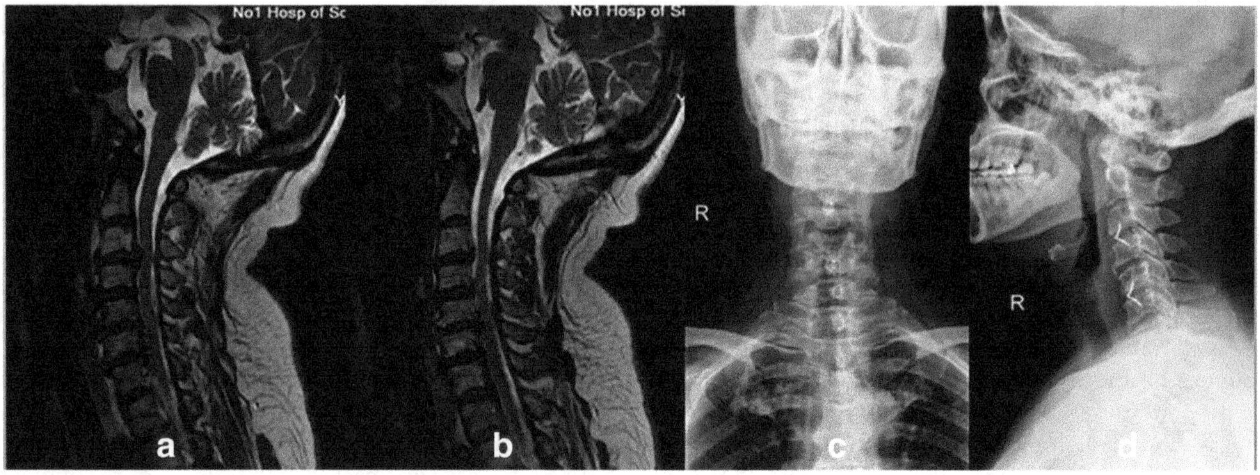

Fig. 2 Preoperative lateral T2-weighted MRI (**a** and **b**) showing a 59-year-old woman with C3-C4 and C5-C6 disc herniation. Anteroposterior (**c**) and lateral (**d**) radiographs showing C3-C4 and C5-C6 anterior cervical discectomy and fusions (ACDF) with the zero-profile anchored spacers

neurological status [13]. Neck Disability Index (NDI; scored from 0 to 100%, with a lower score indicating less severe symptoms) scoring system was used to assess the neck function [14]. The JOA recovery rate (RR) was calculated using the rationale of Hirabayashi [15]: (postoperative score - preoperative score)/(17 - preoperative score) × 100. The incidence of dysphagia was assessed using the Bazaz grading system [16]. Severity of dysphagia was graded as none, mild, moderate, or severe (Table 2).

X-ray and CT scan reconstructions were used to evaluate the bony fusion. Satisfactory fusion include the following conditions [17]: (1) no motion between the spinous processes; (2) no radiolucent gap between the graft and the endplates; (3) continuous bridging bony trabeculae at the graft-endplate interface. The cervical lordosis was assessed by measuring the Cobb angle of C2–C7 from the inferior endplate of C2, to the inferior endplate of C7 in a neutral position (Fig. 4). The radiological evidence of adjacent segment (above, below and intermediate) degeneration included the following radiological manifestations: new osteophyte or enlargement of previous osteophyte; narrowing of a disc space; and increased calcification of anterior longitudinal ligament. Clinical and radiological assessments were conducted and reviewed by two senior spine surgeons and patients were followed up for at least 24 months postoperatively.

Statistical analysis

Data are shown as mean ± standard deviation. Intergroup comparisons were made using *t* test or Chi-square test (Fisher's exact test).The paired data were compared with a paired sample t test. All the analyses were performed

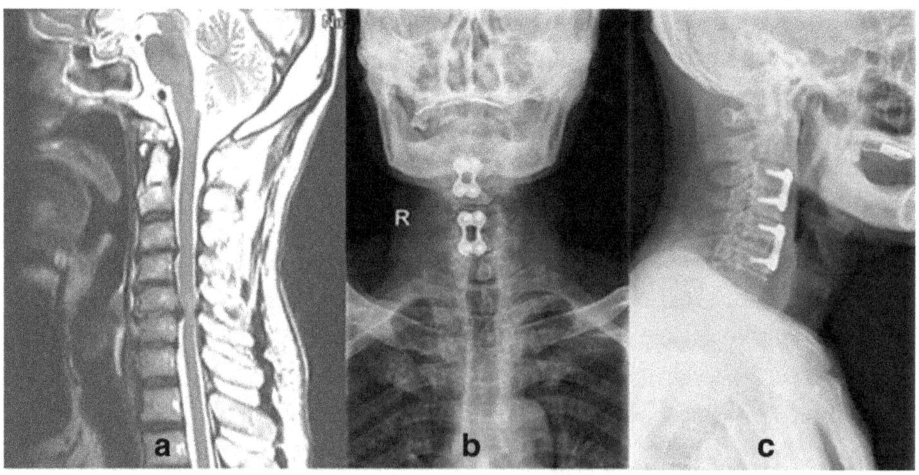

Fig. 3 Preoperative lateral T2-weighted MRI (**a**) showing a 68-year-old man with C3-C4 and C5-C6 disc herniation. Anteroposterior (**b**) and lateral (**c**) radiographs showing C3-C4 and C5-C6 anterior cervical discectomy and fusions (ACDF) with cages and titanium plates

Table 1 Demographic data of patients

	Group NoPlate	Group Plate	*P* value
Patients No	23	21	–
Gender (male: female)	15:8	9:12	0.137
Average age (years)	53.3 ± 8.8 (40–68)	57.8 ± 9.2 (39–70)	0.105
Operated levels	C3-C4 and C5-C6: 13; C4-C5 and C6-C7: 10	C3-C4 and C5-C6: 8; C4-C5 and C6-C7: 13	0.222
Blood loss (ml)	70.0 ± 15.8	75.4 ± 23.0	0.37
Operative time (min)	126.0 ± 13.2	143.4 ± 17.9	0.001
Follow-up period (months)	34.7 ± 7.6 (24–48)	36.2 ± 5.2 (26–48)	0.447

using the Statistical Package for the Social Sciences (version 13.0 SPSS, Chicago, IL, USA) and the difference was considered statistically significant at the $P < 0.05$ level.

Results

Surgical parameters

The operated noncontiguous levels were C3–4 and C5–6 (Group NoPlate, $n = 13$; Group Plate, $n = 8$), and C4–5 and C6–7 (Group NoPlate, $n = 10$; Group Plate, $n = 13$). Group NoPlate had a mean blood loss of 70.0 ± 15.8 ml and the average operative time was 126.0 ± 13.2 min. Group Plate had a mean blood loss of 75.4 ± 23.0 ml and the average operative time was 143.4 ± 17.9 min. No significant difference existed in age, gender, operated levels and blood loss between the 2 groups (Table 1). However, significant differences existed in operative time between the 2 groups ($P < 0.05$).

Clinical outcome

Patients were followed up from 24 to 48 (mean: 35.4 ± 6.5) months. In both groups, the JOA and NDI scores were significantly improved postoperatively ($P < 0.01$, Fig. 5a and b, Table 3). The comparisons of JOA and NDI scores at each follow-up time between the 2 groups showed no statistically significant differences ($P > 0.05$). The mean JOA RR was (62.6 ± 15.1)% in Group NoPlate and (66.8 ± 14.6)% in Group Plate, which was not statistically different ($P > 0.05$).

Radiologic outcomes

The cervical lordosis was significantly corrected postoperatively and the correction was maintained at last follow-up in both groups ($P < 0.01$, Fig. 5c, Table 3). No significant difference in cervical lordosis was found between the two groups at each follow-up time ($P > 0.05$). The fusion rate at 3 months postoperatively was 91.3% (21/23) in Group NoPlate and 95.2% (20/21) in Group Plate, which was not significantly different ($P > 0.05$). All patients achieved solid fusion at final follow-up.

Table 2 Bazaz grading system for dysphagia

Symptom severity	Liquid food	Solid food
None	None	None
Mild	None	Rare
Moderate	None or rare	Occasionally (only with specific food)
Severe	None or rare	Frequent (majority of solids)

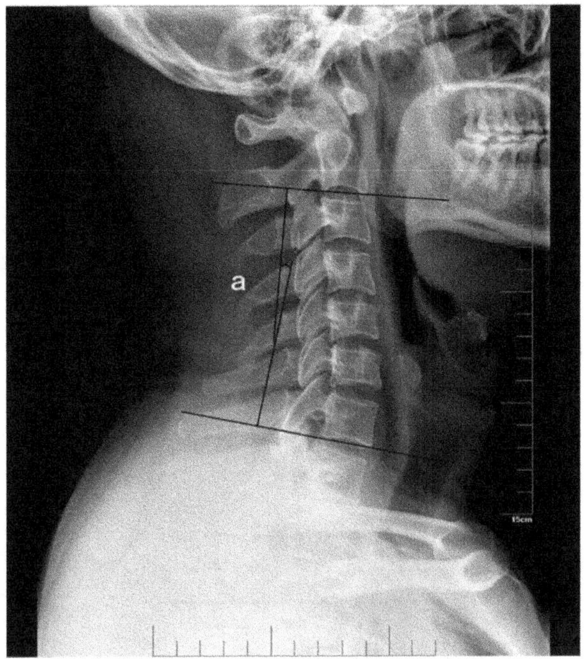

Fig. 4 Lateral radiograph showing cervical lordosis (Cobb angle of C2–C7) calculated by measuring the angle formed by the lines along the inferior endplate of C2 to the inferior endplate of C7 in the neutral position

Complications

All patients tolerated the procedure well and no death was happened during the period of follow-up. No patients complained about dysphagia before operation. In Group NoPlate, 5 patients complained of dysphagia (2 moderate and 3 mild) on 2 weeks postoperatively, 3 patients had dysphagia (1 moderate and 2 mild) 1 month postoperatively, and no patients had dysphagia 3 months after the operation. In Group Plate, 12 patients complained of dysphagia (2 severe, 6 moderate and 4 mild) on 2 weeks postoperatively, 9 patients had dysphagia (4 moderate and 5 mild) 1 month postoperatively, 5 patients had dyphagia (1 moderate and 4 mild) 3 months postoperatively, and 4 patients still suffered from mild dyphagia at the last follow-up. There were significant differences in the presence of dysphagia between the two groups at all follow-up time points (Table 4). There were no adjacent segment degeneration observed in Group NoPlate and 19.0% (4/21) of patients had adjacent segment degeneration in Group Plate (3 patients developed adjacent-level ossification,

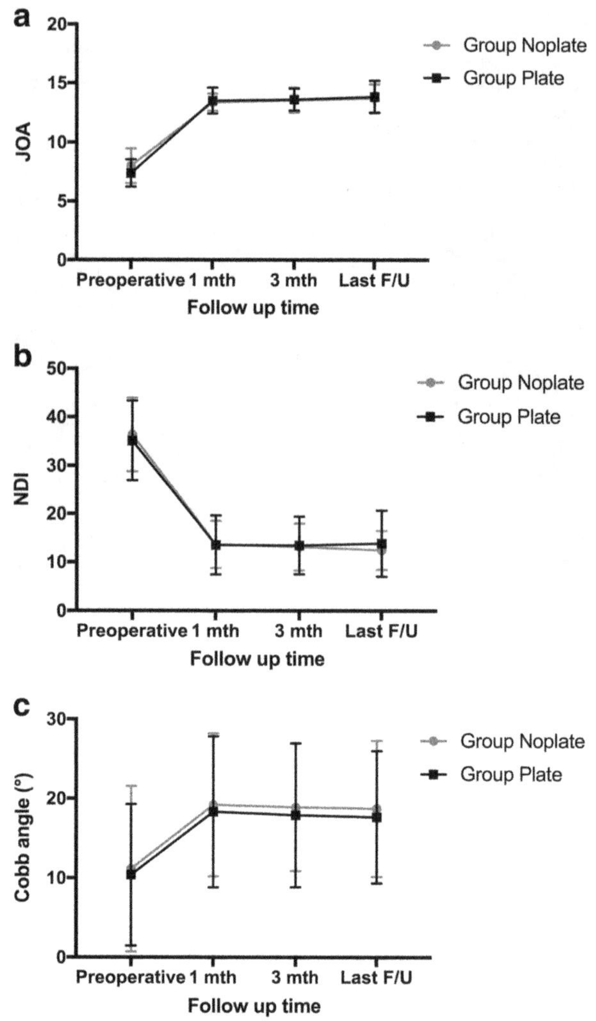

Fig. 5 Line graphs showing a comparison of clinical and radiological results between Group NoPlate and Group Plate. Change trend of the Japanese Orthopaedic Association (JOA) score (**a**); Change trend of the Neck Disability Index (NDI) score (**b**); Change trend of cervical lordosis (**c**)

and 1 patient developed intermediate-level disc space narrowing), and this difference was statistically significant ($P < 0.05$, Table 4).

Discussion

The treatment of two noncontiguous symptomatic levels of CDDD poses a dilemma for spine surgeons. The surgical procedures commonly include anterior cervical corpectomy and fusion (ACCF), 3-level ACDF and 2-level noncontiguous ACDF. Compared with ACDF, ACCF has more bleeding, higher incidences of postoperative complications, and less improvements of cervical lordosis. Three-level ACDF sacrifices an additional motion segment, and has been associated with increased rates of pseudarthrosis and poorer clinical outcomes than shorter constructs [8, 9]. Finn et al. [18], in a cadaveric study, found that the

Table 3 Clinical and radiologic data evaluated before surgery and during follow-up

	Group NoPlate	P value[a]	Group Plate	P value[b]
JOA scores				
Preoperatvie	8.0 ± 1.5	–	7.4 ± 1.2	–
Postoperative 1 month	13.4 ± 0.7	< 0.001	13.5 ± 1.1	0.001
Postoperative 3 month	13.6 ± 1.0	< 0.001	13.6 ± 0.9	0.002
Last follow-up	13.7 ± 1.2	< 0.001	13.9 ± 1.4	0.001
NDI scores				
Preoperatvie	36.3 ± 7.6	–	35.1 ± 8.2	–
Postoperative 1 month	13.7 ± 5.3	< 0.001	13.5 ± 6.1	< 0.001
Postoperative 3 month	13.1 ± 4.9	< 0.001	13.4 ± 6.0	< 0.001
Last follow-up	12.5 ± 4.0	< 0.001	13.9 ± 6.8	< 0.001
Cervical lordosis (°)				
Preoperatvie	11.1 ± 10.4	–	10.4 ± 8.9	–
Postoperative 1 month	19.2 ± 9.0	< 0.001	18.3 ± 9.7	0.001
Postoperative 3 month	18.9 ± 8.0	< 0.001	17.9 ± 9.3	0.002
Last follow-up	18.7 ± 8.6	0.001	17.7 ± 8.3	0.001

[a] P value is given for comparison between pre-operative and post-operative values in Group NoPlate
[b] P value is given for comparison between pre-operative and post-operative values in Group Plate

adjacent levels beared a remarkable increase in stress in the three-level ACDF. However, in the two-level ACDF, the adjacent segments (above, below and intermediate) experienced modest stress relative to intact. Therefore, 2-level noncontiguous ACDF may be the optimal treatment choice.

There is controversy over the use of anterior plate in a single-level ACDF. However, it is beneficial to implant anterior plates in a multilevel ACDF [19], for the fusion rates were reported bo be unacceptably low after multilevel ACDF without plating [8, 20]. To provide immediate postoperative stability and increase the fusion rate, two plates are often applied in 2-level noncontiguous ACDF. However, the procedure of implanting plates at the optional position is very time consuming. On the contrary, the zero-profile anchored spacer, which has two integrated

Table 4 Complications after operations in the two groups

	Group NoPlate	Group Plate	P value
Dysphagia rate			
Postoperative 2 weeks	5/23	12/21	0.029
Postoperative 1 month	3/23	9/21	0.042
Postoperative 3 months	0/23	5/21	0.019
Final follow-up	0/23	4/21	0.044
Adjacent segment degeneration	0/23	4/21	0.044

self-locking and self-directing clips, is simple to implant. In our study, we found the zero-profile anchored spacer was significantly superior to the anterior plate in terms of operative time.

Dysphagia is reported to be the most common postoperative complication after ACDF [21]. In most patients, dysphagia disappears within 3 months. However, there are 12.5–35.1% of cases still have dysphagia 3 months after the operation [16]. In our study, the presence of dysphagia in Group NoPlate is lower compared with that in Group Plate at all follow-up time points, and the duration of dysphagia is shorter. Although the mechanism of dysphagia remains unknown, the irritation of the esophagus by the anterior plate is considered to be a possible cause [16, 22, 23]. At the early stage (2 weeks postoperatively), it could also partly be attributed to longer intraoperative esophagus retraction time and greater retraction extent to fix the anterior plates. The zero-profile anchored spacer can be completely contained in the intervertebral space, avoiding the mechanical irritation of the soft tissue, especially the esophagus, resulting in lower incidence of postoperative dysphagia.

It is reported that the presence of anterior plates increased the incidence of adjacent segment degeneration [24]. Park et al. [11] found that an anterior cervical plate close to the adjacent intervertebral disc may cause adjacent level disc degeneration or surrounding bone formation. In our study, 4 patients in Group Plate developed adjacent segment degeneration, which was significantly higher than that in Group NoPlate. This may occur because the zero-profile anchored spacer can be completely contained in the intervertebral space, minimizing the irritation of the adjacent cervical structures.

This study has several limitations. First, it was retrospective. Second, the number of patients was small. Third, the follow-up period was relatively short. Finally, the final follow-up time was not consistent, which caused variation in adjacent segment degeneration. Thus, the results of this study need to be confirmed by large sample, prospective, randomized studies with long-term follow-up.

Conclusion

ROI-C and cages with plate fixation were both effective in two-level noncontiguous ACDF, and there were no significant difference in clinical outcomes, fusion rate, and cervical lordosis. However, ROI-C was associated with shorter operative time, lower incidence of dysphagia and adjacent segment degeneration.

Abbreviations

ACCF: anterior cervical corpectomy and fusion; ACDF: Anterior cervical discectomy and fusion; CDDD: Cervical disk degenerative disease; CT: Computed tomography; JOA: Japanese Orthopedic Association; MRI: Magnetic resonance imaging; NDI: Neck Disability Index

Funding

No funds were received in support of this work.

Authors' contributions

All authors made substantive intellectual contributions to this study to qualify as authors. WJ contributed to study design, acquisition of data, analysis of data, and interpretation of results. ZZ contributed to study coordination. YL contributed to statistical analysis. ZZ and YL contributed to manuscript preparation. All authors read and approved the final manuscript.

Competing interests

The authors declare that they have no competing interests.

Author details

[1]Department of Orthopaedic Surgery, The First Affiliated Hospital of Soochow University, 899 Pinghai Road, Suzhou, China. [2]Department of Orthopaedic Surgery, Lianyungang Affiliated Hospital of Nanjing University of Chinese Medicine, 148 Chaoyang Road, Lianyungang, China.

References

1. Smith GW, Robinson RA. The treatment of certain cervical-spine disorders by anterior removal of the intervertebral disc and interbody fusion. J Bone Joint Surg Am. 1958;40-a(3):607–24.
2. Gore DR, Sepic SB. Anterior cervical fusion for degenerated or protruded discs. A review of one hundred forty-six patients. Spine. 1984;9(7):667–71.
3. Papadopoulos EC, Huang RC, Girardi FP, Synnott K, Cammisa FP Jr. Three-level anterior cervical discectomy and fusion with plate fixation: radiographic and clinical results. Spine. 2006;31(8):897–902.
4. Bolesta MJ, Rechtine GR 2nd, Chrin AM. Three- and four-level anterior cervical discectomy and fusion with plate fixation: a prospective study. Spine. 2000;25(16):2040–4. discussion 45-6
5. Chang SW, Kakarla UK, Maughan PH, DeSanto J, Fox D, Theodore N, et al. Four-level anterior cervical discectomy and fusion with plate fixation: radiographic and clinical results. Neurosurg. 2010;66(4):639–46. discussion 46-7
6. Kao FC, Niu CC, Chen LH, Lai PL, Chen WJ. Maintenance of interbody space in one- and two-level anterior cervical interbody fusion: comparison of the effectiveness of autograft, allograft, and cage. Clin Orthop Relat Res. 2005;(430):108–16.
7. Kim SW, Limson MA, Kim SB, Arbatin JJ, Chang KY, Park MS, et al. Comparison of radiographic changes after ACDF versus Bryan disc arthroplasty in single and bi-level cases. Eur Spine J. 2009;18(2):218–31.
8. Emery SE, Fisher JR, Bohlman HH. Three-level anterior cervical discectomy and fusion: radiographic and clinical results. Spine. 1997;22(22):2622–4. discussion 25
9. Fraser JF, Hartl R. Anterior approaches to fusion of the cervical spine: a metaanalysis of fusion rates. J Neurosurg Spine. 2007;6(4):298–303.
10. Kim HJ, Kelly MP, Ely CG, Dettori JR, Riew KD. The risk of adjacent-level ossification development after surgery in the cervical spine: are there factors that affect the risk? A systematic review. Spine. 2012;37(22 Suppl):S65–74.
11. Park JB, Cho YS, Riew KD. Development of adjacent-level ossification in patients with an anterior cervical plate. J Bone Joint Surg Am. 2005;87(3):558–63.
12. Wang Z, Jiang W, Li X, Wang H, Shi J, Chen J, et al. The application of zero-profile anchored spacer in anterior cervical discectomy and fusion. Eur Spine J. 2015;24(1):148–54.

13. Yonenobu K, Abumi K, Nagata K, Taketomi E, Ueyama K. Interobserver and intraobserver reliability of the japanese orthopaedic association scoring system for evaluation of cervical compression myelopathy. Spine. 2001; 26(17):1890–4. discussion 95
14. Vernon H, Mior S. The neck disability index: a study of reliability and validity. J Manip Physiol Ther. 1991;14(7):409–15.
15. Hirabayashi K, Miyakawa J, Satomi K, Maruyama T, Wakano K. Operative results and postoperative progression of ossification among patients with ossification of cervical posterior longitudinal ligament. Spine. 1981;6(4):354–64.
16. Bazaz R, Lee MJ, Yoo JU. Incidence of dysphagia after anterior cervical spine surgery: a prospective study. Spine. 2002;27(22):2453–8.
17. Hacker RJ, Cauthen JC, Gilbert TJ, Griffith SL. A prospective randomized multicenter clinical evaluation of an anterior cervical fusion cage. Spine. 2000;25(20):2646–54. discussion 55
18. Finn MA, Samuelson MM, Bishop F, Bachus KN, Brodke DS. Two-level noncontiguous versus three-level anterior cervical discectomy and fusion: a biomechanical comparison. Spine. 2011;36(6):448–53.
19. Resnick DK, Trost GR. Use of ventral plates for cervical arthrodesis. Neurosurg. 2007;60(1 Suppl 1):S112–7.
20. Bohlman HH, Emery SE, Goodfellow DB, Jones PK. Robinson anterior cervical discectomy and arthrodesis for cervical radiculopathy. Long-term follow-up of one hundred and twenty-two patients. J Bone Joint Surg Am. 1993;75(9): 1298–307.
21. Riley LH 3rd, Skolasky RL, Albert TJ, Vaccaro AR, Heller JG. Dysphagia after anterior cervical decompression and fusion: prevalence and risk factors from a longitudinal cohort study. Spine. 2005;30(22):2564–9.
22. Lee MJ, Bazaz R, Furey CG, Yoo J. Influence of anterior cervical plate design on Dysphagia: a 2-year prospective longitudinal follow-up study. J Spinal Disord Tech. 2005;18(5):406–9.
23. Scholz M, Schnake KJ, Pingel A, Hoffmann R, Kandziora F. A new zero-profile implant for stand-alone anterior cervical interbody fusion. Clin Orthop Relat Res. 2011;469(3):666–73.
24. Chung JY, Kim SK, Jung ST, Lee KB. Clinical adjacent-segment pathology after anterior cervical discectomy and fusion: results after a minimum of 10-year follow-up. Spine J Off J North Am Spine Soc. 2014;14(10):2290–8.

9

Anterior cervical discectomy and fusion with stand-alone anchored cages versus posterior laminectomy and fusion for four-level cervical spondylotic myelopathy

Bing Wang, Guohua Lü and Lei Kuang*

Abstract

Background: The optimal treatment for multi-level cervical spondylotic myelopathy (CSM) remains controversial. Posterior approach is most commonly used, but complicated with insufficient decompression and postoperative axial neck pain. The anterior approach is effective in neural decompression with less surgical trauma. However, the profile of the plate or the possible construct failure may cause dysphagia after surgery. Recently, anterior cervical discectomy and fusion (ACDF) with self-anchored cage is reported to have a superior result over ACDF with anterior plates and screws in three-level CSM. The purpose of the study is to compare the clinical and radiological outcomes of ACDF using stand-alone anchored cages to that of laminectomy with fusion (LF) for treating four-level CSM.

Methods: Twenty-six patients underwent four-level ACDF (Group A) and 32 patients with four-level LF (Group B) were retrospectively reviewed and followed-up for 24 months. Clinical efficacy was evaluated by comparing pre- and post-operative Japanese Orthopedic Association (JOA) and Neck Disability Index (NDI) scores. Operative time, blood loss, fusion, lordosis change and complications were evaluated.

Results: There was significantly less blood loss in Group A (163.4 ± 72.1 ml) than Group B (241.0 ± 112.3 ml) ($P < 0.05$). Both groups demonstrated significant improvements in JOA and NDI scores after surgery with similar operative time. Improvements in cervical lordosis and fused segment lordosis were more pronounced in Group A (11.3 ± 5.9°, 9.7 ± 5.3°) than Group B (5.8 ± 4.6°, 5.5 ± 4.5°) ($P < 0.05$). Loss of lordosis in the cervical spine and fused segment was more prominent in Group A (11.7 ± 2.2°, 6.7 ± 3.2°) than Group B (7.5 ± 3.8°, 3.7 ± 3.4°) ($P < 0.05$) at the final follow-up. Complication rate in Group A and Group B was 57.69 and 18.75%, respectively.

Conclusions: ACDF using a stand-alone anchored cage showed similar clinical results to LF for the treatment of four-level CSM, with better lordosis correction and less blood loss. However, ACDF was associated with more loss of lordosis after surgery and more non-unions.

Keywords: Cervical spondylopathy, Stand-alone anchored cage, Anterior cervical discectomy and fusion, Retrospective study

* Correspondence: lei.kuang@csu.edu.cn
Department of Spine Surgery, The Second Xiangya Hospital of Central South University, Changsha City, China

Background

Cervical spondylotic myelopathy (CSM) is a clinically symptomatic degenerative condition resulting from the compression of the spinal cord. The optimal treatment for multi-level CSM (defined as ≥3 levels) remains controversial. Canal decompression can be achieved by posterior strategies; however, the degree of decompression may be insufficient because ventral compression is not resolved [1]. Long-term postoperative axial neck pain may result from surgical invasion of the cervical muscle–ligament complex, and the incidence of C5 nerve root palsy is higher after posterior than anterior surgery due to spinal cord drift [2].

Anterior strategies are effective for neural decompression, especially in cases with preoperative kyphosis, showing better clinical outcomes with less surgical trauma compared to posterior approaches. Traditionally, anterior plating has been used to increase fusion rates and reduce subsidence and postoperative kyphosis. However, complications include screw loosening, screw pullout, dysphagia, and esophageal rupture, especially in multi-level disease [3]. Anterior cervical discectomy and fusion (ACDF) is increasingly performed using stand-alone cages, which overcome the limitations associated with anterior plates and screws [4].

Previous studies showed that ACDF for 3-level CSM using stand-alone cages is technically simpler and involves a shorter operative time, less blood loss, and a lower risk of postoperative dysphagia compared to plate fixation, with satisfactory clinical and radiographic outcomes [5, 6]. To our knowledge, no previous studies have compared the outcomes of ACDF for 4-level CSM using stand-alone cages to laminectomy plus lateral mass fixation and fusion.

Methods

Patient population and indications

Patients from a single institution who underwent cervical decompressive surgery for CSM between January 2012 and January 2014 were eligible for this study. Inclusion criteria were: 1) signs and symptoms of CSM not responsive to conservative therapy; 2) age between 18 and 65 years; 3) disc herniation confirmed by computed tomography (CT) or magnetic resonance imaging with spinal cord compression at 4 contiguous disc levels between C3 and C7 and compression limited to the disc level; and 4) ≥ 24 months of follow-up data. Exclusion criteria were: 1) continuous or combined ossification of the posterior longitudinal ligament; 2) developmental stenosis; 3) history of cervical spine trauma and previous cervical spine surgery; or 4) osteoporosis.

Ethical approval was obtained from the institutional review board (No.S043), and written informed consent was obtained from all study participants.

Surgical procedure

All surgical procedures were conducted by the same senior surgeon (Kuang). In Group A, ADCF was performed using the standard Smith-Robinson approach [7]. The cartilaginous disc endplate was removed, and care was taken to avoid excessive damage to the bony endplate. Posterior osteophytes were removed by curettes and Kerrison rongeurs. After complete decompression of the spinal cord and nerve roots, radiographic-guided trials facilitated selection of correctly sized cages, as previously described [5]. The distance between the two Luschka's joints determined the cage width. Cages that fit tightly in the disc space without over-distraction of the disc space or facet joints were considered the correct height. Synthesized hydroxyapatite-collagen artificial bone (Bonegold®, Allgens, Beijing, China) was used to fill in the cage in all patients. Properly sized devices (ROI-C® or ROI-MC+®, LDR MEDICAL, Troyes, France) and anchorage systems were inserted in vertebral bodies under fluoroscopic guidance (Fig. 1).

In Group B, a midline incision was made followed by a subperiosteal dissection of the paravertebral muscles to expose the spinous processes, laminae, facet joints, and transverse processes of the affected vertebrae. Lateral mass screws (Axon®, Synthes Inc., Raynham, MA, USA) were placed on C3-C5 and pedicle screws (Axon®, Synthes Inc., Raynham, MA, USA) were placed on C7, respectively.Contoured rods (Axon®, Synthes Inc., Raynham, MA, USA) were attached to the screws and locked. Radiographs were obtained to ensure accurate positioning of the screws and rods. Then, the laminae of the planned resection segments were resected using a rongeur and high-speed bur. Prophylactic C4–5 foraminotomy were carried out in patients with foraminal stenosis.Small wedges of auto-graft from the lamina were placed adjacent to bilateral joints to facilitate fusion.

Outcome assessment

Operative time and blood loss were obtained from medical records. Postoperative follow-up visits were performed at 1 week, 3 months, 6 months, 12 months, 18 months, and 24 months after surgery, and every year thereafter. Clinical outcomes were assessed using Japanese Orthopedic Association (JOA) and Neck Disability Index (NDI) scores. Perioperative and postoperative complications, including hardware-related complications, pseudarthrosis, cage subsidence, dysphagia, C5 palsy, axial neck pain, infection were recorded. Cases with reoperation or revision surgery were also recorded. Radiological outcomes, including fusion rate, cervical lordosis, fused segment lordosis, and cage subsidence, were assessed. Nonunion was defined as the presence of a radiolucent gap between the graft and the end plate on radiographs or CT scans in at least one operated level at the last follow-up [8]. Cervical lordosis was defined as the angle formed by the inferior end plate of C2 and C7 in the

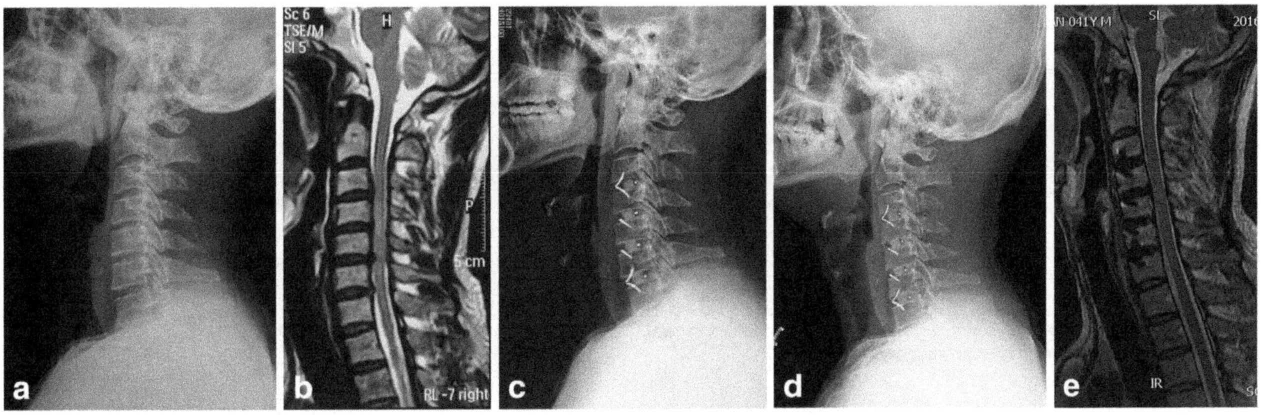

Fig. 1 An illustrative case: A 40-year-old male patient who presented with cervical spondylotic myelopathy was treated by 4-level ACDF using a stand-alone cage. **a** Preoperative lateral radiograph of the cervical spine. **b** Disc herniation at C3/4, C4/5, C5/6, and C6/7 confirmed by MRI. **c** Postoperative radiograph showed the cages were well-positioned and cervical spinal alignment was satisfactory. **d** Postoperative lateral radiograph of the cervical spine at the last follow-up showing maintenance of cervical alignment and restoration of disc height. **e** Postoperative MRI at the last follow-up showed thorough decompression of the spinal cord

neutral position on a plain lateral film [9]. Fused segment lordosis was defined as the angle formed by the superior end plate of C3 and inferior end plate of C7 in the neutral position on a plain lateral film. Improvement in lordosis was defined as an increase in lordosis angle at 1 week after surgery compared to pre-operation. Loss of lordosis was defined as a decrease in cervical lordosis or disc height at the last follow-up compared to 1 week after surgery. Subsidence was defined as loss of > 3 mm disc height at the last follow-up compared to 1 week after surgery [10].

Statistical analysis

All statistical analyses were conducted using SPSS version 19.0 software (SPSS Inc., Chicago, IL, USA). Between-group clinical and radiological outcomes were analyzed using an independent-samples t test. Within-group comparisons of pre- and post-operative parameters were evaluated using a one-way analysis of variance (ANOVA). Categorical variables, such as the incidence of dysphagia and the complication rate, were assessed using the Chi-square test. $P < 0.05$ was considered statistically significant.

Results

Medical records of 58 patients who met all the inclusion criteria and none of the exclusion criteria were reviewed. Of these, 26 patients (12 male, 14 female; mean (±SD) age 55.3 ± 10.1 years) underwent ACDF (Group A) with a stand-alone cage, and 32 patients (16 male, 16 female; mean age 54.4 ± 11.7 years) underwent posterior laminectomy and fixation (Group B). There were no significant differences in demographic variables, including patients' preoperative cervical curvature or JOA and NDI scores, between Groups A and B. Mean follow-up times were 25.1 ± 7.3 months and 25.8 ± 8.9 months in Groups A and B, respectively.

Clinical outcomes

There was significantly less blood loss in Group A (163.4 ± 72.1 ml) compared to Group B (241.0 ± 112.3 ml) ($P < 0.05$). The operative time was similar in both groups (Group A, 138.7 ± 40.2 min; Group B, 153.3 ± 35.1 min) (Table 1). Both groups demonstrated improvements in JOA and NDI scores after surgery with no significant differences between groups. There were no significant differences between groups at each post-operative follow up time point (Table 2).

Radiological outcomes

The fusion rate in Group A and Group B was 86.5 and 100%, respectively. The preoperative cervical lordosis (C2–7) were not significantly different in both groups. The cervical lordosis in both groups improved at postoperative 1 week, 3 months, 6 months, 12 months, but decreased at postoperative 18 months and 24 months (Table 3). Both improvements and loss of lordosis in C2–7 and C3–7 were significantly more pronounced in Group A at the final follow-up ($P < 0.05$). Within each group, there was no significant difference in lordosis improvement between C2–7 and C3–7; however, the loss of lordosis was significantly more pronounced in C2–7 than C3–7 (Table 4).

Table 1 Baseline characteristics of the study population

	Age (years)	Gender (Male/Female)	Follow-up time (months)	Operation time (minutes)	Blood loss (mL)
Group A	55.3 ± 10.1	12/14	25.1 ± 7.3	138.7 ± 40.2	163.4 ± 72.1
Group B	54.4 ± 11.7	16/16	25.8 ± 8.9	153.3 ± 35.1	241.0 ± 112.3
P-value	0.78	0.07	0.73	0.15	0.00

Group A underwent four-level ACDF using a stand-alone anchored PEEK cage and Group B underwent four-level laminectomy and fusion

Table 2 Clinical outcomes of both groups at different time point

	JOA scores			NDI		
	Group A	Group B	*P*-value	Group A	Group B	*P*-value
Preoperative	10.1 ± 1.1	10.0 ± 1.3	0.80	26.6 ± 3.8	26.8 ± 4.8	0.87
Postoperative 3 month	13.7 ± 1.5 *	13.6 ± 1.5 *	0.80	15.5 ± 1.8 *	15.7 ± 1.6 *	0.68
Postoperative 6 month	13.4 ± 1.3 *	13.3 ± 1.1 *	0.92	14.7 ± 1.7 *	15.0 ± 1.2 *	0.40
Postoperative 12 month	13.2 ± 1.3 *	13.1 ± 1.1 *	0.73	14.3 ± 1.6 *	14.9 ± 1.2 *	0.96
Postoperative 18 month	13.0 ± 1.2 *	13.0 ± 1.0 *	0.92	14.1 ± 1.4 *	14.7 ± 1.2 *	0.10
Postoperative 24 month	12.9 ± 1.2 *	12.8 ± 0.9 *	0.80	14.2 ± 1.4 *	14.4 ± 1.2 *	0.61

Group A underwent four-level ACDF using a stand-alone anchored PEEK cage and Group B underwent four-level laminectomy and fusion
*P-value of the time point versus pre-operation was less than 0.05.

Complications

The overall complication rate was significantly higher in Group A (15/26) than in Group B (6/32) ($P < 0.05$). There were no instances of perioperative cerebral fluid leakage, hematoma, cage migration, or hardware-related complications in either group. Six patients (14 levels) did not achieve fusion, and 6 patients (16 levels) had cage subsidence at the last follow-up. Patients with pseudarthrosis or cage subsidence were asymptomatic. Three patients in Group A complained of dysphagia post-surgery, but all recovered spontaneously within 3 months. Two patients in Group B complained of pain and paresis of the unilateral deltoid, which was considered to be C5 palsy, within 1 week postoperatively. Patients were treated conservatively using oral neurotrophic drugs, hyperbaric oxygen therapy, and exercise; all patients' symptoms had resolved by postoperative 3 months. One case of superficial infection was observed in Group B. Three patients in Group B suffered axial neck pain. Symptoms were present at the 6-month follow-up. Two patients had recovered by the final follow-up, while one patient suffered persistent pain. No patients in either group required reoperation (Table 5).

Discussion

To our knowledge, this is the first study to compare the outcomes of ACDF using a stand-alone cage (Group A) with laminectomy plus fixation and fusion (Group B) for multilevel CSM. ACDF using a stand-alone cage was associated with significantly less blood loss compared to laminectomy plus lateral mass fixation. Operative time was similar for both procedures, and all patients demonstrated improvements in JOA and NDI scores after surgery with no significant difference between procedures. Cervical lordosis and fused segment lordosis were both significantly improved at postoperative 1 week in all patients. However, the loss of cervical lordosis and fused segment lordosis at the final follow-up of 24 months was significantly more pronounced and the complication rate was significantly higher in patients who underwent ACDF using a stand-alone cage.

As a well-established procedure, laminectomy has gained widespread acceptance in the treatment of multilevel cervical myelopathy. Following laminectomy alone, indirect decompression of the anterior aspect of the spinal cord is achieved by spinal cord shift. With posterior fixation, complications associated with multi-level cervical laminectomy, including post-operative kyphosis, segmental instability, and subsequent neurologic deterioration, are reduced [11, 12]. However, adverse outcomes, such as axial pain, C5 palsy, restricted neck motion, perineural adhesions, and late neurologic deterioration, continue to occur.

ACDF is also effective for neural decompression in CSM because it corrects kyphotic alignment and preserves the

Table 3 Cervical lordosis in both groups at different time point

Cervical Lordosis (C2–7)	Group A	Group B	*P*-value
Preoperative	8.7 ± 3.1	8.7 ± 4.5	0.98
Postoperative 1 week	20.0 ± 4.5*	14.5 ± 6.0*	0.00
Postoperative 3 month	12.8 ± 4.1*	12.5 ± 4.7*	0.78
Postoperative 6 month	10.2 ± 4.3*	10.3 ± 4.9*	0.90
Postoperative 12 month	9.1 ± 4.7*	8.8 ± 5.0*	0.78
Postoperative 18 month	8.5 ± 4.5*	7.0 ± 4.9*	0.59
Postoperative 24 month	8.3 ± 4.6*	7.8 ± 4.9*	0.30

Group A underwent four-level ACDF using a stand-alone anchored PEEK cage and Group B underwent four-level laminectomy and fusion
*P-value of the time point versus pre operation was less than 0.05.

Table 4 Improvement and Loss of lordosis in both groups

		C2–7	C3–7	*P*-value within a group
Improvement of lordosis	Group A	11.3 ± 5.9	9.7 ± 5.3	0.32
	Group B	5.8 ± 4.6	5.5 ± 4.5	0.83
	P-value between groups	0.00	0.00	
Loss of lordosis	Group A	11.7 ± 2.2	6.7 ± 3.2	0.00
	Group B	7.5 ± 3.8	3.7 ± 3.4	0.00
	P-value between groups	0.00	0.00	

Group A underwent four-level ACDF using a stand-alone anchored PEEK cage and Group B underwent four-level laminectomy and fusion

Table 5 Complications

Subgroup	Group A	Group B
Pseudarthrosis	6	–
Revision surgery	0	0
Hardware-related complications	0	0
Dysphagia	3	0
Infection	0	1
Cage subsidence	6	none
C5 palsy	0	2
Axial neck pain	0	3
Cerebral fluid leakage	0	0
Hematoma	0	0
Total	15	6

Group A underwent four-level ACDF using a stand-alone anchored PEEK cage and Group B underwent four-level laminectomy and fusion

stability of the cervical spine [13]. Traditionally, anterior plating was used as it was thought to increase fusion rates, reduce cage subsidence, and prevent postoperative kyphosis. However, plate-related complications include screw loosening, screw pullout, dysphagia, and esophageal rupture, especially in long fusions. Ning et al. [14] estimated the rate of anterior cervical plate-related complications at 10.7%. Therefore, ACDF using anterior plate fixation is limited to pathology involving 1 or 2 levels. When spinal cord compression involves more than 3 levels, posterior decompression surgery is advocated. Currently, stand-alone cages are widely used to simplify the surgical procedure and avoid complications related to anterior instrumentation. In accordance with the current study, several reports indicate satisfactory clinical outcomes with ACDF using stand-alone cages for the treatment of multi-level cervical degenerative spondylopathy [5, 6].

Primary concerns in multi-level ACDF using stand-alone cages include nonunion and cage subsidence. Although some clinical studies show relatively high rates of union in multi-level stand-alone ACDF (72–100%) (Table 6) [5, 6, 8, 15], evidence suggests that the risk of pseudarthrosis increases with the number of graft–host interfaces. In the current study, 6 of 26 patients (14 levels) in Group A experienced nonunion; all were asymptomatic and none required revision surgery. This is in accordance with a previous report by Pereira [12] et al. in which three patients experienced late kyphosis due to subsidence and pseudarthrosis; all were asymptomatic, with the exception of one who required revision surgery. The bone substitute in Group A of our study was hydroxyapatite, may be attributed to the relative lower fusion rate to auto-graft in Group B.

Cage subsidence is common in multi-level ACDF without anterior plating as the plate curve helps prevent cage subsidence during fusion [16]. Subsidence rates in studies of multi-level ACDF using stand-alone cages range from 8.9 to 16.7% per level [8, 12, 15]. In the current study, the subsidence rate was 6/26 per patient and 13/104 per level in Group A. After reviewing 18 studies of ACDF, including 1468 cases of subsidence, Zajonz et al. suggested that clinical outcomes are unaffected by subsidence [17]. Cage subsidence or loss of disc height may be attributed to loss of cervical lordosis after ACDF. In the current study, patients in group A had a significant improvement in fused segment lordosis at each time point of follow-up compared to pre-operative status. These results are consistent with earlier reports [5, 6]. Postoperative improvements in cervical lordosis and fused segment lordosis were more obvious immediately after surgery in patients in Group A compared to Group B. This suggests that ACDF is more efficacious for restoring cervical disc space and cervical curvature compared to laminectomy and fusion. However, the loss of cervical lordosis at the final follow-up was more pronounced in Group A ($11.7 \pm 2.2°$). This may be due to the use of stand-alone anchored cages. Chen reported that post-operative cage subsidence, loss of disc height, cervical lordosis, and the fused segment angle were relatively higher in multi-level ACDF using stand-alone anchored cages than ACDF using cages and plates [5]. Lee et al. [18] showed that postoperative lordotic changes were 5.85° after ACDF with anterior plating. They proposed that clinical outcomes were unaffected by the loss of cervical lordosis after ACDF. In relation to long-term outcomes, a biomechanical study by Patwardhan et al. showed that cervical spinal sagittal malalignment may play a role in exacerbating adjacent segment degeneration after multilevel fusion as the mechanical burden on the adjacent segment becomes greater due to an imbalanced cervical spine [19]. Therefore, the long-term consequences of cage subsidence and the loss of cervical lordosis after ACDF using a stand-alone cage should be alerted. Interestingly, although improvements in lordosis of the cervical spine (C2–7) and fused segment (C3–7) were similar in both groups, the loss of lordosis was significantly more prominent in the cervical spine (C2–7) than in the fused segment (C3–7). This may be attributed to an acceleration of adjacent segment degeneration in the non-fused C2–3 segment. In that case, measurement of lordosis may not truly reflect the influence of subsidence. As such, the effect of subsidence caused by multi-level ACDF on cervical lordosis may be overestimated.

A previous study shows that C5 nerve root palsy is more likely to happen in patients who undergo laminectomy and fusion compared to ACDF due to excessive spinal cord drift after laminectomy and fusion with preexisting intervertebral foraminal stenosis [20]. A meta-analysis by Shou et al. [2] revealed that the highest prevalence (11.0%) of C5 palsy was found in patients who underwent laminectomy and fusion, while those who received ACDF had

Table 6 Summary of studies reporting multi-level stand-alone ACDF

Author	Study design	Operated levels	Number of cases	Follow-up time (months)	Device	Fusion rate	Subsidence rate per level (%)
Chen [5]	retrospective	3	28	24	ROI-C or ROI-MC+(LDR MEDICAL, Troyes, France)	85.7%	16.7%
Liu [6]	retrospective	3–4	28	24	ROI-C (LDR MEDICAL, Troyes, France)	100%	–
Pereira [12]	prospective	3–4	30	62	Solis (Stryker, Kalamazoo, MI, USA)	–	16.7%
Liu [16]	retrospective	3	25	24	Solis (Stryker, Cestas, France)	72%	4.0%
Zhou [17]	retrospective	3	15	20	ROI-MC+ (LDR MEDICAL, Troyes, France)	93.3%	8.9%
Our study	retrospective	4	26	24	ROI-C or ROI-MC+(LDR MEDICAL, Troyes, France)	86.5%	15.4%

the lowest prevalence (3.3%). In the current study, 6.25% patients (2/32) experienced C5 palsy in Group B. Based on the hypothesis of nerve traction and foraminal stenosis as the mechanism of post-laminoplasty C5 palsy, the use of prophylactic C4–5 foraminotomy to decompress the C5 nerve root has been proposed to eliminating this complication. Evidence suggests that prophylactic bilateral C4/C5 foraminotomy significantly decreases the incidence of postoperative C5 palsy (1.4% in the in the foraminotomy group vs. 6.4% in the non-foraminotomy group) [21]; therefore, all patients with foraminal stenosis who underwent laminectomy and fusion in the current study received prophylactic bilateral C4/C5 foraminotomy in our study. However, C5 palsy may still occur in patients with prolonged duration of symptoms and presence of high intensity cord signal changes at C4–5 [22]. In our study, we had two cases (2/32) of post-laminoplasty C5 palsy. Both of them had symptoms for over 1 year.

Axial neck pain is defined as pain from the nuchal to the periscapular or shoulder region after cervical surgery and may result in decreased range of motion. The reported incidence of axial neck pain after posterior cervical spine surgery ranges from 5.2 to 61.5% [23]. Wada et al. [24] found that patients who had undergone posterior procedures complained more frequently of postoperative posterior neck pain than patients who had undergone anterior fusion. Evidence suggests that axial neck pain that occurs within a few months after surgery is due to surgical trauma to muscles, whereas chronic axial neck pain is caused by an imbalance of flexor and extensor muscle strengths [23, 25]. In the current study, 3/32 patients in Group B developed axial neck pain at postoperative 6 months, two of them had recovered by the final follow-up. Only one patient experienced persistent pain. No patients in Group A developed axial neck pain. This may be because anterior approaches avoid posterior muscle invasion and posterior muscle atrophy, which play a pivotal role in the pathogenesis of axial neck pain.

There were limitations in our study. First, it was a non-randomized controlled trial that included a small sample size. The small sample size may reduce the power to detect a difference between the two groups. In addition, the strict inclusion and exclusion criteria of the retrospective study, some cases of cervical canal stenosis or OPLL case had to be treated with posterior approach were excluded, may lead to a potential selection bias. Second, the influence of the graft material on the fusion rate after ACDF using a stand-alone cage was not analyzed. The difference between auto-graft and hydroxyapatite-collagen artificial bone graft in a 4 level ACDF using a stand-alone cage is known. Whether using artificial bone graft in a 4 level fusion without a plate can achieve similar results to traditional ACDF with a plate an auto-graft/allograft is also unknown. Finally, long-term adverse effects require further consideration, such as adjacent segment degeneration resulting from cage subsidence, nonunion, and loss of correction after multi-level ACDF using a stand-alone cage.

Conclusion

Four-level ACDF using a stand-alone cage appears to be effective compared to laminectomy and fusion when considering clinical outcomes. However, ACDF with a stand-alone cage associated with more non-unions. And loss of correction of cervical lordosis after surgery was more apparent compared to laminectomy and fusion.

Abbreviations

ACDF: Anterior cervical discectomy and fusion; CSM: Cervical spondylotic myelopathy; JOA: Japanese Orthopedic Association; LF: Laminectomy with fusion; NDI: Neck Disability Index

Authors' contributions

BW made substantial contributions to conception and design, and acquisition of data. GL made substantial contributions to manuscript revising. LK made substantial contributions to study design, acquisition, analysis and interpretation of data, and involved in drafting the manuscript and revising it critically for important intellectual content. All authors read and approved the final manuscript.

Consent for publication
Not applicable.

Competing interests
The authors declare that they have no competing interests.

References

1. Lin D, Zhai W, Lian K, Kang L, Ding Z. Anterior versus posterior approach for four-level cervical spondylotic myelopathy. Orthopedics. 2013;36(11):e1431–6. https://doi.org/10.3928/01477447-20131021-28
2. Shou F, Li Z, Wang H, Yan C, Liu Q, Xiao C. Prevalence of C5 nerve root palsy after cervical decompressive surgery: a meta-analysis. Eur Spine J. 2015;24(12):2724–34. https://doi.org/10.1007/s00586-015-4186-5
3. De la Garza-Ramos R, Xu R, Ramhmdani S, Kosztowski T, Bydon M, Sciubba DM, Wolinsky J, Witham TF, Gokaslan ZL, Bydon A. Long-term clinical outcomes following 3- and 4-level anterior cervical discectomy and fusion. J Neurosurg Spine. 2016;24(6):885–91. https://doi.org/10.3171/2015.10.SPINE15795. Erratum in: J Neurosurg Spine. 24(6):996. https://doi.org/10.3171/2016.3.SPINE15795a
4. Song K, Song J, Kim D, Shim DG, Lee K. Efficacy of combined anteroposterior fusion with no plate versus anterior fusion alone with cage and plate for multilevel degenerative cervical disease. Spine J. 2014;14(4):598–603. https://doi.org/10.1016/j.spinee.2013.06.082
5. Chen Y, Lü G, Wang B, Li L, Kuang L. A comparison of anterior cervical discectomy and fusion (ACDF) using self-locking stand-alone polyetheretherketone (PEEK) cage with ACDF using cage and plate in the treatment of three-level cervical degenerative spondylopathy: a retrospective study with 2-year follow-up. Eur Spine J. 2016;25(7):2255–62. https://doi.org/10.1007/s00586-016-4391-x
6. Liu Y, Wang H, Li X, Chen J, Sun H, Wang G, Yang H, Jiang W. Comparison of a zero-profile anchored spacer (ROI-C) and the polyetheretherketone (PEEK) cages with an anterior plate in anterior cervical discectomy and fusion for multilevel cervical spondylotic myelopathy. Eur Spine J. 2016;25(6):1881–90. https://doi.org/10.1007/s00586-016-4500-x
7. Smith GW. Robinson RA (1958) the treatment of certain cervical-spine disorders by anterior removal of the intervertebral disc and interbody fusion. J Bone Joint Surg Am. 1958;40-A(3):607–24.
8. Zhou J, Li X, Dong J, Zhou X, Fang T, Lin H, Ma Y. Three-level anterior cervical discectomy and fusion with self-locking stand-alone polyetheretherketone cages. J Clin Neurosci. 2011;18(11):1505–9. https://doi.org/10.1016/j.jocn.2011.02.045
9. Thom C, Krauss JK, Zevgaridis D. A prospective clinical comparison of rectangular titanium cages and iliac crest autografts in anterior cervical discectomy and fusion. Neurosurg Rev Jan. 2004;27(1):34–41. https://doi.org/10.1007/s10143-003-0297-2
10. Gercek E, Arlet V, Delisle J, Marchesi D. Subsidence of stand-alone cervical cages in anterior interbody fusion: warning. Eur Spine J. 2003;12(5):513–6. https://doi.org/10.1007/s00586-003-0539-6
11. Woods BI, Hohl J, Lee J, Donaldson WR, Kang J. Laminoplasty versus laminectomy and fusion for multilevel cervical spondylotic myelopathy. Clin Orthop Relat Res. 2011;469(3):688–95. https://doi.org/ 10.1007/s11999-010-1653-5
12. Pereira EA, Chari A, Hempenstall J, Leach JC, Chandran H, Cadoux-Hudson TA. Anterior cervical discectomy plus intervertebral polyetheretherketone cage fusion over three and four levels without plating is safe and effective long-term. J Clin Neurosci. 2013;20(9):1250–5. https://doi.org/10.1016/j.jocn.2012.10.028
13. Seng C, Tow BPB, Siddiqui MA, Srivastava A, Wang L, Yew AKS, Yeo W, Khoo SHR, Balakrishnan NMS, Bin Abd Razak HR, Chen JLT, Guo CM, Tan SB, Yue W. Surgically treated cervical myelopathy: a functional outcome comparison study between multilevel anterior cervical decompression fusion with instrumentation and posterior laminoplasty. Spine J. 2013;13(7):723–31. https://doi.org/10.1016/j.spinee.2013.02.038
14. Ning X, Wen Y, Xiao-Jian Y, Bin N, De-Yu C, Jian-Ru X, Lian-Shun J. Anterior cervical locking plate-related complications; prevention and treatment recommendations. Int Orthop. 2008;32(5):649–55. https://doi.org/10.1007/s00264-007-0369-y
15. Liu H, Ploumis A, Li C, Yi X, Li H. Polyetheretherketone cages alone with allograft for three-level anterior cervical fusion. ISRN Neurol. 2012; 2012(452703) https://doi.org/10.5402/2012/452703
16. Chung CK, Kim CH. Anterior plating is better than the stand-alone cage in the restoration of segmental kyphosis. Spine J. 2012;12((9):S100. http://dx.doi.org/10.1016/j.spinee.2012.08.277
17. Zajonz D, Franke A, von der Höh N, Voelker A, Moche M, Gulow J, Heyde C (2014) Is the radiographic subsidence of stand-alone cages associated with adverse clinical outcomes after cervical spine fusion? An observational cohort study with 2-year follow-up outcome scoring. Patient Saf Surg7;8(1): 43.https://doi.org/10.1186/s13037-014-0043-4.
18. Lee J, Park MS, Moon S, Shin J, Kim SW, Kim Y, Lee SJ, Suh B, Lee H. Loss of lordosis and clinical outcomes after anterior cervical fusion with dynamic rotational plates. Yonsei Med J. 2013;54(3):726–31. http://dx.doi.org/10.3349/ymj.2013.54.3.726
19. Patwardhan AG, Khayatzadeh S, Nguyen N, Havey RM, Voronov LI, Muriuki MG, Carandang G, Smith ZA, Sears W, Lomasney LM, Ghanayem AJ. Is cervical sagittal imbalance a risk factor for adjacent segment Pathomechanics after multilevel fusion? Spine (Phila Pa 1976). 2016;41(10): E580–8. http://dx.doi.org/10.1097/BRS.0000000000001316
20. Gu Y, Cao P, Gao R, Tian Y, Liang L, Wang C, Yang L, Yuan W. Incidence and risk factors of C5 palsy following posterior cervical decompression: a systematic review. PLoS One. 2014;9(8):e101933. http://dx.doi.org/10.1371/journal.pone.0101933
21. Katsumi K, Yamazaki A, Watanabe K, Ohashi M, Shoji H (2012) Can prophylactic bilateral C4/C5 Foraminotomy prevent postoperative C5 palsy after open-door Laminoplasty? Spine (Phila Pa 1976) 37(9):748–754. http://dx.doi.org/10.1097/BRS.0b013e3182326957.
22. Liu G, Reyes MR, Riew KD. Why does C5 palsy occur after prophylactic bilateral C4-5 foraminotomy in open-door cervical laminoplasty? A risk factor analysis.Global Spine J 7(7):696–702. http://dx.doi.org/10.1177/2192568217699191.
23. Wang S, Jiang S, Jiang L, Dai L. Axial pain after posterior cervical spine surgery: a systematic review. Eur Spine J. 2011;20(2):185–94. http://dx.doi.org/10.1007/s00586-010-1600-x
24. Wada E, Suzuki S, Kanazawa A, Matsuoka T, Miyamoto S, Yonenobu K. Subtotal corpectomy versus laminoplasty for multilevel cervical spondylotic myelopathy: a long-term follow-up study over 10 years. Spine (Phila Pa 1976). 2001;26(13):1443–7. discussion 1448
25. Nakama S, Nitanai K, Oohashi Y, Endo T, Hoshino Y (2003) Cervical muscle strength after laminoplasty.J Orthop Sci. 2003;8(1):36–40.http://dx.doi.org/https://doi.org/10.1007/s007760300006.

10

Anterior cruciate ligament reconstruction with quadriceps tendon-patellar bone allograft

Yoon-Ho Kwak, Sahnghoon Lee, Myung Chul Lee and Hyuk-Soo Han*

Abstract

Background: Quadriceps tendon-patellar bone (QTPB) autograft is an excellent graft option with good clinical outcome. Use of QTPB autografts have increased because they minimize donor-site morbidity including anterior knee pain, while providing adequate mechanical strength. Although, there were many clinical results about allografts that used in anterior cruciate ligament (ACL) reconstruction, it have never been reported about the clinical outcome of ACL reconstruction with QTPB allograft.

The purpose of this study is to evaluate the clinical outcome of ACL reconstruction with QTPB allograft and to compare with QTPB autograft. We hypothesized that ACL reconstruction with QTPB allograft had good functional outcomes and stability and no significant difference compared to the ACL reconstruction with QTPB autograft.

Methods: From February 2009 to January 2014, 213 cases who received ACL reconstruction with QTPB grafts were included. Forty-five patients who received ACL reconstruction with QTPB allograft were individually matched in age, sex, direction of the injured knee and body mass index (BMI) to a control group of 45 patients who received QTPB autograft. Clinical results were evaluated using International Knee Documentation Committee (IKDC) score, Lysholm score, Tegner scale, Knee injury and Osteoarthritis Outcome Score (KOOS) and ligament laxity. An average follow-up time was 31.2 months.

Results: The functional scores and ligament laxity improved from initial to the last visit in those with ACL reconstruction with QTPB allograft ($p < 0.05$). No significant statistical difference was found in clinical outcomes and complications including re-rupture between the QTPB allograft and autograft groups ($p > 0.05$). Laxity using anterior drawer test, Lachman test and KT-2000 showed no significant difference. No significant difference was found between the two groups in quadriceps peak extension torque, except at 60° per second at 6 months.

Conclusion: QTPB allograft achieved good clinical outcome with no difference compared with QTPB autograft. QTPB allograft for ACL reconstruction is promising alternative to selected and compliant patients. Long-term follow-up needs to further evaluate the clinical outcomes and complications including re-rupture rate.

Keywords: Arthroscopy, Anterior cruciate ligament, Quadriceps tendon-patellar bone, Allograft, Autograft

* Correspondence: oshawks7@snu.ac.kr
Seoul National University Hospital, Seoul, Republic of Korea

Background

ACL reconstruction can be performed using several kinds of autograft or allograft tissue. Although, some recent research showed ACL reconstruction with autograft leads to lower retear rates in younger individuals [1], whether the outcomes of these two graft materials differ significantly is unclear [2–4] and the choice of the optimal graft for ACL reconstruction remains still controversial.

Good clinical results of ACL reconstruction have been achieved using proper graft materials, such as bone-patella tendon-bone (BPTB) or hamstring tendons, as well as quadriceps tendon-patellar bone (QTPB) [5–9]. The QTPB autograft is long established as a viable graft option with good clinical outcome [7, 10–18]. The use of QTPB autografts has increased in recent years because they minimize donor-site morbidity including anterior knee pain, while providing adequate mechanical strength as a graft [7, 12, 19, 20]. Several reports have suggested a biomechanical test for quadriceps tendon is comparable to that for BPTB [21–23]. However, QTPB allograft has been the least studied. Previous studies have compared other allografts with autografts in primary ACL reconstruction with results showing inconsistent clinical equivalency [16, 24, 25] and no study has directly compared QTPB allograft to autograft.

The purpose of this study is to evaluate the clinical outcomes of ACL reconstruction with QTPB allograft regarding anteroposterior knee stability, activity, and functional scores. We also evaluated whether the outcomes differed with QTPB allograft and autograft used for ACL reconstruction. We hypothesized that ACL reconstruction with QTPB allograft had good functional outcomes and stability and no significant difference compared to the ACL reconstruction with QTPB autograft.

Methods

This is a retrospective study with ethically approved by the institutional review board of Seoul National University Hospital (No. H-1604-033-753). From February 2009 to January 2014, 278 patients diagnosed as ACL total ruptures who received ACL reconstruction with QTPB grafts were screened. The choice of the graft was determined by full discussion between the patient and the physician. We included patients followed-up more than 2 years after ACL reconstruction. Exclusion criteria were patients who had previous ligament injury and who had concomitant meniscus or ligament injury of the affected knee, except for a Grade I or II medial collateral ligament injury. Revision ACL reconstructions were also excluded. Finally, 45 patients who had QTPB allografts and 168 patients who had QTPB autografts met these criteria. The 45 patients in the QTPB allograft group were matched for age and body mass index (BMI) with 45 patients in the QTPB autograft group (Fig. 1).

Ligament laxity was evaluated with anterior drawer test, Lachman test, pivot shift test and a KT-2000 arthrometer (MedMetric Inc., San Diego, CA) preoperatively, postoperatively at 1, 3 and 6 months and annually thereafter. Quadriceps peak extension torque was checked at 60° and 180° per second using an isokinetic testing device (Cybex, Ronkonkoma, NY) at 6, 12 and 24 months. Functional outcomes including International Knee Documentation Committee (IKDC) score [26], Lysholm Knee Score [27], Tegner score [28] and Knee Injury and Osteoarthritis Outcome Score (KOOS) [29] were evaluated preoperatively and at the postoperative follow-ups.

QTPB allografts were provided by Community Tissue Services (Kettering, OH), a certified soft tissue bank. Allografts were the non-gamma irradiated fresh frozen type. Serological and microbiological tests were performed on the donors in accordance with American Association of Tissue Bank (AATB) standards. On the day of surgery, the allograft was transported from the local distributor to the operating room adding dry ice for below zero temperature conditions (− 70 to − 60 °C). The state of packaging and expiry dates were checked before use and the grafts soaked in sterile saline, warmed to 37 °C for 30 min. A trapezoidal bone block measuring 10 mm in width, 20- to 25 mm in length and 7 mm in thickness was obtained using an oscillating saw. A strip of the quadriceps tendon measuring 10 mm in width, 6-8 mm in thickness and 6 cm in length was excised from the proximal portion of the patellar bone block (Fig. 2).

The QTPB autograft was harvested through a 4 cm midline incision centered over the patella proximal border and prepared by the same method of used for the QTPB allograft. We were cautioned not to approach the suprapatellar pouch by saving part of the vastus intermedius tendon. If the suprapatellar pouch was damaged, the synovial lining was repaired with an absorbable suture. Superficial layers of the cut surface of the tendon were closed transversely with absorbable sutures and the defect was left as a potential space. The bone defect was left in empty space. A hole was drilled in the bone block from the patella base and two absorbable sutures were passed through. The tendinous portion of the graft was secured with two Number 5 Ethibond™ sutures (Ethicon Inc., Somerville, NJ) using the Krackow method with an extension of approximately 30 mm (Fig. 2).

After a graft had been prepared, ACL reconstruction was performed by the modified transtibial technique [30]. A tibial tunnel 10 mm in diameter was drilled and the intra-articular opening of the tunnel was placed in the center of the ACL attachment using an ACL endoscopic guide system (Smith and Nephew, Inc., Andover, MA). A femoral tunnel that was also 10 mm in diameter was drilled through the tibial tunnel in the 10:30 to 11

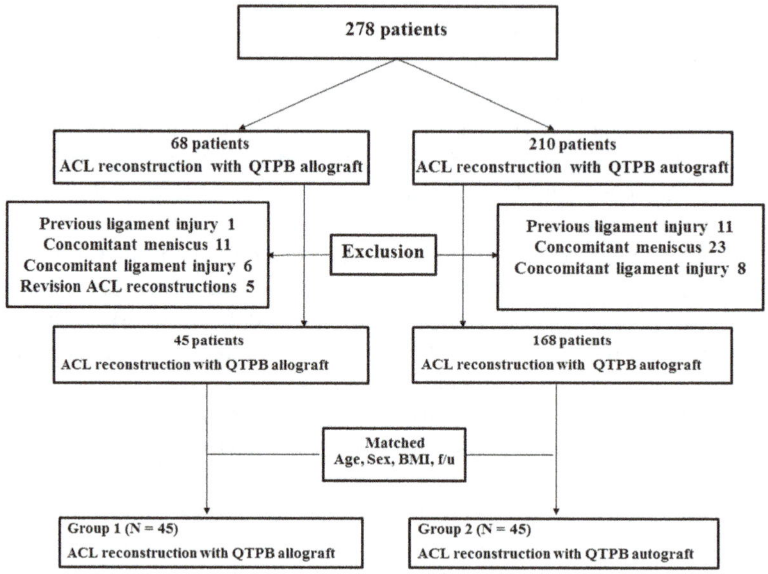

Fig. 1 Flow diagram of patients screened and grouped

o'clock position for the right knee. The posterior cortex of the femoral tunnel was approximately 2 mm thick. Notchplasty was performed to prevent graft impingement if needed. After the graft had been passed through the femoral tunnels, a 8 mm diameter, 25 mm length metal interference screw (Linvatec, Largo, FL) was used to fix the bone block on the femoral side. The ACL reconstructed knee was moved in flexion and extension 15 to 20 times through a full range of motion under tensioning the graft. The tendinous portion was fixed on the tibial side with a 10 mm diameter, 25 mm length metal interference screw (Synthes, West Chester, Pennsylvania) augmented by tying sutures over a cortical screw with the knee extended.

The same rehabilitation protocol was applied for both groups. Patients were taught quadriceps setting exercise and straight leg raising prior to surgery and exercise commenced soon after surgery. Kinetic exercise and weight-bearing progressed as tolerated. Passive range of motion of the ACL reconstructed knee was started from 45° knee flexion and full extension within 3 days after surgery. Patients put on the ACL knee brace 1 week after surgery when swelling decreased. An ACL brace set at 0° to 90° was worn for 3 weeks and then set at 0° to full flexion for an additional 3 weeks postoperatively. Full flexion was allowed at postoperative 7 weeks. Patients usually returned to normal daily activity 3 months after ACL reconstruction and strenuous exercise was approved 6 months postoperatively.

We used SPSS for Windows version 20.0 (SPSS Inc., Chicago, IL) for statistical analyses. The independent t-test was used for the comparison of continuous variables (IKDC score, Lysholm score, Tegner score, KOOS score, extensor strengths and KT-2000 arthrometry), and the chi-squared test was used for the categorical variables (grades of ligament stability including anterior drawer test, Lachman test, pivot shift test). Paired t-test was used for comparing the data before and after the ACL reconstruction. The significance level was set at $P < 0.05$. A post-hoc analysis was performed by G-Power, and confirmed 42 patients in each group to detect one standard deviation difference at 80% power. The ligament laxity

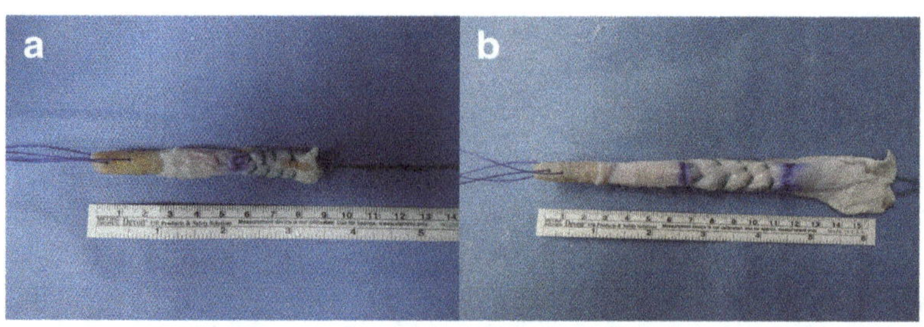

Fig. 2 Quadriceps tendon-patellar bone autograft (**a**) and allograft (**b**)

checked by KT-2000 was primary outcome in which the sample size was based. This study was approved by the institutional review board.

Results

As we mentioned above, 45 patients in each groups were included in this retrospective study. An average follow-up time was 31.2 months.

There were no differences in preoperative demographic data between the two groups (Table 1). Comparisons of knee laxity and clinical outcome between two groups are summarized in Tables 2 and 3. According to the anterior drawer test, Lachman test, and pivot-shift test, there was no significant difference between the two groups preoperatively and at final follow-up (Table 2). All grades of instability were improved from the initial to final visit in both groups ($P < 0.001$). The mean side-to-side differences in anterior laxity during manual maximum testing using KT-2000 arthrometry were similar in the QTPB allograft and autograft groups preoperatively (4.8 ± 1.9 and 4.5 ± 1.8 mm; $P = 0.370$) and postoperatively (1.8 ± 1.6 mm and 1.4 ± 1.2 mm; $P = 0.458$). The KT-2000 measurements at postoperative 2 years follow-up were significantly improved than at preoperative in both groups (both $P < 0.001$).

Forty-one patients, and greater than 5 mm in 12 patients. One patient per group showed grade II in Lachman test, which generally considered clinical failure [31, 32]. However, anterior drawer test, pivot-shift test and KT-2000 measurements showed no instability and had no subjective instability in both 2 patients. Therefore, we decided not to have revision surgery.

No significant differences in functional scores including IKDC score, Lysholm score, Tegner score, KOOS were found between the two groups at preoperative and postoperative 2 years (Table 3). Mean preoperative functional scores in QTPB allografts group and autografts group were improved at postoperative 2 years follow-up ($p < 0.001$).

Quadriceps peak extension torque at 60°and 180° per second increased with time at 6, 12, 24 months in both groups. No significant differences were found the two groups, except the value of the quadriceps peak extension torque at 60° per second at 6 months ($P = 0.042$) (Fig. 3).

In both groups, there were no postoperative complications during follow-ups such as arthrofibrosis, rerupture or infection. In the QTPB autograft group, two patients had paresthesia on the lateral side of the knee. The paresthesia completely disappeared about 2 months after ACL reconstruction. Two patients in the QTPB allograft group and three patients in the QTPB autograft group felt a clicking sensation in the knee during activities, and this symptom was relieved after an average of 3 months.

Table 1 Patient demographic data

	Allograft group ($n = 45$)	Autograft group ($n = 45$)	*p-value*
Age[a]	34.5 ± 12.8	34.5 ± 12.8	1.000
Sex (Male/Female)	38/7	38/7	1.000
Right/Left	20/25	22/23	0.833
BMI (kg/m^2)[a]	25.2 ± 4.0	25.3 ± 4.5	0.905
F/U (months)**	32.6 ± 7.4 (27.5 – 39.5)	29.8 ± 6.5 (24.9 – 44.3)	0.300

Values are expressed as mean ± standard deviation[a] or mean ± standard deviation (range)**

Discussion

This is the first study comparing the knee stability and clinical outcomes of the QTPB allografts and autografts. The most important finding in this study was ACL reconstruction with QTPB allografts showed good clinical outcomes and had no significant differences compared with QTPB autografts. There was no difference about rerupture rate in short-term follow-up. However, 6 months after ACL reconstruction, quadriceps muscle power recovery was relatively good in ACL reconstruction with QTPB allograft.

Several studies have compared ACL reconstruction with QTPB autograft to other autografts and reported comparable results concerning knee stability and functional outcomes [10, 12–14, 19, 20]. Most clinical outcomes about ACL reconstruction with QTPB autograft in these studies were relatively good, which is also shown in our study.

Two studies have compared biomechanical properties of QTPB allograft to other grafts. One study compared the biomechanical properties of 12 QTPB allografts to 11 BPTB allografts [21]. The authors found that the cross-sectional area of the QTPB allografts was nearly twice that of the BPTB allografts and ultimate load to failure and stiffness was significantly higher for the QTPB allografts. The variability in the cross-sectional area was similar in both tendon groups. In the other study, quadriceps and Achilles tendon pairs from nine research-consented donors were tested [33]. All specimens were processed to reduce bioburden and terminally sterilized by gamma irradiation. The authors found that QTPB allografts displayed significantly higher displacement at maximum load and significantly lower stiffness than achilles allografts. Maximum stress, strain at maximum stress, modulus and cyclic elongation exhibited no significant differences between two tendon types. On the basis of these two biomechanical studies, QTPB allograft is judged to be a biomechanically qualified graft for ACL reconstruction.

Several studies have reported allograft rerupture rates were higher than autograft after ACL reconstruction. One study reported a 7% rate of late allograft traumatic

Table 2 Evaluation of knee instability

	Preoperative			Postoperative 2 years		
	Allograft group	Autograft group	*p-value*	Allograft group	Autograft group	*p-value*
Anterior drawer test			0.826			0.652
Grade 0	5 (11.1%)	4 (8.9%)		29 (64.4%)	32 (71.1%)	
Grade 1	16 (35.6%)	15 (33.3%)		16 (35.6%)	13 (28.9%)	
Grade 2	17 (37.8%)	21 (46.7%)		0 (0.0%)	0 (0.0%)	
Grade 3	7 (15.6%)	5 (11.1%)		0 (0.0%)	0 (0.0%)	
Lachman test			0.717			0.404
Grade 0	1 (2.2%)	3 (6.7%)		26 (57.8%)	29 (64.4%)	
Grade 1	17 (37.8%)	14 (31.1%)		18 (40.0%)	15 (33.3%)	
Grade 2	19 (42.2%)	19 (42.2%)		1 (2.2%)	1 (2.2%)	
Grade 3	8 (17.8%)	9 (20.0%)		0 (0.0%)	0 (0.0%)	
Pivot shift test			0.258			0.823
Grade 0	6 (13.3%)	4 (8.9%)		31 (68.9%)	29 (64.4%)	
Grade 1	16 (35.6%)	22 (48.9%)		14 (31.1%)	16 (35.6%)	
Grade 2	21 (46.7%)	14 (31.1%)		0 (0.0%)	0 (0.0%)	
Grade 3	2 (4.4%)	5 (11.1%)		0 (0.0%)	0 (0.0%)	
KT-2000 (mm)[a]	4.8 ± 1.9	4.5 ± 1.8	0.392	1.8 ± 1.6	1.4 ± 1.2	0.235
KT-2000 (No. of patients)						
< 3 mm	2 (4.4%)	5 (11.1%)		39 (86.7%)	34 (75.6%)	
3 – 5 mm	26 (57.8%)	30 (66.7%)		6 (13.3%)	11 (24.4%)	
> 5 mm	17 (37.8%)	10 (22.2%)		0 (0.0%)	0 (0.0%)	

[a]Values are expressed as mean ± standard deviation

rupture versus none in autografts [34]. Another study reported that allograft showed a threefold increase in rerupture rate relative to the autograft (12.7% vs. 4.3%) [35]. There are several possible explanations. Sterilization processes that influence remodeling of the allograft in vivo can cause a higher rate of rerupture in ACL reconstruction done with allograft ACL [36]. In addition, allograft patients may participate in a higher level of activity earlier after surgery, secondary to less pain including donor site pain, with more consequent stress on their grafts, than in autograft patients [37]. In this minimum 2-year follow-up study, there was no rerupture case in ACL reconstruction with QTPB allograft. However, long- term follow-up and further evaluation will be planned.

Although the QTPB autograft has less donor-site morbidity than other autografts, quadriceps graft harvest can cause temporal quadriceps weakness [14, 38–40]. In order to evaluate quadriceps muscle power, we used a Cybex isokinetic testing device. In our study, quadriceps peak extension torque at 60° per second in the QTPB autograft group at postoperative 6 months was less than in the QTPB allograft group. However, there was no significant difference in later follow-up.

In general, unlike primary reconstruction, in revision cases the choice of graft can be determined by the nature of the graft that was previously used, and an allograft may be an appealing situation to use [32]. ACL reconstruction with QTPB allograft showed good clinical

Table 3 Outcomes of functional score

	Preoperative			Postoperative		
	Allograft group	Autograft group	*p-value*	Allograft group	Autograft group	*p-value*
IKDC score	42.3 ± 16.1	42.7 ± 22.6	0.928	70.1 ± 12.5	67.3 ± 16.8	0.366
Lysholm score	65.0 ± 9.1	62.4 ± 8.4	0.166	88.7 ± 6.4	87.0 ± 5.3	0.170
Tegner scale	3.2 [2-4.8]	2.8 [1.8-4]	0.203	7 [6.0-8.0]	7.2 [6.3-8.2]	0.434
KOOS	245.1 ± 87.5	273.8 ± 95.1	0.163	413.2 ± 40.6	423.1 ± 50.9	0.334

Values are expressed as mean ± standard deviation in IKDC score, Lysholm score, KOOS; Values are expressed as the median and interquartile ranges in Tegner scale
IKDC International Knee Documentation Committee, *KOOS* Knee injury and Osteoarthritis Outcome Score

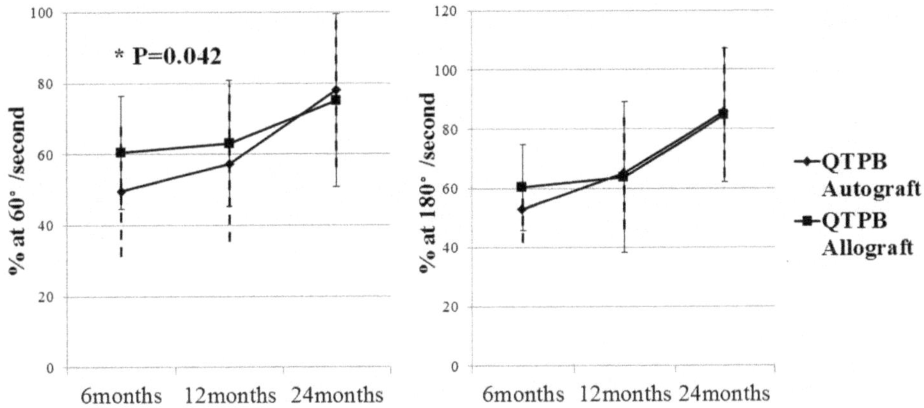

Fig. 3 Side to side ratio of peak torque values by Cybex isokinetic testing at 60° (left) and 180° (right) per second. Vertical full line indicates the standard deviation of the peak extension torque in QTPB allograft group. Vertical dotted line indicates the standard deviation of the peak extension torque in QTPB autograft group. QTPB = quadriceps tendon patellar bone

results in this study, then also possible options in revision ACL reconstruction.

This study has some limitations. First, this study has a retrospective design and the patients were not assigned randomly, increasing selection bias. However, there were several strengths in this study, including the matched demographic features of these patients, same surgical techniques, fixation method and rehabilitation program, which increased the power of statistical results. Furthermore, this is the first study reporting the clinical outcome of QTPB allograft and matched case-control study compared with QTPB allograft. Second, our study includes a relatively small number of patients especially on allograft group and has a short-term follow-up period. According to one study [41], at least 100 patients were required to detect a difference for the majority of outcome measures, and over 800 to detect a difference in return to pre-injury activity level. Comparing to this study, our study has limitations. In order to overcome these limitations, long-term follow up, large scaled, randomized controlled study will be scheduled to confirm the efficacy of this study. Third, our study does not include MRI evaluation of reconstructed ACL to confirm the ligamentizations of ACL. However, we could make an assumption by clinical results including anterior drawer test, Lachman test, pivot shift test and a KT-2000 arthrometer.

Conclusions

ACL reconstruction with QTPB allograft achieves good knee stability and functional outcomes with no difference compared with QTPB autograft at 2 years follow-up. Therefore, QTPB allograft for ACL reconstruction is promising alternative to selected and compliant patients. Long-term follow-up needs to further evaluate the clinical outcomes and complications including re-rupture rate.

Abbreviations

AATB: American Association of Tissue Bank; ACL: Anterior cruciate ligament; BPTB: Bone-patella tendon-bone; IKDC: International Knee Documentation Committee; KOOS: Knee injury and Osteoarthritis Outcome Score; QTPB: Quadriceps tendon-patellar bone

Acknowledgements

Not applicable.

Funding

This study was supported by the Basic Science Research Program through the National Research Foundation of Korea (NRF), funded by the Ministry of Science (NRF-2015R1D1A1A01059785).

Authors' contributions

YHK collected data, performed the statistical analysis with interpretation and wrote the manuscript. SHL and MCL participated in the design of the study and coordination and helped to draft the manuscript. HSH participated in the design of the study and proofread the manuscript as the corresponding author. All authors read and approved the final manuscript.

Consent for publication

Not applicable.

Competing interests

The authors declare that they have no competing interests.

References

1. Kane PW, Wascher J, Dodson CC, Hammoud S, Cohen SB, Ciccotti MG. Anterior cruciate ligament reconstruction with bone-patellar tendon-bone autograft versus allograft in skeletally mature patients aged 25 years or younger. Knee Surg Sports Traumatol Arthrosc. 2016;24(11):3627–33.
2. Foster TE, Wolfe BL, Ryan S, Silvestri L, Kaye EK. Does the graft source really matter in the outcome of patients undergoing anterior cruciate ligament reconstruction? An evaluation of autograft versus allograft reconstruction results: a systematic review. Am J Sports Med. 2010;38(1):189–99.

3. Marrale J, Morrissey MC, Haddad FS. A literature review of autograft and allograft anterior cruciate ligament reconstruction. Knee Surg Sports Traumatol Arthrosc. 2007;15(6):690–704.
4. Carey JL, Dunn WR, Dahm DL, Zeger SL, Spindler KP. A systematic review of anterior cruciate ligament reconstruction with autograft compared with allograft. J Bone Joint Surg Am. 2009;91(9):2242–50.
5. Hertel P, Behrend H, Cierpinski T, Musahl V, Widjaja G. ACL reconstruction using bone-patellar tendon-bone press-fit fixation: 10-year clinical results. Knee Surg Sports Traumatol Arthrosc. 2005;13(4):248–55.
6. Leiter JR, Gourlay R, McRae S, de Korompay N, MacDonald PB. Long-term follow-up of ACL reconstruction with hamstring autograft. Knee Surg Sports Traumatol Arthrosc. 2014;22(5):1061–9.
7. Slone HS, Romine SE, Premkumar A, Xerogeanes JW. Quadriceps tendon autograft for anterior cruciate ligament reconstruction: a comprehensive review of current literature and systematic review of clinical results. Arthroscopy. 2015;31(3):541–54.
8. Streich NA, Reichenbacher S, Barie A, Buchner M, Schmitt H. Long-term outcome of anterior cruciate ligament reconstruction with an autologous four-strand semitendinosus tendon autograft. Int Orthop. 2013;37(2):279–84.
9. Salmon LJ, Russell VJ, Refshauge K, Kader D, Connolly C, Linklater J, Pinczewski LA. Long-term outcome of endoscopic anterior cruciate ligament reconstruction with patellar tendon autograft: minimum 13-year review. Am J Sports Med. 2006;34(5):721–32.
10. Gorschewsky O, Klakow A, Putz A, Mahn H, Neumann W. Clinical comparison of the autologous quadriceps tendon (BQT) and the autologous patella tendon (BPTB) for the reconstruction of the anterior cruciate ligament. Knee Surg Sports Traumatol Arthrosc. 2007;15(11):1284–92.
11. Schulz AP, Lange V, Gille J, Voigt C, Frohlich S, Stuhr M, Jurgens C. Anterior cruciate ligament reconstruction using bone plug-free quadriceps tendon autograft: intermediate-term clinical outcome after 24-36 months. Open Access J Sports Med. 2013;4:243–9.
12. Han HS, Seong SC, Lee S, Lee MC. Anterior cruciate ligament reconstruction : quadriceps versus patellar autograft. Clin Orthop Relat Res. 2008;466(1):198–204.
13. Lee MC, Seong SC, Lee S, Chang CB, Park YK, Jo H, Kim CH. Vertical femoral tunnel placement results in rotational knee laxity after anterior cruciate ligament reconstruction. Arthroscopy. 2007;23(7):771–8.
14. Lee S, Seong SC, Jo H, Park YK, Lee MC. Outcome of anterior cruciate ligament reconstruction using quadriceps tendon autograft. Arthroscopy. 2004;20(8):795–802.
15. DeAngelis JP, Fulkerson JP. Quadriceps tendon–a reliable alternative for reconstruction of the anterior cruciate ligament. Clin Sports Med. 2007;26(4): 587–96.
16. Geib TM, Shelton WR, Phelps RA, Clark L. Anterior cruciate ligament reconstruction using quadriceps tendon autograft: intermediate-term outcome. Arthroscopy. 2009;25(12):1408–14.
17. Akoto R, Hoeher J. Anterior cruciate ligament (ACL) reconstruction with quadriceps tendon autograft and press-fit fixation using an anteromedial portal technique. BMC Musculoskelet Disord. 2012;13:161.
18. Gorschewsky O, Stapf R, Geiser L, Geitner U, Neumann W. Clinical comparison of fixation methods for patellar bone quadriceps tendon autografts in anterior cruciate ligament reconstruction: absorbable cross-pins versus absorbable screws. Am J Sports Med. 2007;35(12):2118–25.
19. Lund B, Nielsen T, Fauno P, Christiansen SE, Lind M. Is quadriceps tendon a better graft choice than patellar tendon? A prospective randomized study. Arthroscopy. 2014;30(5):593–8.
20. Kim SJ, Kumar P, Oh KS. Anterior cruciate ligament reconstruction: autogenous quadriceps tendon-bone compared with bone-patellar tendon-bone grafts at 2-year follow-up. Arthroscopy. 2009;25(2):137–44.
21. Shani RH, Umpierez E, Nasert M, Hiza EA, Xerogeanes J. Biomechanical comparison of quadriceps and patellar tendon grafts in anterior Cruciate ligament reconstruction. Arthroscopy. 2016;32(1):71–5.
22. Staubli HU, Schatzmann L, Brunner P, Rincon L, Nolte LP. Mechanical tensile properties of the quadriceps tendon and patellar ligament in young adults. Am J Sports Med. 1999;27(1):27–34.
23. West RV, Harner CD. Graft selection in anterior cruciate ligament reconstruction. J Am Acad Orthop Surg. 2005;13(3):197–207.
24. Bottoni CR, Smith EL, Shaha J, Shaha SS, Raybin SG, Tokish JM, Rowles DJ. Autograft versus allograft anterior Cruciate ligament reconstruction: a prospective, randomized clinical study with a minimum 10-year follow-up. Am J Sports Med. 2015;43(10):2501–9.
25. Sun K, Tian S, Zhang J, Xia C, Zhang C, Yu T. Anterior cruciate ligament reconstruction with BPTB autograft, irradiated versus non-irradiated allograft: a prospective randomized clinical study. Knee Surg Sports Traumatol Arthrosc. 2009;17(5):464–74.
26. Irrgang JJ, Ho H, Harner CD, Fu FH. Use of the International Knee Documentation Committee guidelines to assess outcome following anterior cruciate ligament reconstruction. Knee Surg Sports Traumatol Arthrosc. 1998;6(2):107–14.
27. Lysholm J, Gillquist J. Evaluation of knee ligament ory results with special emphasis on use of a scoring scale. Am J Sports Med. 1982;10(3):150–4.
28. Tegner Y, Lysholm J. Rating systems in the evaluation of knee ligament injuries. Clin Orthop Relat Res. 1985;198:43–9.
29. Roos EM, Roos HP, Lohmander LS, Ekdahl C, Beynnon BD. Knee Injury and Osteoarthritis Outcome Score (KOOS)–development of a self-administered outcome measure. J Orthop Sports Phys Ther. 1998;28(2):88–96.
30. Lee JK, Lee S, Seong SC, Lee MC. Anatomic single-bundle ACL reconstruction is possible with use of the modified transtibial technique: a comparison with the anteromedial transportal technique. J Bone Joint Surg Am. 2014;96(8):664–72.
31. Crawford SN, Waterman BR, Lubowitz JH. Long-term failure of anterior cruciate ligament reconstruction. Arthroscopy. 2013;29(9):1566–71.
32. Grassi A, Nitri M, Moulton SG, Marcheggiani Muccioli GM, Bondi A, Romagnoli M, Zaffagnini S. Does the type of graft affect the outcome of revision anterior cruciate ligament reconstruction? A meta-analysis of 32 studies. Bone Joint J. 2017;99-B(6):714–23.
33. Mabe I, Hunter S. Quadriceps tendon allografts as an alternative to Achilles tendon allografts: a biomechanical comparison. Cell Tissue Bank. 2014;15(4):523–9.
34. Chang SK, Egami DK, Shaieb MD, Kan DM, Richardson AB. Anterior cruciate ligament reconstruction: allograft versus autograft. Arthroscopy. 2003;19(5): 453–62.
35. Kraeutler MJ, Bravman JT, McCarty EC. Bone-patellar tendon-bone autograft versus allograft in outcomes of anterior cruciate ligament reconstruction: a meta-analysis of 5182 patients. Am J Sports Med. 2013;41(10):2439–48.
36. Gorschewsky O, Klakow A, Riechert K, Pitzl M, Becker R. Clinical comparison of the Tutoplast allograft and autologous patellar tendon (bone-patellar tendon-bone) for the reconstruction of the anterior cruciate ligament: 2- and 6-year results. Am J Sports Med. 2005;33(8):1202–9.
37. Barrett G, Stokes D, White M. Anterior cruciate ligament reconstruction in patients older than 40 years: allograft versus autograft patellar tendon. Am J Sports Med. 2005;33(10):1505–12.
38. Yasuda K, Ohkoshi Y, Tanabe Y, Kaneda K. Quantitative evaluation of knee instability and muscle strength after anterior cruciate ligament reconstruction using patellar and quadriceps tendon. Am J Sports Med. 1992;20(4):471–5.
39. Chen CH, Chuang TY, Wang KC, Chen WJ, Shih CH. Arthroscopic anterior cruciate ligament reconstruction with quadriceps tendon autograft: clinical outcome in 4-7 years. Knee Surg Sports Traumatol Arthrosc. 2006;14(11): 1077–85.
40. Lee S, Seong SC, Jo CH, Han HS, An JH, Lee MC. Anterior cruciate ligament reconstruction with use of autologous quadriceps tendon graft. J Bone Joint Surg Am. 2007;89(Suppl 3):116–26.
41. Guo L, Yang L, Duan XJ, He R, Chen GX, Wang FY, Zhang Y. Anterior cruciate ligament reconstruction with bone-patellar tendon-bone graft: comparison of autograft, fresh-frozen allograft, and gamma-irradiated allograft. Arthroscopy. 2012;28(2):211–7.

11

Comparison of artificial graft versus autograft in anterior cruciate ligament reconstruction

Zhen-Yu Jia[1†], Chen Zhang[1†], Shi-qi Cao[2], Chen-chen Xue[1†], Tian-ze Liu[1†], Xuan Huang[1*] and Wei-Dong Xu[1*]

Abstract

Background: Critically evaluation and summarization for the outcomes between autografts and artificial grafts using in anterior cruciate ligament (ACL) reconstruction have not been performed currently. The purpose of this study is to compare the clinical outcomes between artificial ligaments and autografts at a short- to mid-term follow-up.

Methods: A computerized search of the databases was conducted including Medline, Embase, and the Cochrane library. Only prospective or retrospective comparative studies with a minimum 2-year follow-up and a minimum sample size of 15 for each group were considered for inclusion. Two independent reviewers performed data extraction and methodological quality assessment. A Mantel-Haenszel analysis was used for pooling of results. Sensitivity analysis was performed in order to maintain the stability of results.

Results: Seven studies were included in this study. The total sample size was 403 (autograft group: 206 patients; synthetic graft group: 197 patients). Four studies were randomized controlled trials. Two studies were retrospective comparative studies and one study was non-randomized prospective comparative study. In terms of instrumented laxity, patient-oriented outcomes and complications, no significant difference was occurred between new artificial ligaments and autografts. But the results of IKDC grades and instrumented laxity were worsen in early artificial ligaments compared to autografts.

Conclusions: The outcomes of new generation of artificial ligaments are similar to autografts at a short- to mid-term follow-up. However, the early artificial ligaments are not suggested for ACL reconstruction compared to autografts.

Keywords: Artificial ligament, Autograft, Anterior cruciate ligament, Reconstruction

Background

Anterior cruciate ligament (ACL) injury is a main cause of recurrent knee instability and may result in secondary damages to other structures of the knee, such as meniscal tears and articular cartilage degeneration [1]. Currently, ACL reconstruction is the gold-standard surgical technique for ACL injury [2]. Reconstruction can be performed by using autograft, allograft or synthetic graft [3]. Despite the vast amount of researches, there still have a great deal of debates concentrating on the clinical outcomes of using different grafts in ACL reconstruction.

Autograft is a well-recognized and widely used material for ACL reconstruction due to a good graft stability and a well return to high-level sports [4]. And bone-patella tendon-bone (BPTB) autograft has historically served as the gold standard for ACL reconstruction based not only on widespread global use but also as the first autograft option. Reconstruction with synthetic grafts has the advantage of eliminating both the donor-site morbidity and disease transmission with fast rehabilitation [5]. High graft failures, no so-called ligamentization and severe

* Correspondence: ch_prof_xu@163.com; 9342825@qq.com
† Equal contributors
[1] Department of Orthopedics, Changhai Hospital, Second Military Medical University, Shanghai, China
Full list of author information is available at the end of the article

synovitis have been reported as major disadvantages of synthetic grafts [6–8].

A few conventional narrative reviews have addressed related issues about the graft selection for ACL reconstruction [9–12]. Firm conclusions regarding the clinical outcomes with autografts or synthetic grafts cannot be drawn from those narrative reviews due to some inherent bias. Moreover, there have already been systematic reviews and meta-analysis which compared the clinical outcomes between allografts and autografts using in ACL reconstruction [13–16]. Critically evaluation and summarization for the outcomes between autografts and synthetic grafts using in ACL reconstruction have not been performed currently.

Using the best available evidence, the purpose of this research is to compare synthetic grafts with autografts in ACL reconstruction by evaluation the clinical outcomes including the results of instrumented laxity, patient-oriented outcomes, complications and graft failures.

Methods

Searching strategy

This research was conducted following the Preferred Reporting Items for Systematic Reviews and Meta-Analyses (PRISMA) statement [17]. Two researchers searched the international databases independently up to December 30th, 2016, including Medline, Embase, and the Cochrane library. OpenGrey, the World Health Organization International Clinical Trials Registry Platform, the International Standard Randomised Controlled Trial Number (ISRCTN) registry, and Current Controlled Trials were searched to review the trial registry and grey literature. There was no restriction to years of publication and languages.

Eligibility criteria

Eligibility criteria were as follows: 1) a clinical study with a prospective or retrospective comparative design (Level of Evidence I, II, or III) [18]; 2) patients with no limitation of race and sex undergoing primary ACL reconstruction; 3) a study of ACL reconstruction comparing autografts with synthetic grafts and no restriction for types; 4) the outcomes being evaluated including physical examinations, complications, or patient-oriented outcomes etc.; 5) at least 2 years follow-ups; 6) at least 15 sample size for each group [15]. Knee laxity assessments included the arthrometer test and physical examinations (Lachman test and pivot-shift test). The details were shown in Table 1.

Any researches that failed to meet the inclusion criteria were excluded. In addition, a study was excluded if data from the same patients were reported in another study that had longer follow-up.

Data extraction and quality assessment

Two reviewers independently performed data extraction and quality assessment. In case of discrepancies, any controversy was resolved by further discussion with the corresponding author. The extraction included the following: (1) the characteristics of included researches (author, publication date, study design, participants' demography, sample size, and duration of follow-up); (2) the details of methodology (implant type and drilling technique); (3) the details of outcomes. In our research, Newcastle-Ottawa Scale (NOS) was used to assess quality for cohort study while Jadad scale was used to assess quality for randomized controlled trial (RCT) [19, 20].

Statistical analysis

The meta-analysis was conducted using RevMan Manager 5.3 (Copenhagen: The Nordic Cochrane Centre, The Cochrane Collaboration, 2014). Using the same format, two reviewers independently collected data and crosschecked the results. Disagreements were discussed with the corresponding author and reached consensus in order to ensure accuracy.

Odds ratio (OR) with 95% confidence interval (CI) was calculated for dichotomous while mean difference (MD) with corresponding 95% CI was calculated for continuous outcomes. Statistical heterogeneity was assessed by calculating the heterogeneity index I^2. When heterogeneity was significant (I^2 > 50%), a Mantel-Haenszel analysis utilizing a random-effects model was used; otherwise a fixed-effects model was used when heterogeneity was considered as low ($I^2 \le 0.50$). Funnel plots were used to test publication bias and a relatively symmetric funnel plot indicated inexistence of obvious publication bias. Sensitivity analysis was performed in order to maintain the stability of results.

Results

Article selection results

Three hundred and six relevant articles were initially selected according to the search strategy (Fig. 1). There were 161 articles left after checking for duplicates by using the literature management software Endnote X7. One hundred and forty-five articles were removed by screening the title and abstract. After reviewing the full text, 9 articles were excluded through assessment for eligibility. Eventually, 7 articles were included in qualitative and quantitative synthesis [21–27].

Characteristics of selected articles

All eligible studies were written in English from 1993 to 2013 (Table 2). Two studies were conducted in a North American country, and three studies were conducted in a European country. The other two studies were conducted in China. Among these studies, the synthetic

Table 1 Knee laxity assessment of included studies

Included studies	Arthrometer testing			Physical examination		Time from surgery to test/month
	Equipment	Flexion angle/°	Load level/N	Lachman test	Pivot test	
Engstrom 1993	Knee Laxity Tester; Stryker	20	NR	×	√	12–50
Ghalayini 2010	Stryker laxometer; Stryker	NR	NR	√	×	60
Grøntvedt 1995	KT-1000 arthrometer; MEDmetric	20	89	√	√	24
Liu 2010	KT-1000 arthrometer; MEDmetric	30	134	×	×	48–52
Nau 2002	Instrumented Laxity Tester; Telos	20	250	×	×	24
Pan 2013	KT-1000 arthrometer; MEDmetric	30	134	×	×	48–54
Pritchett 2009	KT-1000 arthrometer; MEDmetric	30	134	×	×	84–228

NR not reported

graft used to compare with autograft included the Ligament Advanced Reinforcement System (LARS) artificial ligament (3 studies), the Leeds-Keio (LK) artificial ligament (2 studies), the Ligament Augmentation Device (LAD) (1 study) and the polyglycolic acid Dacron (PGA-Dacron) graft (1 study). The autograft used for comparison was BPTB (6 studies) and hamstring tendon (1 study). The rate of follow-up was ≥90% and the follow-up periods were ≥24 months in all included studies. The total sample size was 403 patients (autograft group: 206 patients; synthetic graft group: 197 patients). The release source and release date of each artificial ligament were shown in Table 3.

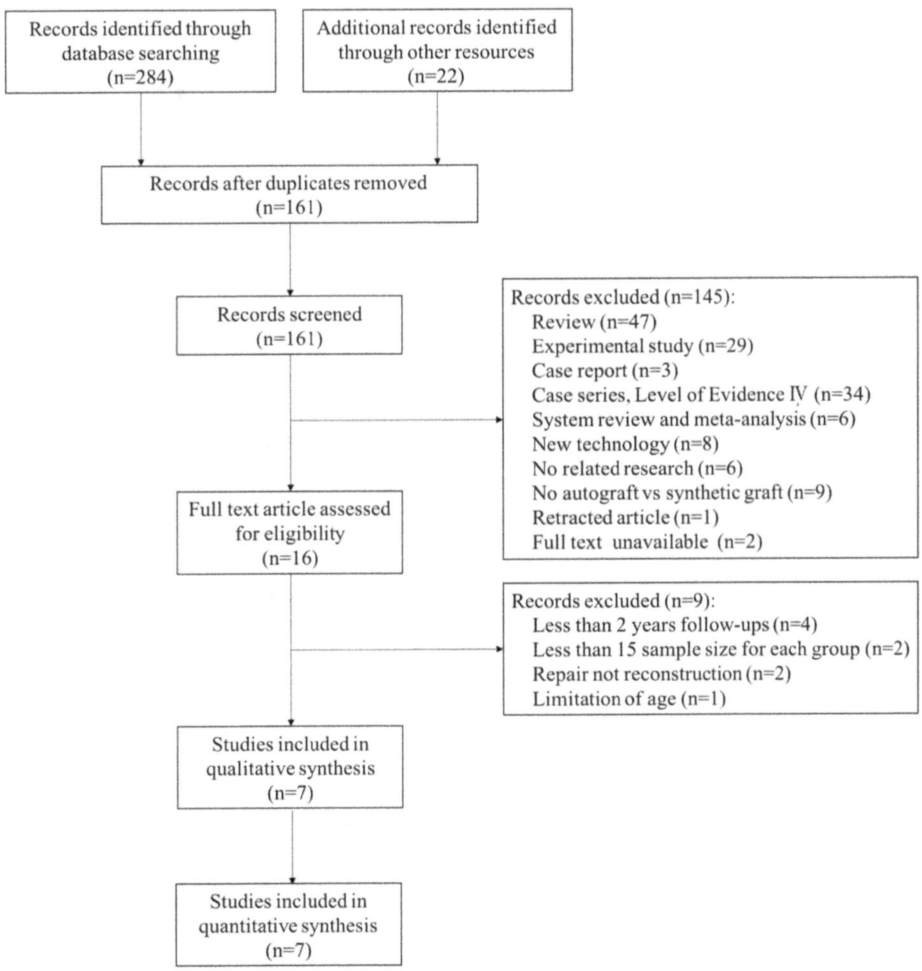

Fig. 1 Flowchart of article selection process

Table 2 Characteristics of Included Comparative Clinical Studies

Study	Journal	Implant		Followups (months)	Autograft			Synthetic graft			Outcome
		Autograft	Synthetic graft		No. of patients	Age	Gender (Male/Female)	No. of patients	Age	Gender (Male/Female)	
Pan 2013	Eur J Orthop Surg Traumatol	BPTB	LARS	50 (48–54)	30	33.9	19/11	32	35.9	25/7	Anterior laxity; IKDC score; Lysholm score; Tegner score
Ghalayini 2010	Knee	BPTB	LK	60	26	30.9	19/7	24	31.7	21/3	Anterior laxity; IKDC score; Lysholm score; Tegner score; one-hop test
Liu 2010	Int Orthop	HT	LARS	49 (48–52)	32	32	24/8	28	36	21/7	Anterior laxity; IKDC score; Lysholm score; Tegner score
Pritchett 2009	J Knee Surg	BPTB	PGADacron	138 (84–228)	35	25	24/11	35	26	23/12	Anterior laxity; IKDC score; Lysholm score; KOOS
Nau 2002	J Bone Joint Surg Br	BPTB	LARS	24	27	30.9	15/12	26	31.0	21/5	Anterior laxity; IKDC score; Tegner score; KOOS
[a]Grøntvedt 1995	Scand J Med Sci Sports	BPTB	LAD	24	26	NR	NR	22	NR	NR	Anterior laxity; Lysholm score; Tegner score; Isokinetic strength
Endstrom 1993	Clin Orthop Relat Res	BPTB	LK	28	30	23.8	14/16	30	23.4	21/9	Anterior laxity; IKDC score; Lysholm score; Tegner score; Muscle performance

BPTB bone-patellar tendon-bone, *LARS* ligament advanced reinforcement system, *LK* Leeds-Keio synthetic graft, *HT* hamstring tendon, *LAD* ligament augmentation device, *PGA-Dacron* polyglycolic acid-Dacron, *IKDC* International Knee Documen- tation Committee, *KOOS* Knee Injury and Osteoarthritis Outcome Score, *NR* not reported

[a]The mean age and the gender distribution were not described separately in this study. The mean age of the patients was 25 years (range 15–42). There were 18 men and 30 women altogether including in this research

Table 3 Details of each artificial ligament in included study

Included studies	Synthetic product name	Release source	Release date
Engstrom 1993	Leeds-Keio graft	Neoligaments, Leeds, UK	1980
Ghalayini 2010	Leeds-Keio graft	Xiros plc formerly Neoligaments Ltd., Leeds, UK	1980
Grøntvedt 1995	LAD	3 M Company, St. Paul, Minnesota, USA	1980
Liu 2010	LARS artificial ligament	Surgical Implants and Devices, Arc-sur-Tille, France	1985
Nau 2002	LARS artificial ligament	Surgical Implants and Devices, Arc-sur-Tille, France	1985
Pan 2013	LARS artificial ligament	Surgical Implants and Devices, Arc-sur-Tille, France	1985
Pritchett 2009	PGA-Dacron graft	Surgitex, Southfield, Mich	NR

LAD ligament augmentation device, *LARS* ligament advanced reinforcement system, *PGA-Dacron* polyglycolic acid-Dacron, *NR* not reported

The synthetic grafts were divided into two groups (Group 1: early generation; Group 2: new generation) for analysis. In this study, the early generation of the artificial ligaments contained the LK artificial ligament and the LAD, while the new generation included the LARS artificial ligament and the PGA-Dacron graft [2, 26]. Among all included articles, 4 articles were related to the new generation and 3 articles were related to the old generation (Table 2).

Quality of selected articles

Assessment of the methodological quality revealed that there were four RCTs (Level I). Two studies were retrospective comparative studies (Level III) and one study was non-randomized prospective comparative study (Level II). Among these four RCTs, only one article was of high quality with scores ≥4 while the other three articles were of low quality with scores ≤3 according to Jadad scale (Table 4). Assessed by NOS scale, two retrospective studies and one prospective study were of high quality. All demographic data were compared between two groups and showed no significant difference in eligible studies.

Meta-analysis

Instrumented laxity

All included studies tested instrumented laxity. The study of Nau et al. was excluded for providing quantitative data other than grade data of instrumented laxity (> 5 mm or ≤5 mm), which could not be compared with other studies [22]. No heterogeneity was found among the studies. Using the fixed-effects model in analysis, the early generation of synthetic grafts had a significant difference in knee laxity compared with autografts and the synthetic graft had a poorer result (OR = 11.44; 95% CI: 2.46, 53.16; $p = 0.98$; $I^2 = 0\%$; Fig. 2a). Conversely, the new generation of synthetic graft showed no significant difference in knee laxity compared with autografts (OR = 0.63; 95% CI: 0.21, 1.93; $p = 0.44$; $I^2 = 0\%$; Fig. 2b).

Table 4 Quality assessment of included studies

Study	Level of evidence	Type	NOS	Jadad scale
Pan 2013	III	Retrospective study	7	
Ghalayini 2010	I	RCT		5
Liu 2010	III	Retrospective study	7	
Pritchett 2009	II	Prospective study	7	
Nau 2002	I	RCT		3
Grøntvedt 1995	I	RCT		1
Endstrom 1993	I	RCT		1

NOS Newcastle-Ottawa Scale, *RCT* randomized controlled trial

Physical examinations

Two studies assessed the anterior stability by Lachman test and two studies evaluated the rotational stability through pivot-shift test (Table 1). All included studies were related to the early artificial ligaments (LK artificial ligament and LAD). The Lachman test showed a poorer result in the early synthetic grafts than in the autografts (OR = 0.02, 95% CI: 0.00, 0.41), indicating a worse anterior stability. The result of pivot-shift test was poor in early synthetic grafts (OR = 0.03, 95% CI: 0.01, 0.16), documenting a worse rotational stability comparing to autografts.

International knee documentation committee (IKDC) grades

Six studies reported postoperative IKDC grades but the study of Nau et al. was excluded for providing the different type of categorical data comparing to other included studies [22]. No heterogeneity was found and a fixed-effects model was used to analysis (Fig. 3). There were 51 patients in the early synthetic graft group and 50 patients in the autograft group. The early synthetic grafts (LK, LAD) had worsen IKDC grades (OR = 3.41; 95% CI: 1.30, 8.89; $p = 0.57$; $I^2 = 0\%$; Fig. 3a). Altogether 95 cases in the new synthetic graft group and 97 cases in the autograft group were reported. The new synthetic grafts (LARS) had no difference in IKDC grades compared to autografts (OR = 0.72; 95% CI: 0.35, 1.48; $p = 0.90$; $I^2 = 0\%$).

a

Study or Subgroup	Synthetic grafts Events	Total	Autografts Events	Total	Weight	Odds Ratio M-H, Fixed, 95% CI
Grontvedt 1995	7	22	1	26	46.2%	11.67 [1.30, 104.34]
Ghalayini 2010	0	22	0	24		Not estimable
Endstrom 1993	9	29	1	26	53.8%	11.25 [1.31, 96.39]
Total (95% CI)		**73**		**76**	**100.0%**	**11.44 [2.46, 53.16]**
Total events	16		2			

Heterogeneity: Chi² = 0.00, df = 1 (P = 0.98); I² = 0%
Test for overall effect: Z = 3.11 (P = 0.002)

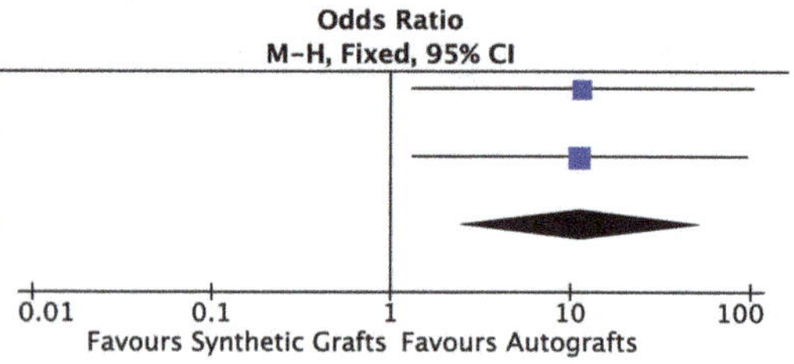

b

Study or Subgroup	Synthetic grafts Events	Total	Autografts Events	Total	Weight	Odds Ratio M-H, Fixed, 95% CI
Liu 2010	0	28	3	32	40.6%	0.15 [0.01, 2.99]
Pan 2013	3	32	2	30	23.6%	1.45 [0.22, 9.33]
Pritchett 2009	2	35	3	35	35.7%	0.65 [0.10, 4.13]
Total (95% CI)		**95**		**97**	**100.0%**	**0.63 [0.21, 1.93]**
Total events	5		8			

Heterogeneity: Chi² = 1.66, df = 2 (P = 0.44); I² = 0%
Test for overall effect: Z = 0.80 (P = 0.42)

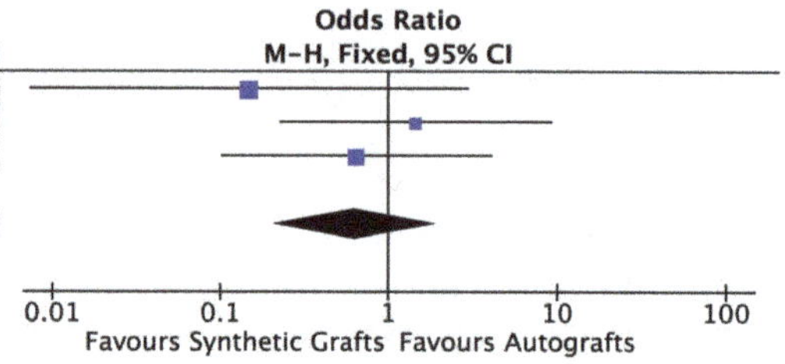

Fig. 2 Forest plot of the instrumented laxity. **a** the early generation of synthetic grafts; **b** the new generation of synthetic grafts

Lysholm scores

Six eligible studies tested postoperative Lysholm scores but the results of two studies could not be analyzed in meta-analysis. One was excluded due to lack of standard deviation and the other was due to suppling Lysholm scores as grade data other than quantitative data [21, 24]. Three studies were in Group 2 while only one study was in Group 1. There were altogether 95 cases in Group 2 and 97 cases in the autograft group. Heterogeneity was not found among these three studies and a fixed-effects model was used (p = 0.88; I^2 = 0%), showing no significant difference in the Lysholm scores between two groups (OR = 1.80; 95% CI: -0.52, 4.13).

Tegner scores

Six studies reported Tegner scores but only 3 studies applied mean scores and standard deviations [23, 25, 27]. The rest three studies documented there was no significant difference between two groups in their longest follow-up time. Two studies were related to the new generation of the synthetic grafts and one study were focused on the old generation. Heterogeneity was not significant and a fixed-effects model was used, no significant difference occurred in new synthetic grafts and autografts (OR = 0.40; 95% CI: -0.09, 0.89).

Complications

Six studies evaluated complications of ACL reconstruction. The study conducted by Endstrom et al. did not report the complications after ACL reconstruction and was excluded for analysis. No heterogeneity was found and a fixed-effects model was used (I^2 = 0%; Fig. 4). Altogether 44 patients were included in the early synthetic graft group and 50 patients were included in

a

Study or Subgroup	Synthetic grafts Events	Total	Autografts Events	Total	Weight	Odds Ratio M-H, Fixed, 95% CI
Endstrom 1993	26	29	17	26	39.6%	4.59 [1.08, 19.42]
Ghalayini 2010	9	22	5	24	60.4%	2.63 [0.72, 9.66]
Total (95% CI)		**51**		**50**	**100.0%**	**3.41 [1.30, 8.89]**
Total events	35		22			

Heterogeneity: Chi² = 0.32, df = 1 (P = 0.57); I² = 0%
Test for overall effect: Z = 2.50 (P = 0.01)

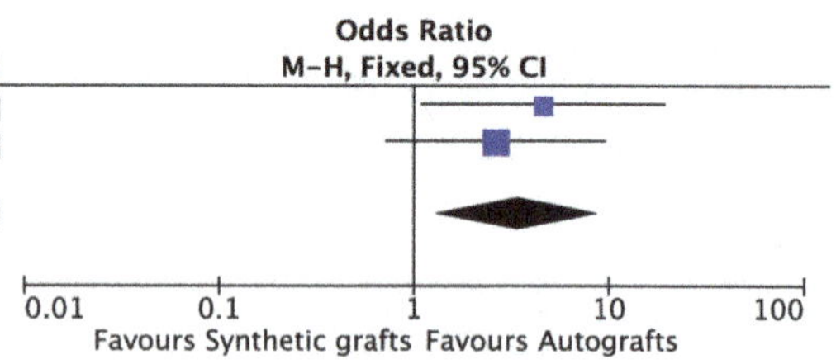

b

Study or Subgroup	Synthetic grafts Events	Total	Autografts Events	Total	Weight	Odds Ratio M-H, Fixed, 95% CI
Liu 2010	2	28	4	32	20.0%	0.54 [0.09, 3.19]
Pan 2013	4	32	4	30	20.8%	0.93 [0.21, 4.10]
Pritchett 2009	17	35	20	35	59.2%	0.71 [0.28, 1.82]
Total (95% CI)		**95**		**97**	**100.0%**	**0.72 [0.35, 1.48]**
Total events	23		28			

Heterogeneity: Chi² = 0.22, df = 2 (P = 0.90); I² = 0%
Test for overall effect: Z = 0.89 (P = 0.37)

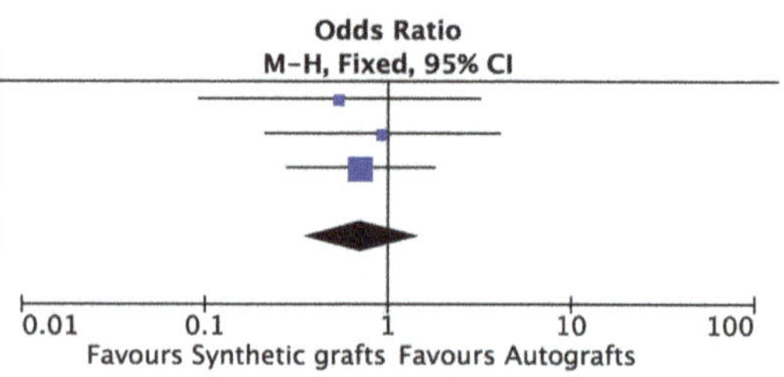

Fig. 3 Forest plot of the IKDC grades. **a** the early generation of synthetic grafts; **b** the new generation of synthetic grafts

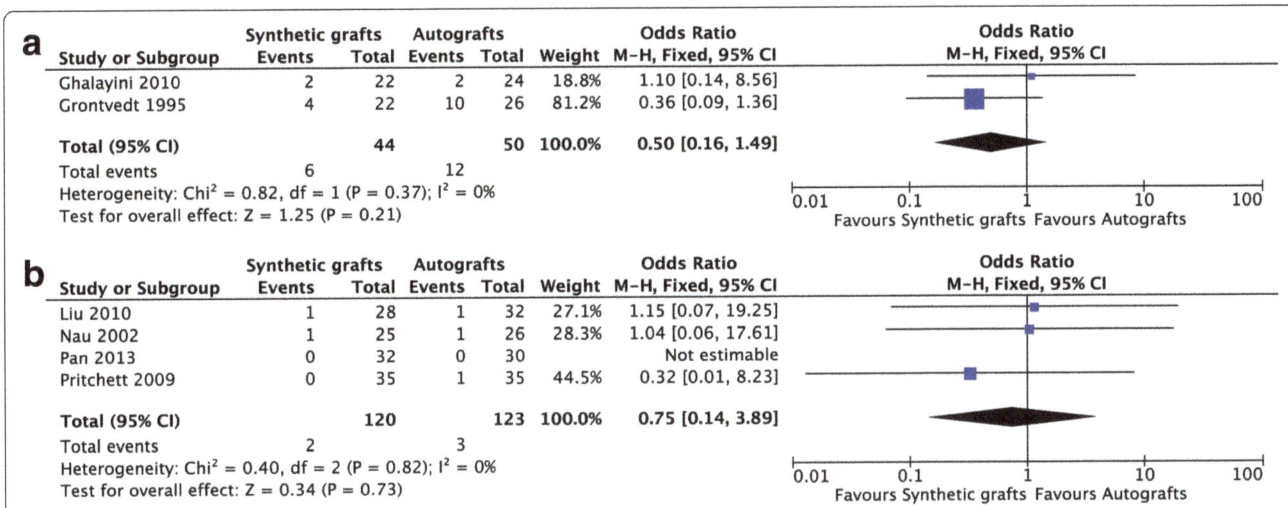

Fig. 4 Forest plot of the complications of anterior cruciate ligament reconstruction. **a** the early generation of synthetic grafts; **b** the new generation of synthetic grafts

the compared group. No significant difference was found in the rate of complications between two groups (OR = 0.50; 95% CI: 0.16, 1.49; Fig. 4a). Similarly, no significant difference occurred in the new synthetic grafts and autografts (OR = 0.75; 95% CI: 0.14, 3.89; Fig. 4b).

Sensitivity analysis indicated that the study with regard to four-strand HT graft had no obvious deviation compared to other studies concerning about BPTB in evaluation of knee laxity, patient-oriented outcomes and the rate of complications.

Publication bias

Funnel plots of instrumented laxity and complications were used to evaluate the publication bias, showing the lack of obvious bias among the eligible studies related to new synthetic grafts according to a relative symmetric funnel plot (Figs. 5 and 6).

Discussion

The key findings of present meta-analysis indicated that, in general, the patient-oriented outcomes and the rate of complications of ACL reconstruction with synthetic grafts were not significantly different from those with autograft, especially for new generation synthetic grafts (LARS and PGA- Dacron). However, with regard to knee laxity, ACL reconstruction with early artificial grafts had obviously poorer knee laxity from those with autografts (95% CI: 1.03, 4.72) while new artificial grafts showed no significant difference with autografts (95% CI: 0.21, 1.93).

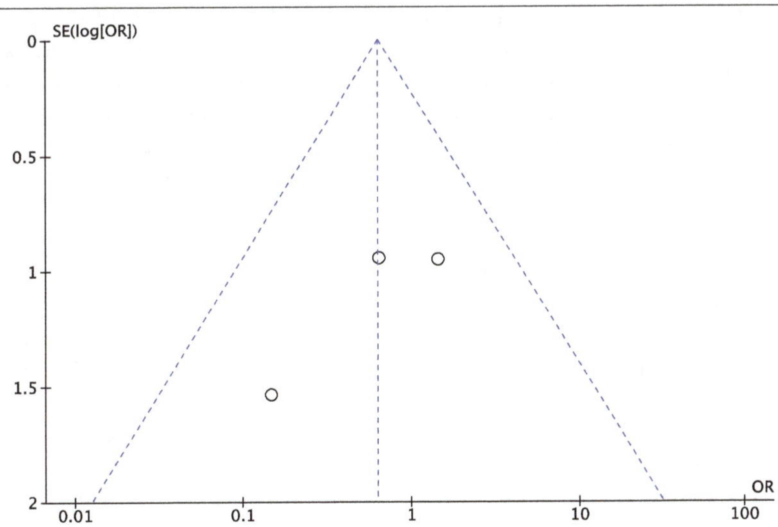

Fig. 5 Funnel plot of publication bias for instrumented laxity in the new generation synthetic graft group

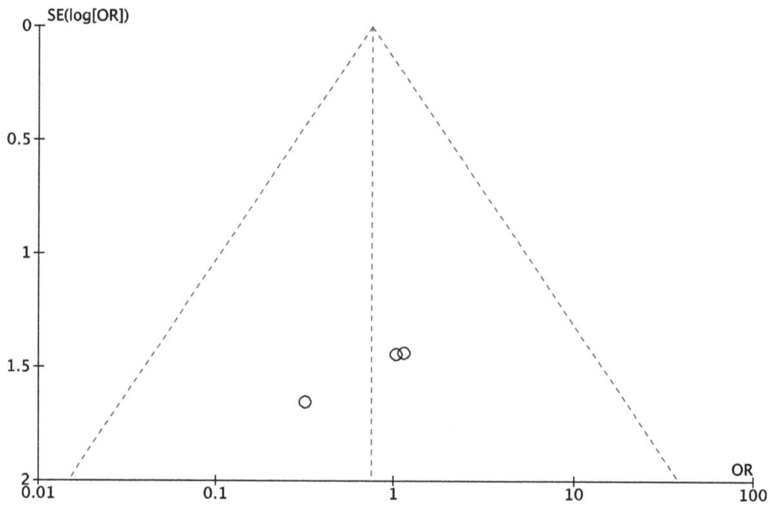

Fig. 6 Funnel plot of publication bias for complications in the new generation synthetic graft group

The LK artificial ligament was a polyester mesh-like structure intended as a scaffold for soft tissue ingrowth [28]. The LAD, a band-like braid of polypropylene, was designed to protect the autogenous graft from excessive stresses [29]. Murray et al. reported that 28% of the group were known to have ruptured the LK ligament and 56% had increased laxity compared to the opposite normal knee at a 10–16 year follow-up [30]. A study conducted since 1983, included 856 patients accepted ACL reconstruction with LAD, showed 63 cases of complications and 73 cases of re-surgery [31]. Long-term follow-up results documented both the LK artificial ligament and the LAD were not suitable as an ACL substitute [30–32]. Moreover, the LAD caused effusions and reactive synovitis in the knee for provoking inflammatory reactions, and was found to delay maturation of autogenous graft [33]. The knee laxity and the IKDC grades were significantly different from autografts and early artificial ligaments, indicating that the short-term outcomes of early artificial ligaments were worsen than autografts. The results of our research for early artificial ligaments were consistent with previous studies. It was not suggested to use early synthetic grafts including the LK artificial ligament and the LAD due to their poor follow-up outcomes.

The LARS artificial ligament was made of polyethylene terephthalate, divided in two parts (intra-articular part and extra-articular part) [34]. Intra-articular part was composed of longitudinal external rotation fibers without transverse fibers as an imitation of ACL anatomic structure while extra-articular part was weaved by longitudinal and transverse fibers in order to avoid ligament deformation. Dericks et al. reported encouraging results in 220 cases of ACL reconstruction used LARS artificial ligament with a mean follow-up of 2.5 years [35]. In 2013, Parchi reported no case of complications and only one case of mechanical graft rupture after using LARS artificial ligament for ACL reconstruction at a mean follow-up of eight years [36]. In 2015, a study with a minimum follow-up of 10 years, showed almost half of the patients (8/18) were subjectively not satisfied with the surgical result using LARS artificial ligament [7]. The clinical outcomes were appealing at short-term but controversy at long-term [36–38]. In our research, 3 studies compared LARS artificial ligament with autografts, showing no significant difference in knee laxity, functions and the rate of complications [22, 25, 27]. The outcomes of LARS artificial ligament used in ACL reconstruction were appealing at least in short-term follow-up. Another new synthetic graft called PGA-Dacron graft, consisted of synthetic braided ligament made of 75% degradable PGA filaments and 25% non-degradable Dacron thread, showed a satisfied result compared to autograft including knee laxity, range of motion, patient-oriented questionnaires, muscle performance, degenerative changes of knee, and the rate of failure and complications [26].

Complications occurred in the autograft group were infection, patellofemoral pain, recurrent effusion and extension loss. In the synthetic graft group, complications included interference screw-related problems (pain and screw loosening), patellofemoral pain and extension loss. There were altogether 12 cases in the autograft group and 8 cases in the synthetic graft group. Extension loss was the most common complication in included studies and it might be associated with graft impingement and a formation of cyclops [39, 40]. Graft impingement was mainly caused by malposition of femoral bone tunnel and a "cyclops" was a fibrous nodule caused by proliferation of fibrovascular tissues similar to a healing scar after

ACL reconstruction [41, 42]. The synthetic grafts were located in a non-anatomic but isometric placement while the autografts were usually located in an anatomic placement. The results of complications showed no significant difference between these two location methods.

Some studies documented that subjective outcomes were not correlated with objective outcomes including instrumented laxity test and clinical examination [43]. Among these included studies, three of them showed difference in objective parameters but no significant difference in patient-oriented outcomes [21, 22, 24]. Meanwhile, the opposite circumstance did not appear (similar in objective outcomes but different in subjective outcomes). Kraeutler et al. suggested that patient satisfaction is the most important measurable index for the outcomes of ACL reconstruction [13]. Only the overall IKDC grades showed better results in the autografts than in the early synthetic grafts and the rest indicators for patient satisfaction showed no significant difference between groups. However, it was still well recognized that a KT-1000 side-to-side difference of >5 mm was defined as a clinical failure [37]. Both objective parameters and subjective outcomes shoulder be considered for assessment of ACL reconstruction.

The limitations of this study were as follows: (1) Until now, there was still lack of high-quality RCT or large-scale multi-center retrospective comparable studies to prove the effectiveness of artificial ligaments compared to autografts. (2) The follow-up time was not sufficiently long for evaluation of ACL reconstruction. (3) In the included studies, the types of grafts used in ACL reconstruction were not the same (Hamstring tendon, BPTB, LK, LAD, LARS and PGA-Dacron). (4) The data included in the research did not cover all included studies due to the lack of relative data.

Conclusions

The outcomes of new generation of artificial ligaments are similar to autografts in terms of knee laxity, patient-oriented outcomes and the rate of complications at a short- to mid-term follow-up. However, the early artificial ligaments (LK, LAD) are not suggested for ACL reconstruction according to worse outcomes in knee laxity and functions compared to autografts.

Abbreviations

ACL: Anterior cruciate ligament; BPTB: Bone-patella tendon-bone; CI: Confidence interval; IKDC: International Knee Documentation Committee; ISRCTN: International Standard Randomised Controlled Trial Number; LAD: Ligament Augmentation Device; LARS: Ligament Advanced Reinforcement System; LK: Leeds-Keio; MD: mean difference; NOS: Newcastle-Ottawa scale; OR: Odds ratio; PGA-Dacron: polyglycolic acid Dacron; PRISMA: Preferred Reporting Items for Systematic Reviews and Meta-Analyses; RCT: Randomized controlled trial

Acknowledgments

The corresponding author wishes to thank all the co-authors for their contributions.

Funding

Scholar Fund of Second Military Medical University (2016JS24).
Tengfei Project (16 T016).
Zonghe Project (2016JS24).

Authors' contributions

JZ and ZC searched the databases and performed data extraction and quality assessment; JZ, HX and XW designed the study; JZ, ZC, CS, XC and LT analyzed the data and wrote the manuscript. JZ, ZC and CS revised the manuscript. All authors read and approved the final content of the manuscript.

Consent for publication

Not applicable.

Competing interests

The authors declare that they have no competing interests.

Author details

[1]Department of Orthopedics, Changhai Hospital, Second Military Medical University, Shanghai, China. [2]Department of Joint Surgery and Sports Medicine, Changzheng Hospital, Shanghai, China.

References

1. Chalmers PN, Mall NA, Moric M, Sherman SL, Paletta GP, Cole BJ, et al. Does ACL reconstruction alter natural history?: a systematic literature review of long-term outcomes. J Bone Joint Surg Am. 2014;96(4):292–300.
2. Mascarenhas R, MacDonald PB. Anterior cruciate ligament reconstruction: a look at prosthetics–past, present and possible future. Mcgill J Med. 2008;11(1):29–37.
3. Kim HS, Seon JK, Jo AR. Current trends in anterior cruciate ligament reconstruction. Knee Surg Relat Res. 2013;25(4):165–73.
4. Shelton WR, Fagan BC. Autografts commonly used in anterior cruciate ligament reconstruction. The Journal of the American Academy of Orthopaedic Surgeons. 2011;19(5):259–64.
5. Vaishya R, Agarwal AK, Ingole S, Vijay V. Current trends in anterior cruciate ligament reconstruction: a review. Cureus. 2015;7(11):e378.
6. Glezos CM, Waller A, Bourke HE, Salmon LJ, Pinczewski LA. Disabling synovitis associated with LARS artificial ligament use in anterior cruciate ligament reconstruction: a case report. Am J Sports Med. 2012;40(5):1167–71.
7. Tiefenboeck TM, Thurmaier E, Tiefenboeck MM, Ostermann RC, Joestl J, Winnisch M, et al. Clinical and functional outcome after anterior cruciate ligament reconstruction using the LARS system at a minimum follow-up of 10 years. Knee. 2015;22(6):565–8.
8. Iliadis DP, Bourlos DN, Mastrokalos DS, Chronopoulos E, Babis GC. LARS artificial ligament versus ABC purely polyester ligament for anterior cruciate ligament reconstruction. Orthop. J Sports Med. 2016;4(6):2325967116653359.
9. Shaerf DA, Pastides PS, Sarraf KM, Willis-Owen CA. Anterior cruciate ligament reconstruction best practice: a review of graft choice. World J Orthop. 2014;5(1):23–9.
10. Sherman OH, Banffy MB. Anterior cruciate ligament reconstruction: which graft is best? Arthroscopy : the journal of arthroscopic & related surgery : official publication of the Arthroscopy Association of North America and the International Arthroscopy Association. 2004;20(9):974–80.

11. Duchman KR, Lynch TS, Spindler KP. Graft selection in anterior cruciate ligament surgery: who gets what and why. Clin Sports Med. 2017;36(1):25–33.
12. Miller SL, Gladstone JN. Graft selection in anterior cruciate ligament reconstruction. The Orthopedic clinics of North America. 2002;33(4):675–83.
13. Kraeutler MJ, Bravman JT, McCarty EC. Bone-patellar tendon-bone autograft versus allograft in outcomes of anterior cruciate ligament reconstruction: a meta-analysis of 5182 patients. Am J Sports Med. 2013;41(10):2439–48.
14. Yao LW, Wang Q, Zhang L, Zhang C, Zhang B, Zhang YJ, et al. Patellar tendon autograft versus patellar tendon allograft in anterior cruciate ligament reconstruction: a systematic review and meta-analysis. Eur J Orthop Surg Traumatol. 2015;25(2):355–65.
15. Carey JL, Dunn WR, Dahm DL, Zeger SL, Spindler KP. A systematic review of anterior cruciate ligament reconstruction with autograft compared with allograft. J Bone Joint Surg Am. 2009;91(9):2242–50.
16. Zeng C, Gao SG, Li H, Yang T, Luo W, Li YS, et al. Autograft versus allograft in anterior cruciate ligament reconstruction: a meta-analysis of randomized controlled trials and systematic review of overlapping systematic reviews. Arthroscopy : the journal of arthroscopic & related surgery : official publication of the Arthroscopy Association of North America and the International Arthroscopy Association. 2016;32(1):153–63. e18
17. Liberati A, Altman DG, Tetzlaff J, Mulrow C, Gotzsche PC, Ioannidis JP, et al. The PRISMA statement for reporting systematic reviews and meta-analyses of studies that evaluate health care interventions: explanation and elaboration. PLoS med. 2009;6(7):e1000100.
18. Wright JG, Swiontkowski MF, Heckman JD. Introducing levels of evidence to the journal. J Bone Joint Surg Am. 2003;85-A(1):1–3.
19. Cota GF, de Sousa MR, Fereguetti TO, Rabello A. Efficacy of anti-leishmania therapy in visceral leishmaniasis among HIV infected patients: a systematic review with indirect comparison. PLoS Negl Trop Dis. 2013;7(5):e2195.
20. Jadad AR, Moore RA, Carroll D, Jenkinson C, Reynolds DJ, Gavaghan DJ, et al. Assessing the quality of reports of randomized clinical trials: is blinding necessary. Control Clin Trials. 1996;17(1):1–12.
21. Engstrom B, Wredmark T, Westblad P. Patellar tendon or Leeds-Keio graft in the surgical treatment of anterior cruciate ligament ruptures. Intermediate results. Clin Orthop Relat Res. 1993;295:190–7.
22. Nau T, Lavoie P, Duval N. A new generation of artificial ligaments in reconstruction of the anterior cruciate ligament. Two-year follow-up of a randomised trial. J Bone Joint Surg Br. 2002;84(3):356–60.
23. Ghalayini SR, Helm AT, Bonshahi AY, Lavender A, Johnson DS, Smith RB. Arthroscopic anterior cruciate ligament surgery: results of autogenous patellar tendon graft versus the Leeds-Keio synthetic graft five year follow-up of a prospective randomised controlled trial. Knee. 2010;17(5):334–9.
24. Grontvedt T, Engebretsen L. Comparison between two techniques for surgical repair of the acutely torn anterior cruciate ligament. A prospective, randomized follow-up study of 48 patients. Scand J Med Sci Sports. 1995;5(6):358–63.
25. Liu ZT, Zhang XL, Jiang Y, Zeng BF. Four-strand hamstring tendon autograft versus LARS artificial ligament for anterior cruciate ligament reconstruction. Int Orthop. 2010;34(1):45–9.
26. Pritchett JW. Assisted reproduction of the anterior cruciate ligament. J Knee Surg. 2009;22(4):325–30.
27. Pan X, Wen H, Wang L, Ge T. Bone-patellar tendon-bone autograft versus LARS artificial ligament for anterior cruciate ligament reconstruction. European journal of orthopaedic surgery & traumatology : orthopedie traumatologie. 2013;23(7):819–23.
28. Fujikawa K, Iseki F, Seedhom BB. Arthroscopy after anterior cruciate reconstruction with the Leeds-Keio ligament. J Bone Joint Surg Br. 1989;71(4):566–70.
29. Kennedy JC, Roth JH, Mendenhall HV, Sanford JB. Presidential address. Intraarticular replacement in the anterior cruciate ligament-deficient knee. Am J Sports Med. 1980;8(1):1–8.
30. Murray AW, Macnicol MF. 10-16 year results of Leeds-Keio anterior cruciate ligament reconstruction. Knee. 2004;11(1):9–14.
31. Riel KA. Augmented anterior cruciate ligament replacement with the Kennedy-LAD (ligament augmentation device)–long term outcome. Zentralbl Chir. 1998;123(9):1014–8.
32. Denti M, Bigoni M, Dodaro G, Monteleone M, Arosio A. Long-term results of the Leeds-Keio anterior cruciate ligament reconstruction. Knee surgery, sports traumatology, arthroscopy : official journal of the ESSKA. 1995;3(2):75–7.
33. Kumar K, Maffulli N. The ligament augmentation device: an historical perspective. Arthroscopy : the journal of arthroscopic & related surgery : official publication of the Arthroscopy Association of North America and the International Arthroscopy Association. 1999;15(4):422–32.
34. Chen J, Gu A, Jiang H, Zhang W, Yu X. A comparison of acute and chronic anterior cruciate ligament reconstruction using LARS artificial ligaments: a randomized prospective study with a 5-year follow-up. Arch Orthop Trauma Surg. 2015;135(1):95–102.
35. Dericks G. Ligament advanced reinforcement system anterior cruciate ligament reconstruction. Op Tech Sports Med. 1995;3:187–205.
36. Parchi PD, Gianluca C, Dolfi L, Baluganti A, Nicola P, Chiellini F, et al. Anterior cruciate ligament reconstruction with LARS artificial ligament results at a mean follow-up of eight years. Int Orthop. 2013;37(8):1567–74.
37. Gao K, Chen S, Wang L, Zhang W, Kang Y, Dong Q, et al. Anterior cruciate ligament reconstruction with LARS artificial ligament: a multicenter study with 3- to 5-year follow-up. Arthroscopy : the journal of arthroscopic & related surgery : official publication of the Arthroscopy Association of North America and the International Arthroscopy Association. 2010;26(4):515–23.
38. Lavoie P, Fletcher J, Duval N. Patient satisfaction needs as related to knee stability and objective findings after ACL reconstruction using the LARS artificial ligament. Knee. 2000;7(3):157–63.
39. Cha J, Choi SH, Kwon JW, Lee SH, Ahn JH. Analysis of cyclops lesions after different anterior cruciate ligament reconstructions: a comparison of the single-bundle and remnant bundle preservation techniques. Skelet Radiol. 2012;41(8):997–1002.
40. van der List JP, Zuiderbaan HA, Nawabi DH, Pearle AD. Impingement following anterior cruciate ligament reconstruction: comparing the direct versus indirect femoral tunnel position. Knee surgery, sports traumatology, arthroscopy : official journal of the ESSKA: p. 2015;
41. Udagawa K, Niki Y, Enomoto H, Toyama Y, Suda Y. Factors influencing graft impingement on the wall of the intercondylar notch after anatomic double-bundle anterior cruciate ligament reconstruction. Am J Sports Med. 2014;42(9):2219–25.
42. Nikolic O, Vanhoenacker FM, Petrovic K, Vandenberk R. Cyclops lesion of the knee. JBR-BTR. 2012;95(5):336.
43. Hyder N, Bollen SR, Sefton G, Swann AC. Correlation between Arthrometric evaluation of knees using KT 1000 and telos stress radiography and functional outcome following ACL reconstruction. Knee. 1997;4(3):121–4.

12

Single cut distal femoral osteotomy for correction of femoral torsion and valgus malformity in patellofemoral malalignment-proof of application of new trigonometrical calculations and 3D-printed cutting guides

Florian B. Imhoff[1,2*], Joscha Schnell[3], Alejandro Magaña[3], Theresa Diermeier[1], Bastian Scheiderer[1,2], Sepp Braun[1], Andreas B. Imhoff[1], Robert A. Arciero[2] and Knut Beitzel[1]

Abstract

Background: The purpose of this study was to perform a derotational osteotomy at the distal femur, as is done in cases of patellofemoral instability, and demonstrate the predictability of three-dimensional (3D) changes on axes in a cadaveric model by the use of a new mathematical approach.

Methods: Ten human cadaveric femurs, with increased antetorsion, underwent a visually observed derotational osteotomy at the distal femur by 20°, as is commonly done in clinics. For surgery, a single cut osteotomy with a defined cutting angle was calculated and given using a simple 3D-printed cutting guide per specimen, based on a newly-created trigonometrical model. To simulate post-operative straight frontal alignment in a normal range, a goal for the mechanical lateral distal femur angle (mLDFA) was set to 87.0° for five specimens (87-goal group) and 90.0° for five specimens (90-goal group). Specimens underwent pre- and post-operative radiographic analysis with CT scan for torsion and frontal plane x-ray for alignment measurements of mLDFA and anatomical mechanical angle (AMA).

Results: Performed derotation showed a mean of 19.69° ±1.08°SD (95% CI: 18.91° to 20.47°). Regarding frontal alignment, a mean mLDFA of 86.9° ±0.66°SD (87-goal-group) and 90.42° ±0.25° SD (90-goal group), was observed ($p = 0.008$). Overall, the mean difference between intended mLDFA-goal and post-operatively achieved mLDFA was 0.14° ±0.56° SD (95% CI: -0.26° to 0.54°).

Conclusion: A preoperative calculated angle for single cut derotational osteotomy at the distal femur leads to a clinically precise post-operative result on torsion and frontal alignment when using this approach.

* Correspondence: f.imhoff@tum.de
[1]Department of Orthopaedic Sports Medicine, Technical University Munich, Ismaninger Str. 22, 81675 Munich, Germany
[2]Department of Orthopaedic Surgery, University of Connecticut, 263 Farmington Ave, Farmington, CT 06030, USA
Full list of author information is available at the end of the article

Background

Increased femoral antetorsion is one important risk factor for patellofemoral instability and anterior knee pain syndrome in teenagers and young adults [1–4]. Correction osteotomy at the distal femur has been shown to be a reliable option for correction of torsional pathologies [4–8]. Increased lateral facet pressure and increased medial retinaculum strain was shown to be correlated with increased femoral antetorsion [9–11]. In the author's clinical observation, valgus deformities often appear in conjunction with torsional deformities in cases of patellofemoral instability. Valgus malalignment is defined as a lateral deviation of the mechanical axis (line from the femoral head to the upper ankle joint), which is referred to the center of the knee joint on a frontal plane radiograph [12]. For more accuracy and confirmability, the amount of valgus deviation is usually measured as the angle between the mechanical axis of the tibia versus the mechanical axis of the femur [13, 14]. Regarding the femur, mechanical and anatomical axes differ on a frontal plane radiograph, whereas the mechanical anatomical angle (AMA) depends on the femoral torsion [15]. While changes of the mechanical and anatomical axes are likely to occur in derotational osteotomy, unintended changes on axes should be minimized. According to previous publications, rotational osteotomies may result in unplanned three-dimensional (3D) effects, such as aggravation of valgus malalignment [1, 16].

Thus, a reliable anatomical reference of the cutting plane is the most important surgical step to prevent these complications. Mathematical models, commonly used in robotics for calculating transformations for serial kinematics, allow for a prediction of the resulting 3D changes when rotation of a limb is performed with a defined angle of the rotation-joint [17]. When these models are transferred to derotational osteotomies, prediction of the exact changes of axes can be made when there is a known angle of the cutting plane and the tubular bone is rotated on its axis. However, these calculations are not easily applicable in the OR. Therefore, easy to handle tools, such as pre-calculated tables and individual cutting guides, could help surgeons increase the precision of their surgical procedure.

The purpose of this study was to perform a derotational osteotomy at the distal femur, as it is done in cases of patellofemoral instability, and demonstrate the predictability of three-dimensional (3D) changes on axes in a cadaveric model. We hypothesized that a distal femoral derotational osteotomy with a defined inclination of the cutting plane can correct the frontal alignment due to correction of torsion according to the preoperative calculated values.

Methods

Experimental design

For proof of concept, a standardized protocol was developed to investigate mathematical predictions in a clinical cadaver model. Human cadaveric femurs with individual increased antetorsion and valgus imitating mechanical axes, were radiographically analyzed for exact angle calculations. A derotation of 20° was defined across all specimens, which in terms of consistency is clinically applicable [2, 4]. In this femur cadaver model, it was not possible to obtain the corrective goal on a total leg axis to achieve a straight frontal alignment, as it would be done in clinical practice. Therefore, the goal for frontal alignment correction was based on the femoral mechanical axis, and the mechanical lateral distal femur angle (mLDFA) was set to mLDFA = 87.0° for five specimens (87-goal group), and mLDFA = 90.0° for five specimens (90-goal group). These angles were chosen as they represent normal range angles and allow for statistical comparison of two groups within a clinical significant 3° difference [15]. Femurs were assigned to a group, based on their preoperative mLDFA, to achieve homogenous corrective angles for both groups. Based on a new trigonometrical model for single cut rotational osteotomy, tables with practical values were created for future implementation into clinical use. Then, an individual defined cutting angle from a lateral approach was given for each specimen to correct rotational and frontal axis. This unique inclined single-cut was provided by a simple 3D-printed cutting guide. Postoperatively, achieved angles were measured radiographically and compared to their intended goal.

Specimens

Ten cadaveric femurs, five left and five right, were used in this study, which had been obtained from MedCure (MedCure, Inc., Cumberland, RI, USA). Specimens had served for an Orthopaedic Residency Training Program for total hip (THA). Each femur was dissected free from all its soft tissue and muscle, and all implants were taken out. Femoral heads, which were previously removed for THA, were then fixed with k-wires on the corresponding femoral neck with an individual increased antetorsion (25° - 45°) with regards to clinical observed values [2–4]. At the distal femur, joint lines were artificially cut oblique from lateral to medial to create a slight valgus malalignment, which was measured as a decreased mLDFA. Next, these prepared specimens underwent radiographic analysis. This study was reported to the institutional review board (IRB). It was documented that de-identified specimens do not constitute human subjects research, and no IRB approval was required.

Radiographic imaging

If increased maltorsion is suspected in clinics, magnetic resonance imaging is usually performed to avoid additional radiation. However, attention must be given to different techniques and thresholds [18]. Due to the biomechanical nature of this proof of concept study, computer tomographic (CT) scans were performed using a standardized bone protocol preserving 3 mm axial slices (Osteo window b50s kernel algorithm, Siemens Somatom Definition Dual Energy 64 slice). For x-ray imaging, specimens were clamped on a x-ray-grit in a supine position, making sure that the distal femoral condyles were levelled perpendicular to the path of rays. Antero-posterior radiographs were taken with a C-arm (GE Medical Systems Inc.) and, according to the x-ray-grit, precisely combined to generate a panoramic view of the entire femur. CT scans, x-ray and measurements were repeated postoperatively. Measurement of the angles were repeated three times by one observer and the average was taken.

Imaging analysis

Torsion measurement of the femur was done as described by Waidelich et al. [19], a CT-based method, which is used according to several clinical publications [4, 20, 21]. The center of the femoral head was determined on one image and the center of the greater trochanter was marked with an ellipse on a second image. The third image showed a tangential line at the posterior condyles. When all three images were merged, the positive angle between a line from the femoral head to the trochanter versus the posterior condyles equaled femoral antetorsion.

The frontal plane x-ray provided measurement of mLDFA and AMA according to Strecker [13]. The mechanical femoral axis is a line from the center of the femoral head to the center of the distal femoral joint line (Fig. 1a). The anatomical axis was drawn as a line from the middle of the proximal femur shaft to the middle of the distal shaft. This point was defined 7 cm from the distal joint line, where the cutting plane of the distal femoral osteotomy was assumed. Usually, anatomical and mechanical axes cross at the middle of the condyles and not at the joint line [12]. The angle between the anatomical and mechanical axis (AMA) was measured. The mechanical lateral distal femur angle is the angle between the mechanical axis and the distal femoral joint line.

In order to decrease valgus alignment, the femoral head was virtually planned to be medialized (Fig. 1b). As a result, mLDFA increased as well. The intended postoperative position of the femoral head was set in a manner that resulted in a mLDFA of 87.0°, and 90.0°, respectively. Then, the angle between the center of the femoral head, middle of the assumed cutting plane, and intended center of the femoral head was measured. This angle is also known as the corrective angle at the cutting point (Fig. 1c) [13]. A DICOM Imaging software (OsiriX Lite, PIXMEO SARL, Switzerland) was used for all measurements. Measurements and planning was done by the

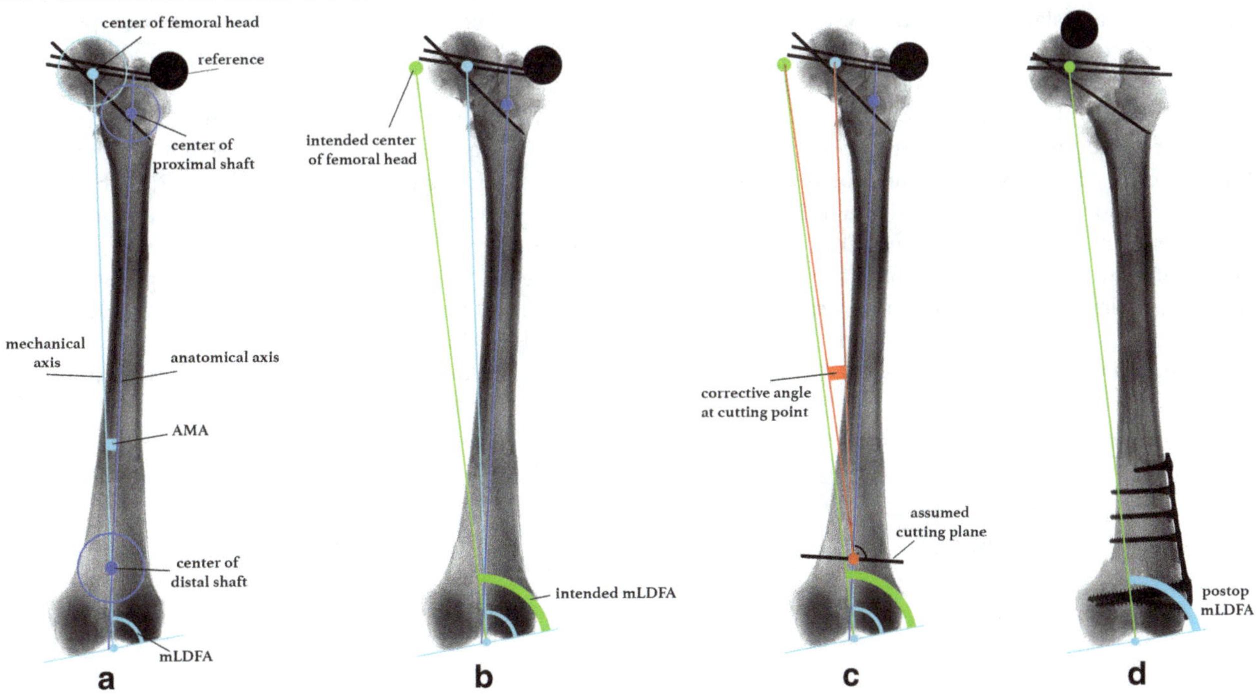

Fig. 1 Planning of correction of frontal alignment (x-ray-grit is vanished for better visualization): **a** preoperative measurements and reference; **b** drawing of intended mechanical axis/center of femoral head; **c** measuring corrective angle at assumed cutting plane; **d** postoperative result

first author. Postoperative measurements were done at two different time periods with 6 weeks in between and average values were taken. All measurements were made to the tenth of a degree.

The following calculation had to be done to receive the remaining corrective angle (Fig. 2): Torsion angle and intended derotation angle changed the AMA, which was observed on the frontal plane x-ray, by a certain amount. This change of the AMA was subtracted from the corrective angle at cutting point, which resulted in the remaining corrective angle at cutting point. In order to achieve the amount of the remaining corrective angle on the frontal plane by means of a derotation, the cutting plane had to be inclined from a sagittal view. The precise value was determined using a trigonometrical formula, obtained from the robotics.

Mathematical model

Derotation is defined as an external rotation of the distal limb, which equals an internal rotation of the proximal limb. The Pythagorean Theorem was used to calculate angular changes between the anatomical and mechanical axes of the femur. Measurement of the AMA on a coronal view at different torsion angles will result in a change of AMA when a derotation is performed (Fig. 3a, b). Then, an approach commonly known from robotics was applied [17]. The Denavit-Hartenberg transformation matrix calculates in a cartesian coordinate system (XYZ) the sagittal and coronal changes of axis when defining an oblique cutting angle on one plane and a rotation through its central axis (Fig. 3c). For transition into clinical practice, an inverse equation was derived: Intended change of axis on the coronal view and planned rotation equals an individual inclined cutting plane from the sagittal view. The mathematical model calculated change on frontal, sagittal, and axial axis. Trigonometrical formulas were processed with Matlab (MathWorks, Version R2017a) and Mathematica (Wolfram, Version 11.1).

3D printed cutting guide

In order to provide a precise cutting angle in a clinical setup, a new simple cutting guide was self-designed using open-source parametric 3D modeling software (FreeCAD, Version 0.16). The basic concept of the guide was to provide the exact cutting angle from a lateral approach and did not have to be adapted to the individual bone when overall orientation was maintained. This cutting guide provides two fixation holes for 2.0 mm k-wires and a proximal spacer to adjust the guide to the shaft in line with the anatomic axis on the coronal plane. A guiding slot on the lateral side was virtually mounted on top, allowing for the use of an oscillating saw. For each specimen, an individual cutting angle needed to achieve the proposed axis effect was imported to the designed guide. Printing of the common standard tessellation language files (*.stl) for each individualized guide was performed on a 3D printer (Ultimaker2+ extended, Ultimaker B.V., Netherlands) using simple PLA (polyactic acid) material.

Surgical technique

Surgical procedure specimens were clamped in a supine position on a table. For rotational osteotomy from the lateral side, the entry point of the single cut was set at 70 mm proximal to the knee joint line with regards to the plate design. A 3D-printed cutting guide was then fixed with two 2.0 mm k-wires on the lateral side of the femur (Fig. 4a). The guide was aligned parallel to the virtual anatomic axis from a coronal view and parallel to the virtual anatomical axis from a sagittal view. The virtual anatomical axis is a line from the middle of the proximal shaft at the greater trochanter to the middle of the distal shaft at the assumed height of the cutting plane, on a frontal and a sagittal view [22]. For rotational control, two 2.5 mm k-wires were inserted from anterior to posterior, one proximal to the assumed osteotomy and one on the distal side. An oscillating saw provided the perfect single cut with an individualized oblique angle (Fig. 4b, c). The cutting guide was removed, followed by derotation of 20° (external rotation of the

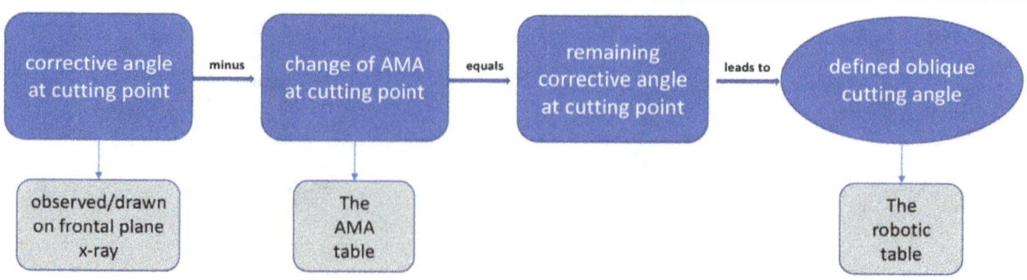

Fig. 2 Calculation for clinical practice: Processing radiographically observed corrective angle and change of AMA to the remaining corrective angle, which leads to a defined oblique cutting angle

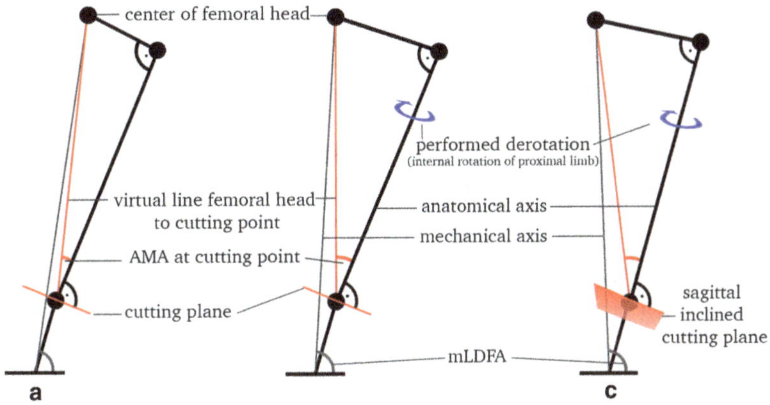

Fig. 3 Elementary mathematical approach: **a** Increased antetorsion, decreased mLDFA; **b** If cutting plane is perpendicular, derotation leads to normal antetorsion and slight increased mLDFA; **c** If the cutting plane is oblique from a sagittal view, derotation leads to normal antetorsion and significant increased mLDFA

distal limb). This was observed with a goniometer from an axial perspective regarding two k-wires, as is routinely done in clinical practice [23]. Osteotomies were fixed with a lateral distal femur plate (Fa. Arthrex, Naples, USA) (Fig. 4d).

Statistical analysis

A 95% confidence interval with limits of ±1° was deemed to be clinically appropriate. A standard deviation of 1° in alignment correction, as observed with goniometric measurement, was assumed across specimens. Based on this desired level of precision using these estimates, a sample size calculation was performed which determined that at least eight specimens were required. Descriptive statistics including mean, range, and standard deviation (SD) were calculated to characterize the specimens. The results of the analysis are presented as mean values with corresponding 95% confidence intervals. Differences between pre- and post-operative measurements were analyzed with the Wilcoxon sign rank test, the non-parametric equivalent of the paired *t* test. The alpha level was 0.05 for all statistical tests. The analysis was conducted with STATA (Stata/IC 14.2, StataCorp LP).

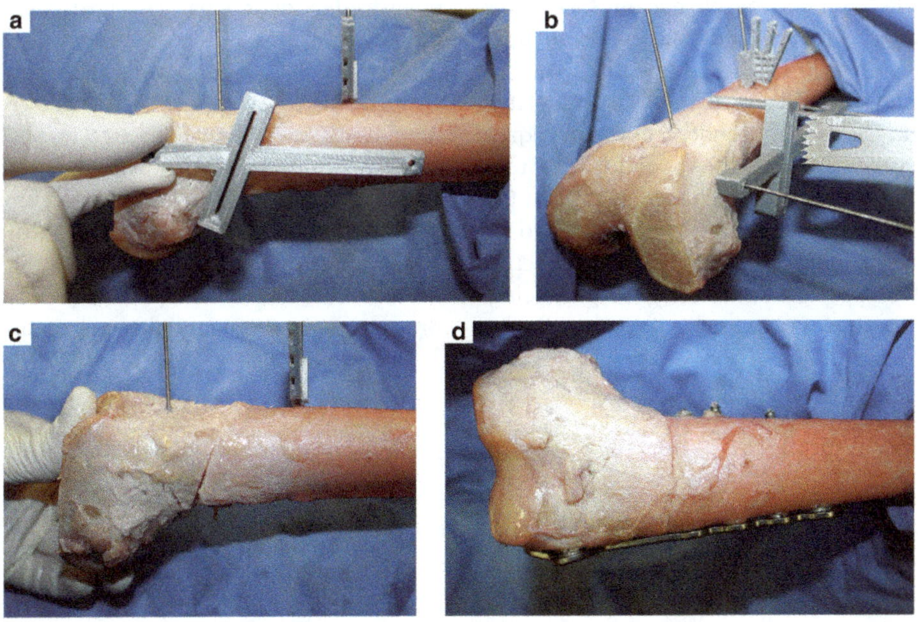

Fig. 4 Surgery of specimens: **a** Cutting guide aligned parallel to the virtual shaft axis (distal: middle of the shaft; proximal: middle of the shaft at height of the greater trochanter), **b** Single cut osteotomy through the cutting guide, **c** Derotation by 20°, **d** plate fixation, resulting in slight varus change on the coronal axis

Results

Radiographic outcome and statistical analysis

Pre-operatively, specimens showed mean antetorsion of 37.1° (range 27.6° - 48.7°) and a mean mLDFA of 84.5° (range 80.4° - 87.5°). Post-operatively, mean performed derotation was 19.69° ± 1.08°SD (95% CI: 18.91° to 20.47°). Post-operative frontal alignment in the 87-goal group was observed as a mean mLDFA of 86.9° ± 0.66°SD, and a mean mLDFA of 90.42° ± 0.25° SD in the 90-goal group. Overall, difference between post-operatively achieved mLDFA compared to intended mLDFA-goal showed a mean of 0.14° ± 0.56° SD (95% CI: -0.26° to 0.54°). When both groups were compared based on their post-operative achieved mLDFA (87-goal-group versus 90-goal-group), two sample Wilcoxon (Mann-Whitney) test showed a significant difference ($p = 0.008$). Detailed information is given in Table 1.

The mean sagittal inclination of the cutting plane was 10.3° (range 3.5° – 19.3°). Ten cutting guides were 3D-printed, giving an individual oblique cutting plane from antero-proximal to postero-distal from a sagittal point of view. Duration of 3D-printing took approximately 60 min and had a filament cost of about $0.50 per guide. The doubled postoperative measurements showed an averaged standard deviation of ±0.25°.

Mathematical model

Trigonometric calculations showed varus producing effects after a simple internal rotation of the proximal limb when the cutting plane was 90 degrees to the proximal virtual anatomical axis (regarding the greater trochanter) [22]. Table 2 shows the change of AMA at a defined torsion angle, which is independent from limb length, (formula is shown in Fig. 5 in Appendix).

The inclination of the cutting plane was calculated with the use of the Denavit-Hartenberg notation (equations are shown in Figs. 6 and 7 in Appendix). In order to receive a significant ($p = 0.0001$) change of axis on the coronal view, inclination of the cutting plane had to be angled from a sagittal point of view (varus producing: anterior-proximal to posterior-distal, valgus producing: anterior-distal to posterior-proximal), if perpendicular from a coronal view, when internal rotation of the proximal limb (external rotation of the distal limb) is performed (Table 3). In addition to the change on frontal axis, the simultaneous change of the axis from a sagittal view (extension/flexion of the femur) is given in parentheses and shows only marginal change on axis. An example of calculations with the specimen's mean values is given in the Appendix. According to the mathematical model, length of the limb changed with a shortening by only 0.2% when derotation of 20° is performed at an inclined cutting angle of a mean of 10.3°.

Discussion

The most important findings of the study were that when a pre-calculated inclined osteotomy is performed, which is referred to the virtual anatomical axis by use of a simple 3D printed cutting guide, a precise postoperative result on frontal and torsional angle can be achieved in distal femur rotational osteotomy. The objective of this study was to develop simplified charts for angle calculations based on precise mathematical models and provide a proof of concept in a cadaveric model to demonstrate the predictability of 3D correction in the clinical setting with the use of simple individual cutting guides.

Derotational osteotomy is the gold standard for the treatment of torsional deformities in the lower extremity, as Dickschas et al. postulate by regards of their clinical cases [4]. Little is known about correlation of valgus malalignment and patellofemoral instability. According to the literature, combining a distal femoral lateral open-wedge or medial closing-wedge osteotomy to a derotational osteotomy is rarely done because of its complexity [7]. But, several studies suggest that increased valgus deformity is considered to be an additional risk factor in such cases [4, 7, 24]. Furthermore, different studies have shown the correlation of valgus alignment and increase of patellofemoral arthritis [25–28]. Yet it is unknown if correction of valgus malalignment may necessarily correct tracking abnormalities at the patellofemoral joint [28]. The proposed Q-angle by Brattström in 1964 and his annotations grounded the

Table 1 Results of measurements, mean and SD, values in degrees

		Preoperative			Calculations			Postoperative	
		Torsion	mLDFA	AMA at cut	Corrective angle	Resulting corrective angle	Oblique cutting angle	Torsion	mLDFA
87-goal-group	mean	41.24	82.92	5.396	4.68	3.44	10.14	21.52	86.86
	SD	4.75	1.88	1.15	2.08	2.04	6.10	5.22	0.66
90-goal-group	mean	32.88	85.98	6.634	4.6	3.54	10.44	13.22	90.42
	SD	6.08	1.27	0.89	1.37	1.57	4.66	6.63	0.25
All specimens combined	mean	37.06	84.45	6.015	4.64	3.49	10.29	17.37	
	SD	6.77	2.21	1.17	1.66	1.72	5.12	7.12	

Table 2 The AMA table; a certain antetorsion and an intended derotation will give a specific additional change on AMA at a specific measured AMA, reprinted from Imhoff et al. [22]

Antetorsion (°)	25	30	30	35	35	40	40	40	45	45	45
Derotation (°)	10	10	15	15	20	20	25	30	20	25	30
AMA (°)											
3	0.2	0.3	0.3	0.4	0.5	0.7	0.8	0.9	0.8	1.0	1.1
3.5			0.4	0.5	0.6	0.8	0.9	1.0	1.0	1.1	1.3
4	0.3	0.3	0.5	0.6	0.7	0.9	1.0	1.1	1.1	1.3	1.5
4.5			0.5	0.7	0.8	1.0	1.2	1.3	1.3	1.5	1.6
5	0.3	0.4	0.6	0.7	0.9	1.1	1.3	1.4	1.4	1.6	1.8
5.5			0.6	0.8	1.0	1.2	1.4	1.6	1.5	1.8	2.0
6	0.4	0.5	0.7	0.9	1.1	1.3	1.5	1.7	1.7	2.0	2.2
6.5			0.7	0.9	1.2	1.5	1.7	1.8	1.8	2.1	2.3
7	0.5	0.6	0.8	1.0	1.2	1.6	1.8	2.0	1.9	2.3	2.5
7.5			0.9	1.1	1.3	1.7	1.9	2.1	2.1	2.4	2.7
The AMA table				Change of AMA (°) = varus increase							

Table 3 The robotic table: An intended derotation angle and an intended change on the coronal axis, equals a specific inclined cutting angle from the sagittal view

Change on coronal axis	Derotation = external rotation of the distal limb / internal rotation of proximal limb							
	10°	15°	20°	25°	30°	35°	40°	
1	5.8	3.9	2.9	2.4	2.0	1.7	1.6	*Additional change on sagittal axis in []*
1.5	8.7	5.8	4.4	3.6	3.0	2.6	2.3	
2	11.6 [0.2]	7.8	5.9	4.7 [0.4]	4.0	3.5	3.1 [0.7]	
2.5	14.5	9.7	7.3	6.0	5.0	4.4	3.9	
3	17.5	11.7	8.8	7.1	6.0	5.2	4.7	
3.5	20.6	13.6	10.3	8.3	7.0	6.1	5.4	
4	23.7 [0.3]	15.6	11.8	9.5 [0.9]	8.0	7.0	6.2 [1.4]	
4.5	26.9	17.6	13.3	10.7	9.0	7.9	7.0	
5	30.1	19.7	14.8	11.9	10.0	8.7	7.8	
5.5	33.5	21.7	16.3	13.1	11.0	9.6	8.6	
6	37.0 [0.4]	23.8	17.8	14.3 [1.3]	12.1	10.5	9.4 [2.2]	
6.5	40.7	26.0	19.3	15.5	13.1	11.4	10.1	
7	44.6	28.1	20.9	16.8	14.1	12.3	10.9	
7.5	48.7	30.3	22.4	18.0	15.1	13.1	11.7	
8	53.3 [0.4]	32.5	24.0	19.2 [1.7]	16.2	14.0	12.5 [2.7]	
8.5	58.4	34.8	25.6	20.5	17.2	14.9	13.3	
9	64.3	37.2	27.2	21.7	18.2	15.8	14.1	
9.5	71.9	39.6	28.8	23.0	19.3	16.7	14.9	
10	89.0 [.01]	42.1	30.5	24.3 [2.0]	20.3	17.6	15.6 [3.5]	
The Robotic Table	Inclination of cutting plane from sagittal view							All values in degrees (°)
	Ant.-prox. to post.-dist. = varus producing							
	Ant.-dist. to post.-prox. = valgus producing							

idea of alignment tracking [29]. He suggested that muscular vectors might be improved due to derotation, although the Q-angle may not be reliable and very accurate in clinics [30]. We believe that a combined correction of alignment, which is a derotation of an increased antetorsion and correction of valgus malalignment, improves patellar stability and patellar tracking. Therefore, our single cut approach in distal femoral derotational osteotomy can avoid aggravating frontal malalignment and can even be used for an intended change on axes.

Single-cut correction for torsional and angular deformity has been described many years ago by the French D'Aubigne in 1952 [31]. There is even a European patent from 1996 held by a French inventor Du Toit for surgical instruments to "guide a saw while it makes an oblique cut in a long bone" (EP 0570187). Subsequently the planning of the osteotomy angle with mathematical models and tables was improved in the 80's for example by Sangeorzan et al. [32] Despite the mathematical calculations to achieve the correct osteotomy plane, Gürke and Strecker et al. showed a graphical approach to define the plane of the single-cut osteotomy in 1999 [33]. However, our approach does not address the center of deformity and we aimed to achieve a reproducible technique for cases of patellofemoral instability and indicated derotational osteotomy. Therefore, only one plane is inclined, given by an easy-to-read table, from the lateral view versus the shaft, as this reflects the standard surgical approach.

It is known that any rotational osteotomy will have changes on frontal and sagittal axes as described by Paley et al. in principles of deformity corrections, and as shown by Kim et al. and Lee et al. in their computed mathematical articles [15, 16, 34]. In order to receive reproducible results in a clinical cadaver model, a new mathematical approach for calculation of the cutting plane was chosen. Our findings show that a correct reference of the cutting plane versus the anatomical shaft is elementary. Using a cutting plane perpendicular to the virtual anatomic axis will lead to a slight increase of AMA and will not aggravate a valgus malalignment. Trigonometrical calculations from the robotics show that inclination of the cutting plane from the sagittal view will have the most change on axis on the coronal view, and only slight change of axis on the sagittal view. Based on the presented table (Table 3), change on varus (cutting plane: antero-proximal to postero-distal) or valgus (cutting plane: antero-distal to postero-proximal) alignment can be performed.

This presented "robotic formula" and the provided table (Table 3) with common values for clinical use show that an inclination of the cutting plane between 8.8° and 11.8° (3° difference) will have a change in the coronal change of axis from 3.5° to 4° (0.5° difference), when rotation by 20° is performed. In terms of clinical accuracy this may be acceptable; however, this can be improved by more exact surgical guides as it is shown in this study and has been described for distal femur open wedge osteotomy by Victor et al. in 2013 [35].

The current study may help to explain why reference of the osteotomy plane to the shaft is one of the most important step in such procedures in order to avoid unintended changes on axes. Bowing of the femur can lead to increased or decreased mLDFA, dependent whether osteotomy is proximal or distal as Nelitz et al. showed in a computed model [1]. In that study, the cutting plane was always set to be perpendicular to the actual anatomic shaft, which differs distally versus proximally. We believe that our approach is able to simplify derotational osteotomy and to avoid postoperative malalignment. Angulation of the cutting plane to the virtual anatomical axis is key to an exact reproducible result in our study.

It is likely that other factors lead to a certain margin of error when measuring angles. To improve accuracy in calculations, an exact frontal plane radiograph of the knee joint is important. As coronal CT reconstructions may help to improve accuracy regarding correct plane of views, we normally perform MRI images for torsion measurement to reduce radiation to young patients. Methods for torsion measurement are well investigated and show reliable results in terms of intraobserver and interobserver agreement as Kaiser et al. describe [36]. But different threshold values depending on the measurement technique should be considered in clinical use. We used the method from Waidelich et al. for exact pre- and postoperative measurements because of the iatrogenic prepared proximal femur bones [19]. These had passed through different femoral neck removals due to the THA workshop, but fully preserved femoral heads and trochanters. Therefore, this method was suitable for our model, and with regards to the virtual anatomical axis, this method supports our model even more.

The performed derotation of 20°, which is visually controlled by two k-wires, shows acceptable results (mean 19.69°). Regarding the mathematic formula, if cutting plane is 10° oblique, derotation between 19° and 21° results in a difference of change of coronal axis by only 0.4°. In order to gain perfection for rotational control, an electromagnetic tracking device processing in real-time as Geisbuesch et al. describe, could be added [37]. The height of the osteotomy (7 cm from the distal joint line) which was chosen due to plate design should not affect the overall outcome, if planning of the osteotomy with its corrective angle is done at this same height. If the osteotomy is supposed to be more proximal, the corrective angle will increase and the inclination of the cut will have to be increased, as well. The mathematical model does not have an angular limitation. However, as shown in Table 3 (the robotic table), a derotation of 20° and an accompanied frontal alignment correction of 10° equals an oblique cutting angle of 30°, which has to be considered in practice.

The principal limitations of this work lie in the perfect anatomical overview from the frontal and lateral view in order to navigate the perfect osteotomy cut. The removed soft tissue helped to perfectly rotate and handle the osteotomy. In vivo, this can be very challenging regarding medial-lateral translation or missed hinge of the osteotomy. The biomechanical nature of the study contains iatrogenic prepared specimen, which showed common pathologic angle values (increased torsion and slight decreased mLDFA). We produced antetorsion artificially in the femoral neck after THA by k-wire fixation. However, the problem of antetorsion of the femur is not only located at the femoral neck. It can occur at the proximal, diaphyseal or distal side of the femur, which was shown by Seitlinger et al. [18] Moreover, this simplified model does not involve any form of dysplasia of the condyles, trochlea, and shaft, which may be observed in patellofemoral instability cases. Another limitation is that surgery was performed by only one surgeon, in order to receive consistent data and proof the concept. But when the calculations and surgical approach are taken into clinics and performed by several surgeons, accuracy may be decreased. 3D-printed cutting guides are used in several publications, and even in osteotomy surgery [35, 38, 39]. But, its practicality and understanding are not widespread. Therefore, stainless steel cutting guide assemblies with intraoperative adjustments of the inclination may help surgeons as well. For a consecutive study, we suggest to perform the analysis and surgery on total leg cadavers with soft tissue for proof of its feasibility in a clinical setup.

Conclusion

A preoperative calculated angle for single cut derotational osteotomy at the distal femur led to a clinically precise post-operative result on torsion and frontal alignment when using this approach. 3D-changes were mathematically predicted and provided by the use of an individualized cutting guide, based on angle measurements from standard two-dimensional radiograph and axial CT slicing.

Appendix

Example calculation of cutting angle (mean values of specimens)

Each specimen underwent specific radiographic analysis, giving an intended mean corrective angle of 4.64° observed on frontal plane x-ray, and a mean change of AMA at cutting point of 1.15° when derotation of 20° was intended. This results in a mean remaining corrective angle of 3.49°. Converting the remaining corrective angle resulted in a mean sagittal inclination of the cutting plane of 10.06°. Aside from intended change on the coronal view (increased varus), additional calculations showed a mean simultaneous change on the sagittal view (increased extension) of only 0.59° ($p = .0001$).

Change of AMA at cutting

Trigonometrical calculations were done to forecast the angular changes on "AMA at cutting point" when internal rotation of the proximal limb is performed at a cutting plane perpendicular to the virtual anatomical shaft from a coronal and a sagittal view. No actual lengths are needed when calculations are done with at least two known angles in a perpendicular triangle (Fig. 5 in Appendix) [22].

Denavit-Hartenberg Transformation

In order to calculate the position of the rotated end point after definition of a cutting plane and a rotation angle, an approach commonly used in from robotics was applied [17]. Hereby, a combination of translational and rotational matrices was used to calculate the position of a robot joint. The coordinates x_n, y_n, z_n of a joint number n can be calculated using a standardized transformation of the coordinate system of the joint number $n-1$ with the axes x_{n-1}, y_{n-1}, z_{n-1}. The Denavit-Hartenberg transformation matrix for the transition from position $n-1$ to position n can be described (Fig. 6 in Appendix, Step 1):

Here, d_n describes a translation along the original z_{n-1} axis. The angle θ_n defines a rotation around the original z_{n-1} axis, from original x_{n-1} to new x_n. The distance r_n denotes an offset perpendicular to the original z_{n-1} axis, which can be set to zero in this case. Finally, the angle α_n describes a rotation around the new x_n axis.

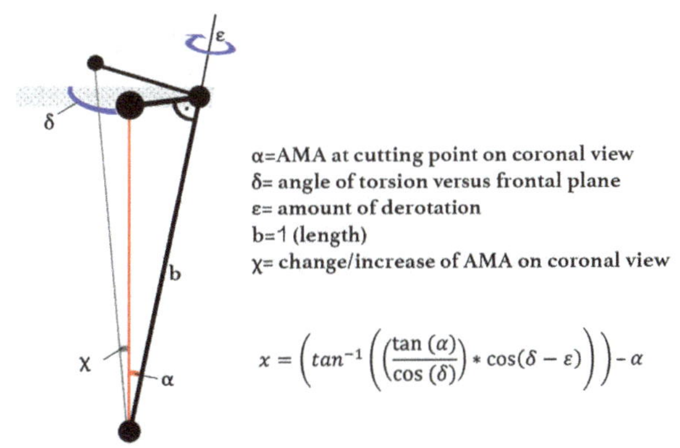

$$x = \left(tan^{-1}\left(\left(\frac{\tan(\alpha)}{\cos(\delta)}\right) * \cos(\delta - \varepsilon)\right)\right) - \alpha$$

Fig. 5 Illustration and Equation for change of AMA at cutting point

Step 1:

$$^{n-1}T_n = \begin{pmatrix} \cos\theta_n & -\sin\theta_n\cos\alpha_n & \sin\theta_n\sin\alpha_n & r_n\cos\theta_n \\ \sin\theta_n & \cos\theta_n\cos\alpha_n & -\cos\theta_n\sin\alpha_n & r_n\sin\theta_n \\ 0 & \sin\alpha_n & \cos\alpha_n & d_n \\ 0 & 0 & 0 & 1 \end{pmatrix} = \begin{pmatrix} & R & & T \\ & & & \\ 0 & 0 & 0 & 1 \end{pmatrix}$$

Step 2:

$$^{0}T_1 = \begin{pmatrix} 1 & 0 & 0 & 0 \\ 0 & \cos\alpha_1 & -\sin\alpha_1 & 0 \\ 0 & \sin\alpha_1 & \cos\alpha_1 & 0 \\ 0 & 0 & 0 & 1 \end{pmatrix}$$

$$^{1}T_2 = \begin{pmatrix} \cos\theta_2 & -\sin\theta_2\cos\alpha_2 & \sin\theta_2\sin\alpha_2 & 0 \\ \sin\theta_2 & \cos\theta_2\cos\alpha_2 & -\cos\theta_2\sin\alpha_2 & 0 \\ 0 & \sin\alpha_2 & \cos\alpha_2 & 0 \\ 0 & 0 & 0 & 1 \end{pmatrix}$$

$$^{2}T_3 = \begin{pmatrix} 1 & 0 & 0 & 0 \\ 0 & 1 & 0 & 0 \\ 0 & 0 & 1 & d_3 \\ 0 & 0 & 0 & 1 \end{pmatrix}$$

Step 3:

$$^{0}T_3 = {}^{0}T_1 \cdot {}^{1}T_2 \cdot {}^{2}T_3 =$$

$$\begin{pmatrix} \cos\theta & -\sin\theta\cos\alpha & -\sin\theta\sin\alpha & -d\sin\theta\sin\alpha \\ \sin\theta\cos\alpha & \cos\theta\cos^2\alpha + \sin^2\alpha & \cos\theta\sin\alpha\cos\alpha - \sin\alpha\cos\alpha & d(\cos\theta\sin\alpha\cos\alpha - \sin\alpha\cos\alpha) \\ \sin\theta\sin\alpha & \cos\theta\sin\alpha\cos\alpha - \sin\alpha\cos\alpha & \cos\theta\sin^2\alpha + \cos^2\alpha & d(\cos\theta\sin^2\alpha + \cos^2\alpha) \\ 0 & 0 & 0 & 1 \end{pmatrix}$$

Step 4:

$$T = d\begin{pmatrix} -\sin\theta\sin\alpha \\ \cos\theta\sin\alpha\cos\alpha - \sin\alpha\cos\alpha \\ \cos\theta\sin^2\alpha + \cos^2\alpha \end{pmatrix}$$

Fig. 6 Mathematical equation, Denavit-Hartenberg Transformation: Development of equation for change of axis due to rotation and an oblique cutting angle

In the particular case presented in this paper, the following three transformations are required to describe the position of the rotated end point relative to the center of the rotational plane: At first, the angle $\alpha_1 \equiv \alpha$ is used to define the cutting plane. Subsequently, the actual rotation around the cutting plane is described by $\theta_2 \equiv \theta$, followed by a reverse rotation around $\alpha_2 = -\alpha_1 = -\alpha$ to account for proper positioning of the end point with respect to the cutting plane. Finally, the translation $d_3 \equiv d$ denotes the length of the piece to be rotated, i.e. the distance of the rotated end point from the rotational plane.

Hence, the three respective transformation matrices can be constructed (Fig. 6 in Appendix, Step 2). The final transformation matrix is the result of the three matrices multiplications (Fig. 6 in Appendix, Step 3). The cartesian position of the rotated end point is given by the first three row elements of the fourth column (Fig. 6 in Appendix Step 4). When given a defined inclination angle and a defined rotation angle, resulting changes on XYZ-axis can be calculated in distance (Fig. 7 in Appendix). Adding trigonometric equations will also help calculate angles for coronal (XZ-plane) and sagittal (YZ-plane) changes of axes.

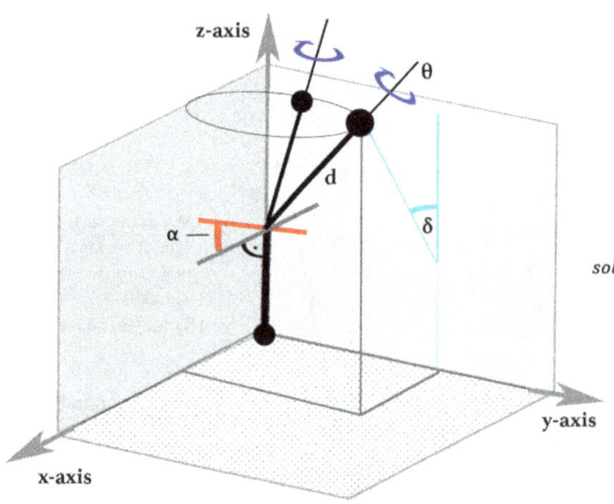

α = inclination of cutting plane
θ = rotation
d = length of limb (=1cm)
δ = angle of coronal change

$$solve\left[\delta = tan^{-1}\left\{\frac{(\sin\alpha * \sin\theta) * d}{(\cos\theta * \sin^2\alpha + \cos^2\alpha) * d}\right\}, \alpha\right]$$

Fig. 7 Illustration of schematic XYZ-coordinate for calculations of three dimensional effects; reverse equation for angle of coronal change (XZ-plane)

Abbreviations
3D: Three-dimensional; aLDFA: Anatomical lateral distal femur angle; AMA: Anatomical mechanical axis; mLDFA: Mechanical lateral distal femur angle

Acknowledgements
The authors thank Mark P. Cote, PT, DPT, MCTR for his advice on statistical analyses.

Funding
The University of Connecticut Health Center/UConn Musculoskeletal Institute has received direct funding and material support from Arthrex Inc. (Naples. Fl). The company had no influence on study design, data collection or interpretation of the results or the final manuscript.

Authors' contributions
IFB had the initial idea of the present study, developed the mathematical approach, executed the specimens, xray and analysis, as well as the majority of the writing. SJ and MA are engineers, specialized in robotics, and helped to develop the mathematical approach. DT and SB helped with specimen preparation, x-ray analysis and served as internal reviewer of the manuscript. BS had the elementary idea of developing a 3D-printed Guide as single usage for every surgery. IAB made substantial contributions to conception of the clinical background and improved the methods with his intellectual content. ARA added critical intellectual content regarding clinical educational aims, helped writing the final manuscript and served as a critical internal reviewer with his clinical experience. KB is a cofounder of the basic idea and was a major contributor to the methodology section. All authors had read and approved the final manuscript.

Authors' information
Florian B. Imhoff, MD; Specialist Orthopaedic and Trauma Surgery; German Board Certified Currently: Postdoctoral Research Fellow at Uconn Health, Department of Orthopaedic Surgery 263 Farmington Avenue, Farmington, CT 06030, USA.

Consent for publication
Not applicable.

Competing interests
Authors IFB, SJ, MA, DT, SB declare that they have no conflict of interest and nothing to disclose.
Author BS is a consultant for Arthrex.
Author IAB is a consultant for Arthrosurface, Arthrex, and mediBayreuth.
Author ARA received an educational and institutional grant from Arthrex and is a consultant for Biorez.
Author BK is a consultant for Arthrex.
No-one of the above-mentioned authors has received personal financial support related to this study.

Author details
[1]Department of Orthopaedic Sports Medicine, Technical University Munich, Ismaninger Str. 22, 81675 Munich, Germany. [2]Department of Orthopaedic Surgery, University of Connecticut, 263 Farmington Ave, Farmington, CT 06030, USA. [3]Department of Mechanical Engineering, Institute for Machine Tools and Industrial Management, Technical University Munich, Boltzmannstr. 15, 85748 Garching, Munich, Germany.

References

1. Nelitz M, Wehner T, Steiner M, Durselen L, Lippacher S. The effects of femoral external derotational osteotomy on frontal plane alignment. Knee Surg Sports Traumatol Arthrosc. 2014;22:2740–6. https://doi.org/10.1007/s00167-013-2618-5.
2. Nelitz M, Dreyhaupt J, Williams SR, Dornacher D. Combined supracondylar femoral derotation osteotomy and patellofemoral ligament reconstruction for recurrent patellar dislocation and severe femoral anteversion syndrome: surgical technique and clinical outcome. Int Orthop. 2015;39:2355–62. https://doi.org/10.1007/s00264-015-2859-7.
3. Eckhoff DG, Montgomery WK, Kilcoyne RF, Stamm ER. Femoral morphometry and anterior knee pain. Clin Orthop Relat Res. 1994;(302):64–8.
4. Dickschas J, Harrer J, Pfefferkorn R, Strecker W. Operative treatment of patellofemoral maltracking with torsional osteotomy. Arch Orthop Trauma Surg. 2012;132:289–98. https://doi.org/10.1007/s00402-011-1303-8.
5. Delgado ED, Schoenecker PL, Rich MM, Capelli AM. Treatment of severe torsional malalignment syndrome. J Pediatr Orthop. 1996;16:484–8.
6. Staheli LT. Torsion–treatment indications. Clin Orthop Relat Res. 1989;(247): 61–6. Review.
7. Petersen W, Forkel P. Medial closing wedge osteotomy for correction of genu valgum and torsional malalignment. Oper Orthop Traumatol. 2013;25: 593–607; quiz 608. https://doi.org/10.1007/s00064-013-0258-z.
8. Brinkman JM, Freiling D, Lobenhoffer P, Staubli AE, van Heerwaarden RJ. Supracondylar femur osteotomies around the knee: patient selection, planning, operative techniques, stability of fixation, and bone healing. Orthopade. 2014;43(Suppl 1):S1–10. https://doi.org/10.1007/s00132-014-3007-6.
9. Lee TQ, Anzel SH, Bennett KA, Pang D, Kim WC. The influence of fixed rotational deformities of the femur on the patellofemoral contact pressures in human cadaver knees. Clin Orthop Relat Res. 1994;(302):69–74.
10. Lee TQ, Morris G, Csintalan RP. The influence of tibial and femoral rotation on patellofemoral contact area and pressure. J Orthop Sports Phys Ther. 2003;33:686–93. https://doi.org/10.2519/jospt.2003.33.11.686.
11. Souza RB, Draper CE, Fredericson M, Powers CM. Femur rotation and patellofemoral joint kinematics: a weight-bearing magnetic resonance imaging analysis. J Orthop Sports Phys Ther. 2010;40:277–85. https://doi.org/10.2519/jospt.2010.3215.
12. Paley D, Pfeil J. Principles of deformity correction around the knee. Orthopade. 2000;29:18–38. https://doi.org/10.1007/PL00003691.
13. Strecker W. Planning analysis of knee-adjacent deformities. I. Frontal plane deformities. Oper Orthop Traumatol. 2006;18:259–72. https://doi.org/10.1007/s00064-006-1175-1.
14. Dickschas J, Harrer J, Reuter B, Schwitulla J, Strecker W. Torsional osteotomies of the femur. J Orthop Res. 2015;33:318–24. https://doi.org/10.1002/jor.22758.
15. Paley D, Herzenberg JE. Principles of deformity correction. Berlin Heidelberg: Springer; 2002.
16. Lee SY, Jeong J, Lee K, Chung CY, Lee KM, Kwon SS, Choi Y, Kim TG, Lee JI, Lee J, Park MS. Unexpected angular or rotational deformity after corrective osteotomy. BMC Musculoskelet Disord. 2014;15:175. https://doi.org/10.1186/1471-2474-15-175.
17. Hartenberg RS, Denavit J. Kinematic synthesis of linkages. New York; Toronto: McGraw-Hill; 1964.
18. Seitlinger G, Moroder P, Scheurecker G, Hofmann S, Grelsamer RP. The contribution of different femur segments to overall femoral torsion. Am J Sports Med. 2016;44:1796–800. https://doi.org/10.1177/0363546516639945.
19. Waidelich HA, Strecker W, Schneider E. Computed tomographic torsion-angle and length measurement of the lower extremity. The methods, normal values and radiation load. Rofo. 1992;157:245–51. https://doi.org/10.1055/s-2008-1033007.
20. Strecker W, Dickschas J. Torsional osteotomy: operative treatment of patellofemoral maltracking. Oper Orthop Traumatol. 2015;27:505–24. https://doi.org/10.1007/s00064-015-0430-8.

21. Dickschas J, Harrer J, Bayer T, Schwitulla J, Strecker W. Correlation of the tibial tuberosity-trochlear groove distance with the Q-angle. Knee Surg Sports Traumatol Arthrosc. 2016;24:915–20. https://doi.org/10.1007/s00167-014-3426-2.
22. Imhoff FB, Scheiderer B, Zakko P, Obopilwe E, Liska F, Imhoff AB, Mazzocca AD, Arciero RA, Beitzel K. How to avoid unintended valgus alignment in distal femoral derotational osteotomy for treatment of femoral torsional malalignment - a concept study. BMC Musculoskelet Disord. 2017;18:553. https://doi.org/10.1186/s12891-017-1904-7.
23. Hinterwimmer S, Minzlaff P, Saier T, Niemeyer P, Imhoff AB, Feucht MJ. Biplanar supracondylar femoral derotation osteotomy for patellofemoral malalignment: the anterior closed-wedge technique. Knee Surg Sports Traumatol Arthrosc. 2014;22:2518–21. https://doi.org/10.1007/s00167-014-2993-6.
24. O'Malley MP, Pareek A, Reardon PJ, Stuart MJ, Krych AJ. Distal femoral osteotomy: lateral opening wedge technique. Arthrosc Tech. 2016;5:e725–30. https://doi.org/10.1016/j.eats.2016.02.037.
25. Teichtahl AJ, Wluka AE, Cicuttini FM. Frontal plane knee alignment is associated with a longitudinal reduction in patella cartilage volume in people with knee osteoarthritis. Osteoarthr Cartil. 2008;16:851–4. https://doi.org/10.1016/j.joca.2007.12.002.
26. Cahue S, Dunlop D, Hayes K, Song J, Torres L, Sharma L. Varus-valgus alignment in the progression of patellofemoral osteoarthritis. Arthritis Rheum. 2004;50:2184–90. https://doi.org/10.1002/art.20348.
27. Elahi S, Cahue S, Felson DT, Engelman L, Sharma L. The association between varus-valgus alignment and patellofemoral osteoarthritis. Arthritis Rheum. 2000;43:1874–80. https://doi.org/10.1002/1529-0131(200008)43:8<1874::AID-ANR25>3.0.CO;2-2.
28. McWalter EJ, Cibere J, MacIntyre NJ, Nicolaou S, Schulzer M, Wilson DR. Relationship between varus-valgus alignment and patellar kinematics in individuals with knee osteoarthritis. J Bone Joint Surg Am. 2007;89:2723–31. https://doi.org/10.2106/JBJS.F.01016.
29. Brattström H. Shape of the intercondylar groove normally and in recurrent dislocation of patella: a clinical and X-ray anatomical investigation. Acta Orthop Scand. 1964;35:1–148. https://doi.org/10.3109/ort.1964.35.suppl-68.01.
30. Greene CC, Edwards TB, Wade MR, Carson EW. Reliability of the quadriceps angle measurement. Am J Knee Surg. 2001;14:97–103.
31. Merle d'Aubigné R, Descamps L. L'ostéotomie plane oblique dans la correction des deformations des membres. Bull Mem Arch Chirurgie. 1952;8:271–6.
32. Sangeorzan BP, Judd RP, Sangeorzan BJ. Mathematical analysis of single-cut osteotomy for complex long bone deformity. J Biomech. 1989;22:1271–8.
33. Gurke L, Strecker W, Martinoli S. Graphical analysis and operative technique of single-cut osteotomy for complex femur deformities. Unfallchirurg. 1999; 102:684–90.
34. Kim SS. Three-dimensional effect of the single plane proximal femur osteotomy. Hip Pelvis. 2015;27:23–9. https://doi.org/10.5371/hp.2015.27.1.23.
35. Victor J, Premanathan A. Virtual 3D planning and patient specific surgical guides for osteotomies around the knee: a feasibility and proof-of-concept study. Bone Joint J. 2013;95-B:153–8. https://doi.org/10.1302/0301-620X.95B11.32950.
36. Kaiser P, Schmoelz W, Schoettle P, Zwierzina M, Heinrichs C, Attal R. Increased internal femoral torsion can be regarded as a risk factor for patellar instability - a biomechanical study. Clin Biomech (Bristol, Avon). 2017;47:103–9. https://doi.org/10.1016/j.clinbiomech.2017.06.007.
37. Geisbusch A, Auer C, Dickhaus H, Niklasch M, Dreher T. Electromagnetic bone segment tracking to control femoral derotation osteotomy-a saw bone study. J Orthop Res. 2017;35:1106–12. https://doi.org/10.1002/jor.23348.
38. Hoekstra H, Rosseels W, Sermon A, Nijs S. Corrective limb osteotomy using patient specific 3D-printed guides: a technical note. Injury. 2016;47:2375–80. https://doi.org/10.1016/j.injury.2016.07.021.
39. Zheng P, Xu P, Yao Q, Tang K, Lou Y. 3D-printed navigation template in proximal femoral osteotomy for older children with developmental dysplasia of the hip. Sci Rep. 2017;7:44993. https://doi.org/10.1038/srep44993.

13

Nanotechnology in orthopedics: a clinically oriented review

Walter Ryan Smith[1], Parke William Hudson[1], Brent Andrew Ponce[1] and Sakthivel Rajan Rajaram Manoharan[2*]

Abstract

The utility of nanotechnology in medicine, specifically within the field of orthopedics, is a topic of extensive research. Our review provides a unique comprehensive overview of the current and potential future uses of nanotechnology with respect to orthopedic sub-specialties. Nanotechnology offers an immense assortment of novel applications, most notably the use of nanomaterials as scaffolds to induce a more favorable interaction between orthopedic implants and native bone. Nanotechnology has the capability to revolutionize the diagnostics and treatment of orthopedic surgery, however the long-term health effects of nanomaterials are poorly understood and extensive research is needed regarding clinical safety.

Background

Disruptive technology and innovation have long held the promise of improving patient outcomes. The field of nanotechnology is one of these domains with breakthrough potential to aid in diagnosing and treating complex medical problems. Nanotechnology was originally defined by the National Nanotechnology Initiative as the study and controlled manipulation of individual atoms and molecules of size between 1 and 100 nm, however the definition has since evolved to include a broader spectrum of research endeavors and applications [1]. Richard Feynman was the first to conceptualize the potential of nanotechnology nearly six decades ago. In 1959, he described it as "a field in which little has been done, but in which an enormous amount can be done in principle [2]." Since then, the applications of nanotechnology have vastly expanded into fields such as food packaging, cosmetics, water filtration, and medicine [3].

The application of nanotechnology to medicine, known as "nanomedicine," has been utilized in a number of novel therapies in the field of orthopedics. A few clinical applications include targeted drug delivery, implantable materials, vertebral disk regeneration, and diagnostic modalities [4]. Previous reviews of nanotechnology in orthopedics have provided extensive summaries regarding the use of different biomaterials that have been studied and implemented [5, 6]. Our review is unique in the sense that it is structured by orthopedic sub-specialty with a specific focus on the clinical aspects of nanotechnology in orthopedics. While specialty designations are arbitrary, they are useful to highlight the clinical relevance of certain innovations with appreciation that cross over applications into other sub-specialties are likely in the future. Our main objective is to provide orthopedic surgeons and musculoskeletal researchers with knowledge regarding the current impact and future potential of nanotechnology. We will also identify nanotechnology studies with ongoing clinical trials in each respective section.

Basics of nanotechnology

Nanotechnology exists as a collaboration among multiple scientific disciplines including surface science, molecular biology, microelectronics, and tissue engineering. When conventional macro-materials are engineered into much smaller nanosized particles, they may possess completely different physical and chemical properties in certain instances. Specifically, as the size of particulate matter decreases to 100 nm or smaller, phenomena such as the quantum size effect become more prominent [7]. This principle is observed when the electrical properties of a material change as a result of significant reductions in particle size. For example, materials that are insulators at the macroscale may possess conductive properties when reduced to the nanoscale. In addition to alterations in electrical properties, changes in mechanical properties may take place as well due to an increased surface area to volume ratio as particle size is reduced. This bears significance as nanophase materials are able to maintain relatively large surface

* Correspondence: srajaram@uabmc.edu
[2]Department of Orthopaedic Surgery, University of Alabama at Birmingham, FOT 950, 20 Street South, Birmingham, AL 35294, USA
Full list of author information is available at the end of the article

area to volume ratios allowing for more favorable interactions with surrounding structures. In the example of orthopedic implants, this allows for a greater degree of interaction between an implant and native bone, leading to more effective osseointegration [8]. Much of nanotechnologies' potential benefit with regards to medicine rests in the fact that nanotechnology may allow for more precise therapeutic applications at the subcellular level [9]. Given that many molecules involved in cellular processes exist and interact fundamentally at the nanometer scale, nanoengineered materials have the theoretical ability to target and modify these processes [10]. Applying this principle to orthopedics, bone when broken down to the nanoscale is naturally a nanostructure composite of collagen and hydroxyapatite [11]. The practical application of these principles and appreciation of these relationships has allowed for improvements in functionality and performance of a wide variety of products both in and outside of the medical field. Figure 1 summarizes the potential utilities of nanotechnology among different orthopedic sub-specialties.

Spine

Tissue regeneration

Surgical treatments for degenerative disc disease such as discectomy and fusion are often associated with the loss of spinal mobility, degenerative post-discectomy spondylosis, and disc herniation recurrence [12]. Inconsistent outcomes and complications with current treatments have created a role for nanotech research involving novel cell-based therapies, including tissue engineering for intervertebral disc (IVD) regeneration. These experimental therapies have demonstrated the ability of progenitor cells, such as mesenchymal stem cells (MSCs) to undergo differentiation into a nucleus pulposus-like phenotype [13–16]. Injection therapy with poly (γ-glutamic acid) nanocomplexes has been shown in multiple studies to enhance recovery of native IVD matrix [13, 14]. Additionally, these nanocomplexes have demonstrated anti-inflammatory properties in ex vivo models. Growth factors are often used concurrently to promote proliferation and differentiation. However, one of the underlying problems with this technique is that short lives in vivo limit their utility. To address this issue, current studies are aiming to develop nanofibrous scaffolds to help sustain biologically active growth factors and maximize the potential of MSCs. The combination of these scaffolds with growth factors such as TGF-β under certain conditions has shown promising results in achieving a functional graft for IVD regeneration [15]. These advances in scaffold engineering, while still relatively new, may offer an efficient method for nucleus pulposus regeneration.

Surgical interventions for peripheral nerve injuries have been criticized in the past as inefficient and cost-defective. Neuron regeneration using nanoengineering may offer an attractive method for management of peripheral nerve injuries by eliminating the morbidity associated with surgical interventions to harvest an autograft. Synthetic conduits using carbon nanotubes and nanoscaffolds offer more tunable mechanical properties than autografts and may enhance nerve regeneration through augmented surface topographical interactions [17]. Carbon nanotubes have demonstrated the ability to promote axonal growth and even mimic some electrical properties of myelin (Fig. 2) [9]. Electrospinning techniques have been paramount in allowing for the creation of nanoscaffolds, which closely resemble

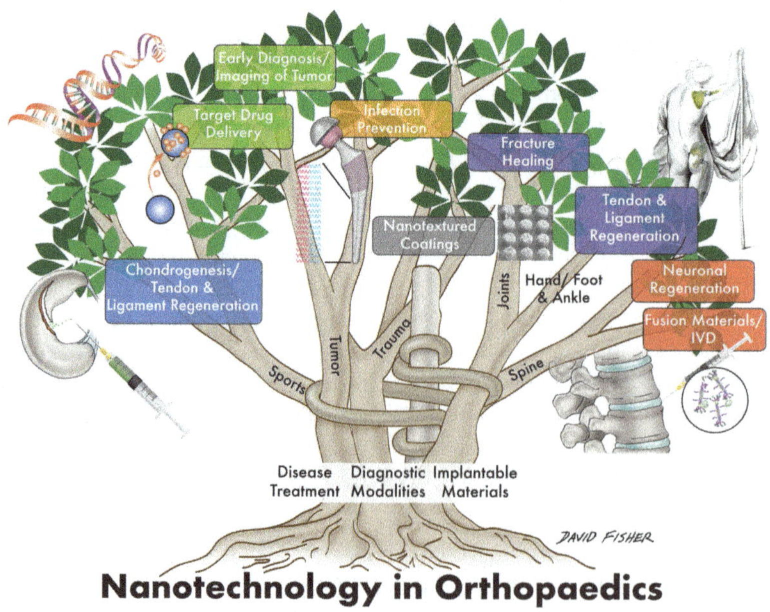

Fig. 1 Diagram outlining the domains and applications of nanotechnology within orthopedics

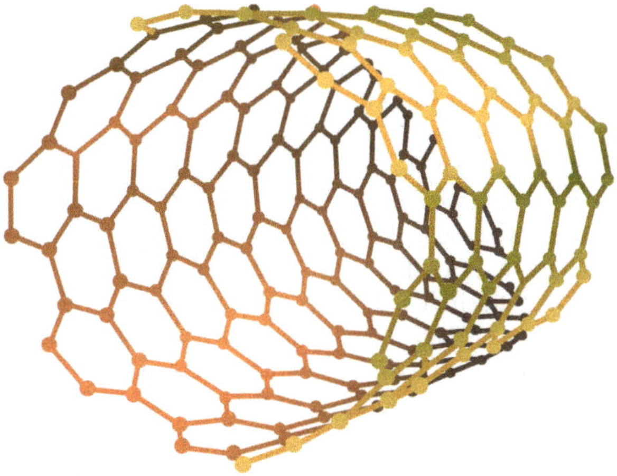

Fig. 2 Illustration showing the basic structure of a carbon nanotube. These materials are of significant interest in multiple realms of orthopedics including nerve regeneration, implant scaffold engineering, and drug delivery

native extracellular environments. [18] The nanoscale fibers that comprise these conduits have increased area available for protein absorption, stem cell migration, and axonal regeneration and guided growth in addition to being easily and cheaply manufactured [17]. Commonly used materials in conduit composition include collagen and silicone. Although not yet clinically mainstream, nanoscale synthetic nerve conduits appear to be the future of nerve regeneration therapy. Artificial conduits have the potential to replace autografting as first-line therapy and may even allow surgeons to tailor conduits according to the type of nerve, sensory, motor or mixed, needed.

Spinal implants

In addition to disc and nerve regeneration, nanotechnology may potentially facilitate spinal fusion and avoid the cost and potential complications associated with recombinant human bone morphogenetic protein (rhBMP). Surface modifications to titanium spinal implants through the addition of nanoparticles such as titanium oxide and zirconia have shown promise in promoting increased bone formation and decreased resorption compared to conventional smooth implants. [19] Additionally, cervical cages enhanced with silicone nitride nanoparticles have demonstrated multiple biomechanical advantages over standard PEEK (poly-ether-ether-ketone) and are currently on the market [20]. In 2014, the FDA approved the first interbody fusion device to feature nanotechnology [21]. The nanoLOCK™ by Titan Spine technology has been shown to induce a greater amount of osteogenic and angiogenic growth factors compared to conventional titanium PEEK cages [22]. This breakthrough demonstrates the potential that nanotech offers in improving the topographical interaction between implant and bone to increase osteogenesis.

Use of rhBMP-2 is commonly associated with side effects due to supraphysiologic dosing [23]. Nanotechnology efforts are underway to address these limitations. One particular strategy uses nanofiber structures known as peptide amphiphile (PA) molecules to mimic extracellular filaments and induce cellular regeneration. Studies found that the use of PA nanofibers in the form of a gel scaffold showed overall superior fusion rates while allowing for reduction of therapeutic doses of BMP-2 by up to 10-fold [24, 25]. Further efforts are investigating the reliability of this technique in promoting osteogenesis in vivo and ultimately its potential use as a growth-factor substitute in spinal fusion surgery [24].

Orthopedic oncology

Therapeutic applications - drug delivery

Substantial progress has been made in the treatment of osteosarcoma and Ewing sarcoma in terms of prolonging survivorship, but major challenges still remain including cytotoxicity and decreased selectivity of chemotherapies, drug-resistance, and pharmacokinetic problems [26]. Nanotechnology may offer a solution to some of these issues through the use of unique carrier molecules that aid in drug delivery. The principle behind nanotechnology drug delivery as a treatment modality begins with the creation of a drug-loaded nanomolecule (Fig. 3). Next, this structure is attached to a specific ligand such as a monoclonal antibody, which is able to bind and enter the cancer cell. This allows for direct action of the chemotherapy on the desired target with reduced collateral toxicity to non-cancerous cells [27]. There are a wide variety of carrier materials including titanium, gold, calcium phosphate, and chitosan that are under investigation for use as nanoparticle drug carriers [28]. Lipid nanoparticle carriers offer an attractive method of treatment against osteosarcoma, as they have been shown to have excellent bioavailability and can be orally administered [29]. Conventional chemotherapeutic agents such as etoposide have been investigated using this technique in treating other types of cancer and have shown promising

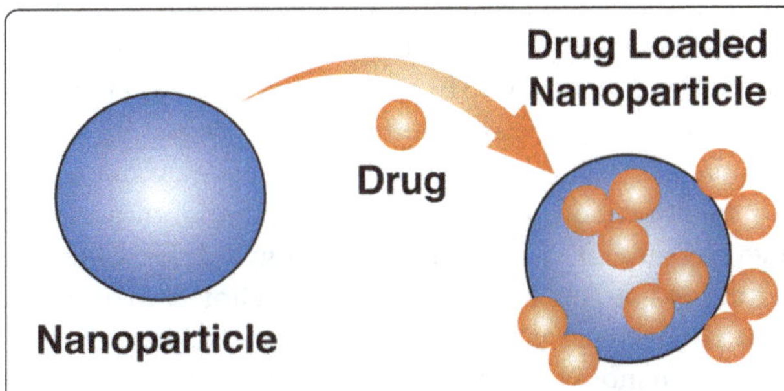

Fig. 3 Diagram demonstrating the fundamental principle of drug delivery using nanoparticles. This method not only allows for more precise drug targeting, but also greater control of drug release in treating bone cancer, prosthetic joint infections, and osteomyelitis

results against bone metastases [30, 31]. Silica nanocarriers enhanced with Zoledronate and loaded with doxorubicin exhibited significant cytotoxic activity against boney metastasis as well [32]. Most recently, Liu et al. developed a gambogic acid and retinoic acid loaded nanoparticle that induced a remarkably higher rate (28%) of apoptosis in osteosarcoma cells than conventional drug delivery [33]. Additionally, Zhou et al. demonstrated that the use of tailored nanocarriers loaded with cisplatin resulted in reduced renal accumulation and side effects compared to the free form while maintaining optimal anti-tumor activity against osteosarcoma cells [34]. Despite the encouraging results demonstrated by these novel drug carrier methods using nanotechnology, this research is very much still in its early stages.

Therapeutic applications - anti-cancerous materials

It is common for patients who have undergone bone cancer resections to receive orthopedic implants. However, standard materials are not designed to inhibit the growth or recurrence of cancer. Therefore, efforts are underway to design implants that will encourage normal bone growth while preventing cancer growth. Selenium has been shown to exhibit these properties in the past, and nano-selenium implants have been demonstrated to inhibit the growth of malignant osteoblasts while promoting healthy bone function at the implant-tissue interface [35]. It was identified that the selenium nanomaterial, unlike untreated titanium implants, increased bone adhesion, calcium deposition, bone proliferation, and alkaline phosphatase activity. More recently, nanostructured magnesium alloy implants demonstrated anti-tumor properties after being enhanced through grain refinement. Human osteosarcoma cells were less viable and adhesive to this material [36].

Diagnostic applications

The role of nanotechnology in cancer diagnosis is based on the binding of nanoparticle-ligand complexes to specific genetic mutations that allow for detailed imaging at the cellular level. The addition of a contrast agent to these complexes allows for visualization of the tumor cells that express the specific mutation [27]. This technique has been studied using the p15 gene, a tumor marker mutation commonly associated with lung metastasis in osteosarcoma [37]. Utilization of this practice may allow for early identification of the metastatic potential of a malignancy. Coupled with nanotechnology drug delivery, chemotherapy can be initiated before clinical symptoms appear to decrease patient morbidity. Additionally, the detection of nanomaterials using fluorescent probes may aid in the assessment of cancer response after therapy [38]. This method potentially offers higher accuracy in the calculation of the amount of tumor remaining than histologic analysis after tumor resection [39].

Arthroplasty

Implant material

Although primary joint replacement surgery is highly successful, its longevity remains limited. Nanotechnology in arthroplasty is focusing on the development of implantable materials that can function safely and effectively while extending the average lifespan of implants and preventing infection. Through the modification of specific surface characteristics on the implant, a more favorable interaction can be induced between the implant and native bone (Fig. 4). Nanotextured implant surfaces have augmented the function and growth of osteoblasts to increase implant osseointegration [5]. Specifically, the technique of severe plastic deformation (SPD), which breaks down the coarse grains of metals into the nanoscale range by exposing the metal to a complex high stress state, has demonstrated the ability to improve the biocompatibility and mechanical properties of titanium implants [40]. The use of ultra-high molecular weight polyethylene (UHMWPE)

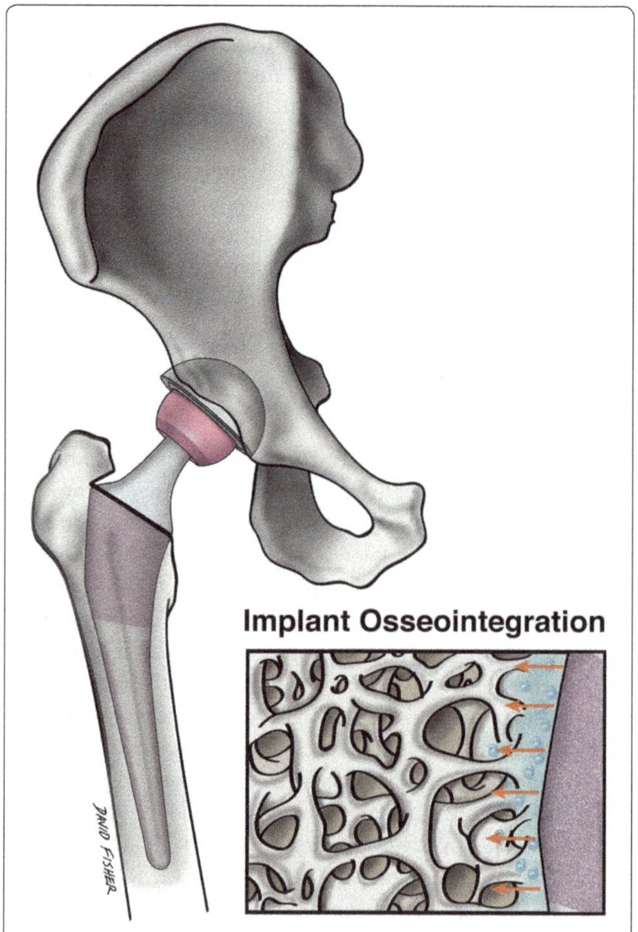

Fig. 4 Nanostructured implants may better mimic the environment of native bone, and stimulate implant osseointegration and surrounding osteogenesis to a greater degree than conventional implants. This illustration shows a magnified nanoengineered implant surface and its topographical interaction with adjacent bone

implants has been limited in the field of arthroplasty due to concern for potential fracture. However, due to its favorable biocompatibility properties and wear resistance, there has been increased interest in improving the mechanical strength of UHMWPE through nanotechnology. The addition of carbon nanotubes to this material to create a novel composite has demonstrated translational success and may eventually have utility as an acetabular lining or tibial component [41]. Altering an implant's surface nanostructure has the potential to increase resistance to static and dynamic fatigue, improve functionality, and increase implant survivorship.

Cements

Efforts to improve commonly used bone cements such as polymethyl methacrylate (PMMA) using nanotechnology are currently underway. Addition of antibiotics to bone cement is common practice, however it is well known that antibiotics often persist for only a short period of time ([42] Swearingen). Nanotechnology-based antibiotic carriers such as lipid nanoparticles [43], silica [44], and clay nanotubes [45] added to common cement material such as polymethyl methacrylate (PMMA) may enhance drug delivery and allow for timed release. Other types of non-antibiotic based nanotechnology cement additives such as chitosan, silver, and dendrimer are also under investigation for their antimicrobial properties [46]. Additionally, PMMA is well-known for eliciting an autoimmune response that can potentially lead to implant failure through fibrous encapsulation and inflammation [47]. Studies have found that the addition of nanostructured additives to PMMA demonstrated increased osseointegration and osteoblast activity [48, 49]. Ceramic particles such as zirconia and barium sulfate are often added to cements to allow for x-ray visualization, but these particles have a negative impact on the biocompatibility at the bone-implant interface [50]. Gilliani et al. showed that nanoscale modification of these particles added to bone cements increased cytocompatibility and decreased mechanical failure [50]. Collectively, these results demonstrate the positive impact nanotechnology may have on improving the efficacy of bone cements.

Sports medicine

Chondrogenesis

Repair of cartilage defects is a topic that has been under extensive investigation in the field of regenerative medicine. Adult cartilage tissue lacks the proper repair response needed for complete regeneration, which if left untreated will undergo progressive degeneration to osteoarthritis. Preclinical efforts using nanotechnology to augment MSC therapy (Fig. 5) by developing a biomcompatible scaffold that enhances native cartilage repair have seen early success. [51–56] Yaylaci et al. designed a hyaluronic acid analogue using nanofibers to facilitate MSC differentiation towards the proper chondrogenic lineage without associated toxicities of natural scaffolds [53]. Liu et al. designed a nanofibrous scaffold composed of polycaprolactone and gelatin that enhanced articular cartilage repair and subchondral bone regeneration using pluripotent stem cells [54]. Recently, Mahboudi et al. demonstrated that the use

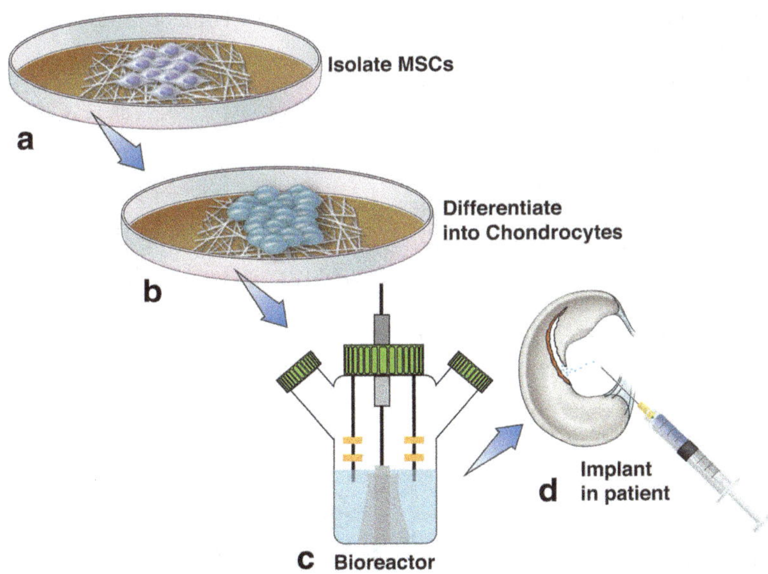

Fig. 5 Regenerative techniques using human MSCs to treat osteochondral defects have had limited success, however nanotechnology may enhance the efficacy of these therapies. This diagram demonstrates the typical sequence of events for MSC treatment using nanotechnology. MSCs are first harvested from the patient and cultured in a growth medium (**a**). Once differentiated into chondrocytes (**b**), these cells are implanted onto the desired scaffold material, cultured in a bioreactor (**c**), and reimplanted into the patient (**d**)

of nanofiber-based polyethersulfone scaffold significantly enhanced chondrogenic differentiation of MSCs [51]. Aside from the aforementioned studies, a wide variety of other scaffolds including injectable hydrogels [57] and peptide-based materials [52] are under investigation for treatment of cartilage defects. One pilot study involving 28 patients with osteochondral defects showed 70% of defects were completely filled at two-year follow-up using an osteochondral nanoscaffold graft [56]. Other clinical trials have demonstrated mixed results at 3 years follow-up [58], however further studies are underway to investigate the efficacy and safety of these scaffolds. Although nanotechnology in cartilage regeneration has not yet achieved widespread clinical use, the utilization of nanomaterials as scaffolds for regenerative tissue engineering has been shown to favorably affect cell adhesion, proliferation, and phenotypic selection of chondrocytes [59].

Tendon healing

Adhesion formation after tendon surgery remains a significant problem even with recent advances in surgical technique and post-operative care. Advances in nanotechnology and drug delivery may offer an appealing alternate to improve extrinsic and intrinsic tendon healing. Zhao et al. developed a strategy to allow for controlled release of mitomycin-C, a chemotherapy agent with the ability to decrease post-operative adhesions using hydrosol nanoparticles as drug carriers [60]. This allowed for reduction of tendon adhesion formation in vivo while maintaining comparable mechanical strength to naturally healed tendons. Tendon tissue engineering, particularly the through use of nanocomposite scaffolds, is another innovation that highlights the potential clinical value of nanotechnology in tendon healing. A plethora of different scaffolding materials are under investigation. Studies have shown that these scaffolds facilitate improved healing and mechanical stability and presentably fit the needs of regenerating tendons better than allografts [61–65]. Sharif-Aghdam et al. prepared a modified silk nanoscaffold that demonstrated excellent collagen content production and viability [66]. Huegel et al. showed that rat shoulders treated with autologous nanoscaffolds during supraspinatus repair surgery exhibited improved healing and mechanical stability [61]. Although tendon healing using nanotechnology has not yet reached the stage of clinical trials, research studies using tissue engineering techniques to simulate the bone-to-tendon interface are rampant [67–69].

Musculoskeletal trauma

Osteogenic properties of materials

Similar to arthroplasty, nanotechnology research in the field of orthopedic trauma is focused on improving osseointegration of implants and promotion of healthy bone growth following fracture or non-union treatment. The key to the potential success of nanostructured implants in trauma is surface modifications that allow for better simulation of natural bone environment than conventional implants. The goal of many research efforts is to engineer a bioactive scaffold for bone regeneration that will allow for faster healing time and recovery of function (Fig. 6). Nanofiber scaffolds have been observed to improve cell migration and growth during bone healing and many studies have demonstrated the osteogenic capability of these nanomaterials [70–74]. Nanostructuring of an array of materials including polymers, ceramics, composites, and metals are under immense investigation but are not yet used clinically due to unanswered concerns regarding clinical safety. Nanotechnology may also have the ability to aid in the management of nonunion defects by providing an acceptable alternative to bone allografting. Nanoengineered synthetic grafts that mimic native bone structure have shown pre-clinical success in their ability to provide adequate mechanical stability and enhance osteoblast adhesion [75, 76]. Nanosilicates, an ultra-thin nanomaterial, may also be helpful in the healing of bony defects. They have demonstrated excellent bone stiffness, porosity, and mineralization when added to collagen-based hydrogels [77]. The capability of nanomaterials to improve osseointegration of orthopedic implants and enhance osteogenesis highlights the potential future utility of these materials in the clinical setting.

Orthopedic infections

Infection remains a significant problem in the field of orthopedics and can lead to delayed healing, implant failure, and repeat surgery. Bacterial biofilms are often the source of infection and are definitively treated with

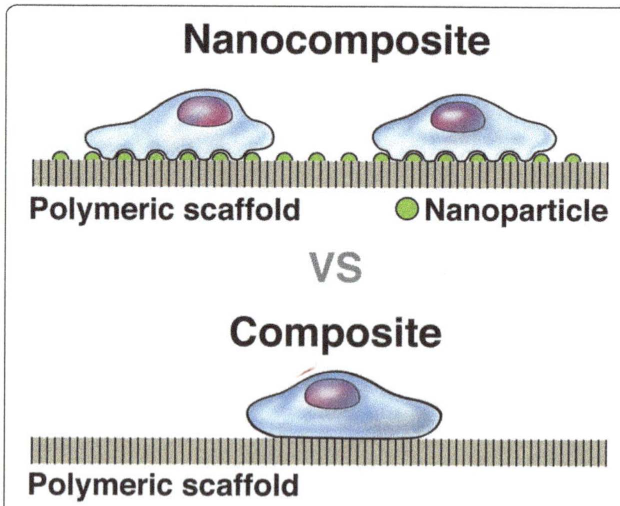

Fig. 6 This illustration highlights the elemental layout of a nanocomposite scaffold compared to a conventional composite. The addition of nanoparticles to the general structure allows for more effective adhesion of surrounding osteoblasts

implant removal. Therefore, recent efforts have focused on development of novel anti-biofilm implants equipped with nanoparticles. For example, titanium femoral stems incorporated with a novel vancomycin drug delivery system demonstrated sustained release for as long as 100 h [78]. Additionally, Besheli et al. showed that silk fibroin nanoparticles are effective in treating severe osteomyelitis in a controlled animal study [79].

Nanophase silver has become of significant interest in orthopedics over the past decade and is used clinically in wound care. Anti-microbial nanophase silver dressings have proven to be more effective at infection prevention and healing than conventional dressings [80]. Kose et al. developed a silver nanopowder coating that led to a decrease in bacterial colonization on coated titanium implants compared with uncoated [81]. Novel efforts investigating IL-12 as nanocoatings have shown promise in preventing open fracture-related infections, and may modulate immune responses to prevent infection [82]. Most recently, researchers developed a titanium pedicle screw coated with silver nanoparticles which has inhibited biofilm formation on the implanted screws in rabbits [83]. Overall, nanotechnology infection control efforts have demonstrated substantial promise to prevent acute post-operative infections in trauma and spinal implants in addition to joint replacements.

Potential concerns

Though early translational research efforts have demonstrated the incredible potential of nanomedicine, major barriers exist to its widespread implementation into orthopedic clinical practice. First, the long-term effect of nanomaterials on human health is poorly understood. Early research has shown that nanomaterials may be associated with brain and lung cytotoxicity, systemic inflammation, and oxidative stress [84]. However, other studies suggest that the products of nanomaterial metabolism may actually benefit bone and lung tissue health at the cellular level [85]. With such uncertainty comes the intense regulatory processes of clinical trials set forth by the United States Food and Drug Administration (FDA). In addition to the rigorous process of approval for human use, the monetary cost of clinical trials can amass hundreds of millions of dollars. The combination of these two obstacles may cause many medical device companies to be reluctant to invest millions of dollars in capital when adequate implants already exist on the market [86]. In total, only 3% of nanotechnology research funding since 2008 has gone towards investigating its health effects [3]. Taking these issues into consideration, extensive research will be needed to investigate potential toxicities of nanomaterials before they can become widely used clinically.

Another challenge is the mass production of nanomaterials. Some experts argue that the high volume manufacturing of materials less than three nanometers is not consistently reproducible due to the complex structural properties. Kelly et al. demonstrated that when these materials are mass-produced on such a small scale, there can be variation in the size of certain components as well as variation in the physical properties [87]. Hence, the low-cost, high-volume model of manufacturing may not be accomplishable with certain nanomaterials without sacrificing some degree of reproducibility.

Conclusion

Although still in its infancy, nanotechnology has the potential to revolutionize diagnostics, treatment, and research in orthopedics. The success of nanotech in commercial and service industries supports the expectation that the field will eventually play a significant role in clinical practice. Nanotechnology has the capability to inexpensively replace many conventional therapies and provide a multitude of novel applications. Nanotechnology offers more precise treatment modalities that may lead to more effective and longer lasting implants, decreased infection rates, and improved bone and tendon healing. Through immense basic science research efforts, the theoretical benefits of nanomedicine are beginning to be realized, specifically within the field of orthopedics. However, further investigations are needed to fully understand the safety and potential of this exciting technology.

Acknowledgements

The authors would like to thank and acknowledge David Fisher for contributing illustrations for our manuscript.

Funding

Not applicable.

Authors' contributions

WRS gathered and synthesized literature included in the manuscript and was a major contributor in writing the majority of the manuscript. PWH gathered and synthesized literature included in the manuscript and was a major contributor in writing the manuscript. BAP was a contributor in writing and editing the manuscript. SRRM was a contributor in writing and editing the manuscript. All authors read and approved the final manuscript.

Consent for publication

Not applicable.

Competing interests

SRRM is a member of the Editorial Board of BMC Musculoskeletal Disorders. The other authors declare that they have no competing interests.

Author details

[1]Department of Orthopaedic Surgery, University of Alabama at Birmingham, 1313 13 St. South, Birmingham, AL 35205, USA. [2]Department of Orthopaedic Surgery, University of Alabama at Birmingham, FOT 950, 20 Street South, Birmingham, AL 35294, USA.

References

1. Health Quality Ontario. Nanotechnology: an evidence-based analysis. Ontario Health Tech Assessment Series. 2006;6(19):1–43.
2. Feynman R. There's plenty of room at the bottom. Eng Sci. 1960;23:22–36.
3. Sullivan MP, McHale KJ, Parvizi J, Mehta S. Nanotechnology: current concepts in orthopaedic surgery and future directions. Bone Joint J. 2014; 96-B(5):569–73.
4. Pleshko N, Grande DA, Myers KR. Nanotechnology in orthopaedics. J Am Acad Orthop Surg. 2012;20(1):60–2.
5. Gusić N, Ivković A, VaFaye J, Vukasović A, Ivković J, Hudetz D, Janković S. Nanobiotechnology and bone regeneration: a mini-review. Int Orthop. 2014; 38(9):1877–84.
6. Zhang ZG, Li ZH, Mao XZ, Wang WC. Advances in bone repair with nanobiomaterials: mini-review. Cytotechnology. 2011;63(5):437–43.
7. Sichert JA, Tong Y, Mutz N, Vollmer M, Fischer S, Milowska KZ, García Cortadella R, Nickel B, Cardenas-Daw C, Stolarczyk JK, Urban AS, Feldmann J. Quantum Size Effect in Organometal Halide Perovskite Nanoplatelets. Nano Lett 2015; 15(10):6521–6527. https://doi.org/10.1021/acs.nanolett.5b02985. Epub 2015 Sep 3. PubMed PMID: 26327242.
8. Karazisis D, Ballo AM, Petronis S, Agheli H, Emanuelsson L, Thomsen P, Omar O. The role of well-defined nanotopography of titanium implants on osseointegration: cellular and molecular events in vivo. Int J Nanomedicine 2016;11:1367–1382. doi: https://doi.org/10.2147/IJN.S101294. eCollection 2016. PubMed PMID: 27099496.
9. Mattei TA, Rehman AA. 'Extremely minimally invasive': recent advances in nanotechnology research and future applications in neurosurgery. Neurosurg Rev 2015;38(1):27–37; discussion 37. https://doi.org/10.1007/s10143-014-0566-2. Epub 2014 Aug 31. Review. PubMed PMID: 25173621.
10. Wong KK, Liu XL. Nanomedicine: a primer for surgeons. Pediatr Surg Int 2012;28(10):943–951. Epub 2012 Aug 15. Review. PubMed PMID: 22892910.
11. Korkusuz F. Editorial comment: Nanoscience in musculoskeletal medicine. Clin Orthop Relat Res. 2013;471(8):2530–1.
12. Yorimitsu E, Chiba K, Toyama Y, Hirabayashi K. Long-term outcomes of standard discectomy for lumbar disc herniation: a follow-up study of more than 10 years. Spine (Phila Pa 1976). 2001;26(6):652–7.
13. Antunes JC, Pereira CL, Teixeira GQ, Silva RV, Caldeira J, Grad S, Gonçalves RM, Barbosa MA. Poly(γ-glutamic acid) and poly(γ-glutamic acid)-based nanocomplexes enhance type II collagen production in intervertebral disc. J Mater Sci Mater Med 2017;28(1):6. Epub 2016 Nov 24. PubMed PMID: 27885573.
14. Teixeira GQ, Leite Pereira C, Castro F, Ferreira JR, Gomez-Lazaro M, Aguiar P, Barbosa MA, Neidlinger-Wilke C, Goncalves RM. Anti-inflammatory chitosan/poly-γ-glutamic acid nanoparticles control inflammation while remodeling extracellular matrix in degenerated intervertebral disc. Acta Biomater. 2016; 42:168–79. https://doi.org/10.1016/j.actbio.2016.06.013.
15. Cui X, Liu M, Wang J, Zhou Y, Xiang Q. Electrospun scaffold containing TGF-β1 promotes human mesenchymal stem cell differentiation towards a nucleus pulposus-like phenotype under hypoxia. IET Nanobiotechnol. 2015;9(2):76–84.
16. Richardson SM, Kalamegam G, Pushparaj PN, Matta C, Memic A, Khademhosseini A, Mobasheri R, Poletti FL, Hoyland JA, Mobasheri A. Mesenchymal stem cells in regenerative medicine: focus on articular cartilage and intervertebral disc regeneration. Methods. 2016;99:69–80.
17. Dalamagkas K, Tsintou M, Seifalian A. Advances in peripheral nervous system regenerative therapeutic strategies: a biomaterials approach. Mater Sci Eng C Mater Biol Appl. 2016;65:425–32.
18. Kwak S, Haider A, Gupta KC, Kim S, Kang IK. Micro/Nano multilayered scaffolds of PLGA and collagen by alternately electrospinning for bone tissue engineering. Nanoscale Res Lett 2016;11(1):323. https://doi.org/10.1186/s11671-016-1532-4. Epub 2016 Jul 4. PubMed PMID: 27376895.
19. Hsu WK, Goldstein CL, Shamji MF, Cho SK, Arnold PM, Fehlings MG, Mroz TE. Novel Osteobiologics and biomaterials in the treatment of spinal disorders. Neurosurgery 2017;80(3S):S100-S107. doi: https://doi.org/10.1093/neuros/nyw085. Review. PubMed PMID: 28350951.
20. Ganau M, Holly LT, Mizuno J, Fehlings MG. Future directions and new Technologies for the Management of degenerative cervical myelopathy. Neurosurg Clin N Am. 2018;29(1):185–93. https://doi.org/10.1016/j.nec.2017.09.006.
21. Titan Spine Initiates Full U.S. Launch of New nanoLOCK® Surface Technology. Business Wire (2016). Available at: https://www.businesswire.com/news/home/20161013006094/en/Titan-Spine-Initiates-Full-U.S.-Launch-New. (Accessed: 10 Jan 2017).
22. Olivares-Navarrete R, Hyzy SL, Slosar PJ, Schneider JM, Schwartz Z, Boyan BD. Implant materials generate different peri-implant inflammatory factors: poly-ether-ether-ketone promotes fibrosis and microtextured titanium promotes osteogenic factors. Spine (Phila Pa 1976). 2015;40(6):399–404.
23. Hsu WK, Polavarapu M, Riaz R, Larson AC, Diegmueller JJ, Ghodasra JH, Hsu EL. Characterizing the host response to rhBMP-2 in a rat spinal arthrodesis model. Spine (Phila Pa 1976) 2013;38(12):E691–E698. https://doi.org/10.1097/BRS.0b013e31828cb977. PubMed PMID: 23429681.
24. Kannan A, Dodward SN, Hsu WK. Biologics in spine arthrodesis. J Spinal Disord Tech. 2015;28(5):163–70.
25. Lee SS, Hsu EL, Mendoza M, et al. Gel scaffolds of BMP-2 binding peptide amphiphile nanofibers for spinal arthrodesis. Adv Healthc Mater. 2015;4(1): 131–41.
26. Li L, Liang S, Wasylishen AR, Zhang Y, Yang X, Zhou B, Shan L, Han X, Mu T, Wang G, Xiong S. PLA2G16 promotes osteosarcoma metastasis and drug resistance via the MAPK pathway. Oncotarget. 2016;7(14):18021–18035. doi: https://doi.org/10.18632/oncotarget.7694. PubMed PMID: 26933804.
27. Savvidou OD, Bolia IK, Chloros GD, Goumenos SD, Sakellariou VI, Galanis EC, Papagelopoulos PJ. Applied nanotechnology and nanoscience in orthopedic oncology. Orthopedics. 2016;39(5):280–6.
28. Cheng H, Chawla A, Yang Y, Li Y, Zhang J, Jang HL, Khademhosseini A. Development of nanomaterials for bone-targeted drug delivery. Drug Discov Today 2017;22(9):1336–1350. doi: https://doi.org/10.1016/j.drudis.2017.04.021. Epub 2017 May 6. Review. PubMed PMID: 28487069.
29. Susa M, Milane L, Amiji MM, Hornicek FJ, Duan Z. Nanoparticles: a promising modality in the treatment of sarcomas. Pharm Res. 2011;28(2):260–72.
30. Patlolla RR, Vobalaboina V. Folate-targeted etoposide-encapsulated lipid nanospheres. J Drug Target. 2008;16(4):269–75.
31. Athawale RB, Jain DS, Singh KK, Gude RP. Etoposide loaded solid lipid nanoparticles for curtailing B16F10 melanoma colonization in lung. Biomed Pharmacother. 2014;68(2):231–40.
32. Sun W, Han Y, Li Z, Ge K, Zhang J. Bone-targeted mesoporous silica Nanocarrier anchored by Zoledronate for cancer bone metastasis. Langmuir. 2016;32(36):9237–44. https://doi.org/10.1021/acs.langmuir.6b02228.
33. Liu L, Qi XJ, Zhong ZK, Zhang EN. Nanomedicine-based combination of gambogic acid and retinoic acid chlorochalcone for enhanced anticancer efficacy in osteosarcoma. Biomed Pharmacother. 2016;83: 79–84. https://doi.org/10.1016/j.biopha.2016.06.001.
34. Zhou H, Wang G, Lu Y, Pan Z. Bio-inspired cisplatin nanocarriers for osteosarcoma treatment. Biomater Sci. 2016;4(8):1212–8. https://doi.org/10.1039/c6bm00331a.
35. Tran PA, Sarin L, Hurt RH, Webster TJ. Differential effects of nanoselenium doping on healthy and cancerous osteoblasts in coculture on titanium. Int J Nanomedicine. 2010;5:351–8.
36. Nayak S, Bhushan B, Jayaganthan R, Gopinath P, Agarwal RD, Lahiri D. Strengthening of mg based alloy through grain refinement for orthopaedic application. J Mech Behav Biomed Mater. 2016;59:57–70. https://doi.org/10.1016/j.jmbbm.2015.12.010.
37. Yu C, Wang W. Relationship between P15 gene mutation and formation and metastasis of malignant osteosarcoma. Med Sci Monit. 2016;22:656–61.
38. Hennig S, van de Linde S, Lummer M, Simonis M, Huser T, Sauer M. Instant live-cell super-resolution imaging of cellular structures by nanoinjection of fluorescent probes. Nano Lett. 2015;15(2):1374–81.

39. Young JK, Figueroa ER, Drezek RA. Tunable nanostructures as photothermal theranostic agents. Ann Biomed Eng. 2012;40(2):438–59.
40. Serra G, Morais L, Elias CN, Semenova IP, Valiev R, Salimgareeva G, Pithon M, Lacerda R. Nanostructured severe plastic deformation processed titanium for orthodontic mini-implants. Mater Sci Eng C Mater Biol Appl. 2013;33(7):4197–202.
41. Puértolas JA, Kurtz SM. Evaluation of carbon nanotubes and graphene as reinforcements for UHMWPE-based composites in arthroplastic applications: a review. J Mech Behav Biomed Mater. 2014;39:129–45.
42. Swearingen MC, Granger JF, Sullivan A, Stoodley P. Elution of antibiotics from poly(methyl methacrylate) bone cement after extended implantation does not necessarily clear the infection despite susceptibility of the clinical isolates. Pathog Dis. 2016;74(1):ftv103.
43. Ayre WN, Birchall JC, Evans SL, Denyer SP. A novel liposomal drug delivery system for PMMA bone cements. J Biomed Mater Res B Appl Biomater. 2016;104(8):1510–24.
44. Shen SC, Ng WK, Dong YC, Ng J, Tan RB. Nanostructured material formulated acrylic bone cements with enhanced drug release. Mater Sci Eng C Mater Biol Appl. 2016;58:233–41.
45. Wei W, Abdullayev E, Hollister A, Mills D, Lvov YM. Clay nanotube/poly(methyl methacrylate) bone cement composites with sustained antibiotic release. Macromol Mater Eng. 2012;297:645–53. https://doi.org/10.1002/mame.201100309.
46. Al Thaher Y, Perni S, Prokopovich P. Nano-carrier based drug delivery systems for sustained antimicrobial agent release from orthopaedic cementous material. Adv Colloid Interf Sci. 2017;249:234–47.
47. Frick C, Dietz AC, Merritt K, Umbreit TH, Tomazic-Jezic VJ. Effects of prosthetic materials on the host immune response: evaluation of polymethyl-methacrylate (PMMA), polyethylene (PE), and polystyrene (PS) particles. J Long-Term Eff Med Implants. 2006;16(6):423–33.
48. No YJ, Roohani-Esfahani SI, Zreiqat H. Nanomaterials: the next step in injectable bone cements. Nanomed (Lond). 2014;9(11):1745–64.
49. Ricker A, Liu-Snyder P, Webster TJ. The influence of nano MgO and BaSO4 particle size additives on properties of PMMA bone cement. Int J Nanomedicine. 2008;3(1):125–32.
50. Gillani R, Ercan B, Qiao A, Webster TJ. Nanofunctionalized zirconia and barium sulfate particles as bone cement additives. Int J Nanomedicine. 2010;5:1–11.
51. Mahboudi H, Kazemi B, Soleimani M, Hanaee-Ahvaz H, Ghanbarian H, Bandehpour M, Enderami SE, Kehtari M, Barati G. Enhanced chondrogenesis of human bone marrow mesenchymal stem cell (BMSC) on nanofiber-based polyethersulfone (PES) scaffold. Gene. 2018;643:98–106. https://doi.org/10.1016/j.gene.2017.11.073.
52. Hastar N, Arslan E, Guler MO, Tekinay AB. Peptide-based materials for cartilage tissue regeneration. Adv Exp Med Biol 2017;1030:155–166. doi: https://doi.org/10.1007/978-3-319-66095-0_7. PubMed PMID: 29081053.
53. Ustun Yaylaci S, Sardan Ekiz M, Arslan E, Can N, Kilic E, Ozkan H, Orujalipoor I, Ide S, Tekinay AB, Guler MO. Supramolecular GAG-like self-assembled Glycopeptide nanofibers induce Chondrogenesis and cartilage regeneration. Biomacromolecules. 2016;17(2):679–89.
54. Liu J, Nie H, Xu Z, Niu X, Guo S, Yin J, Guo F, Li G, Wang Y, Zhang C. The effect of 3D nanofibrous scaffolds on the chondrogenesis of induced pluripotent stem cells and their application in restoration of cartilage defects. PLoS One. 2014;9(11):e111566.
55. Tampieri A, Sandri M, Landi E, Pressato D, Francioli S, Quarto R, Martin I. Design of graded biomimetic osteochondral composite scaffolds. Biomaterials. 2008;29(26):3539–46.
56. Kon E, Delcogliano M, Filardo G, Busacca M, Di Martino A, Marcacci M. Novel nano-composite multilayered biomaterial for osteochondral regeneration: a pilot clinical trial. Am J Sports Med. 2011;39(6):1180–90.
57. Liu M, Zeng X, Ma C, Yi H, Ali Z, Mou X, Li S, Deng Y, He N. Injectable hydrogels for cartilage and bone tissue engineering. Bone Res. 2017;5:17014. https://doi.org/10.1038/boneres.2017.
58. Christensen BB, Foldager CB, Jensen J, Jensen NC, Lind M. Poor osteochondral repair by a biomimetic collagen scaffold: 1- to 3-year clinical and radiological follow-up. Knee Surg Sports Traumatol Arthrosc. 2016;24(7):2380–7.
59. Parchi PD, Vittorio O, Andreani L, Piolanti N, Cirillo G, et al. How nanotechnology can really improve the future of orthopedic implants and scaffolds for bone and cartilage defects. J Nanomed Biotherapeutic Discov. 2013;3:114.
60. Zhao X, Jiang S, Liu S, Chen S, Lin ZY, Pan G, He F, Li F, Fan C, Cui W. Optimization of intrinsic and extrinsic tendon healing through controllable water-soluble mitomycin-C release from electrospun fibers by mediating adhesion-related gene expression. Biomaterials. 2015;61:61–74.
61. Huegel J, Kim DH, Cirone JM, Pardes AM, Morris TR, Nuss CA, Mauck RL, Soslowsky LJ, Kuntz AF. Autologous tendon-derived cell-seeded nanofibrous scaffolds improve rotator cuff repair in an age-dependent fashion. J Orthop Res. 2017;35(6):1250–1257.
62. Verdiyeva G, Koshy K, Glibbery N, Mann H, Seifalian AM. Tendon reconstruction with tissue engineering approach–a review. J Biomed Nanotechnol. 2015;11(9):1495–523.
63. Nezakati T, Tan A, Seifalian AM. Enhancing the electrical conductivity of a hybrid POSS-PCL/graphene nanocomposite polymer. J Colloid Interface Sci. 2014;435:145–55.
64. Ahmed M, Hamilton G, Seifalian AM. The performance of a small-calibre graft for vascular reconstructions in a senescent sheep model. Biomaterials. 2014;35(33):9033–40.
65. Nayyer L, Birchall M, Seifalian AM, Jell G. Design and development of nanocomposite scaffolds for auricular reconstruction. Nanomedicine. 2014;10(1):235–46.
66. Sharifi-Aghdam M, Faridi-Majidi R, Derakhshan MA, Chegeni A, Azami M. Preparation of collagen/polyurethane/knitted silk as a composite scaffold for tendon tissue engineering. Proc Inst Mech Eng H. 2017;231(7):652–62.
67. Silva ED, Babo PS, Costa-Almeida R, Domingues RMA, Mendes BB, Paz E, Freitas P, Rodrigues MT, Granja PL, Gomes ME. Multifunctional magnetic-responsive hydrogels to engineer tendon-to-bone interface. Nanomedicine. 2017: S1549-S9634(17)30108-9. doi: https://doi.org/10.1016/j.nano.2017.06.002.
68. Baldino L, Cardea S, Maffulli N, Reverchon E. Regeneration techniques for bone-to-tendon and muscle-to-tendon interfaces reconstruction. Br Med Bull. 2016;117(1):25–37. https://doi.org/10.1093/bmb/ldv056.
69. Gonçalves AI, Rodrigues MT, Carvalho PP, Bañobre-López M, Paz E, Freitas P, Gomes ME. Exploring the potential of starch/Polycaprolactone aligned magnetic responsive scaffolds for tendon regeneration. Adv Healthc Mater. 2016;5(2):213–22. https://doi.org/10.1002/adhm.201500623.
70. Schofer MD, Roessler PP, Schaefer J, Theisen C, Schlimme S, Heverhagen JT, Voelker M, Dersch R, Agarwal S, Fuchs-Winkelmann S, Paletta JR. Electrospun PLLA nanofiber scaffolds and their use in combination with BMP-2 for reconstruction of bone defects. PLoS One. 2011;6(9):e25462.
71. Schiavi J, Keller L, Morand DN, De Isla N, Huck O, Lutz JC, Mainard D, Schwinté P, Benkirane-Jessel N. Active implant combining human stem cell microtissues and growth factors for bone-regenerative nanomedicine. Nanomedicine (Lond). 2015;10(5):753–63.
72. Cao X, Yu WQ, Qiu J, Zhao YF, Zhang YL, Zhang FQ. RGD peptide immobilized on TiO2 nanotubes for increased bone marrow stromal cells adhesion and osteogenic gene expression. J Mater Sci Mater Med. 2012;23(2):527–36.
73. Minardi S, Corradetti B, Taraballi F, Sandri M, Van Eps J, Cabrera FJ, Weiner BK, Tampieri A, Tasciotti E. Evaluation of the osteoinductive potential of a bio-inspired scaffold mimicking the osteogenic niche for bone augmentation. Biomaterials. 2015;62:128–37.
74. Nair M, Nancy D, Krishnan AG, Anjusree GS, Vadukumpully S, Nair SV. Graphene oxide nanoflakes incorporated gelatin-hydroxyapatite scaffolds enhance osteogenic differentiation of human mesenchymal stem cells. Nanotechnology. 2015;26(16):161001.
75. Zhang L, Ramsaywack S, Fenniri H, Webster TJ. Enhanced osteoblast adhesion on self-assembled nanostructured hydrogel scaffolds. Tissue Eng Part A. 2008;14(8):1353–64.
76. Zhang L, Rodriguez J, Raez J, Myles AJ, Fenniri H, Webster TJ. Biologically inspired rosette nanotubes and nanocrystalline hydroxyapatite hydrogel nanocomposites as improved bone substitutes. Nanotechnology. 2009;20(17):175101.
77. Xavier JR, Thakur T, Desai P, Jaiswal MK, Sears N, Cosgriff-Hernandez E, Kaunas R, Gaharwar AK. Bioactive nanoengineered hydrogels for bone tissue engineering: a growth-factor-free approach. ACS Nano. 2015;9(3):3109–18.
78. Bezuidenhout MB, Dimitrov DM, van Staden AD, Oosthuizen GA, Dicks LM. Titanium-based hip stems with drug delivery functionality through additive manufacturing. Biomed Res Int 2015;2015:134093. doi: https://doi.org/10.1155/2015/134093. Epub 2015 Oct 4. Review. PubMed PMID: 26504776.

79. Hassani Besheli N, Mottaghitalab F, Eslami M, Gholami M, Kundu SC, Kaplan DL, Farokhi M. Sustainable release of vancomycin from silk fibroin nanoparticles for treating severe bone infection in rat tibia osteomyelitis model. ACS Appl Mater Interfaces. 2017;9(6):5128–38.
80. Jia Z, Xiu P, Li M, Xu X, Shi Y, Cheng Y, Wei S, Zheng Y, Xi T, Cai H, Liu Z. Bioinspired anchoring AgNPs onto micro-nanoporous TiO2 orthopedic coatings: trap-killing of bacteria, surface-regulated osteoblast functions and host responses. Biomaterials. 2016;75:203–22.
81. Kose N, Çaylak R, Pekşen C, Kiremitçi A, Burukoglu D, Koparal S, Doğan A. Silver ion doped ceramic nano-powder coated nails prevent infection in open fractures: in vivo study. Injury. 2016;47(2):320–4.
82. Li B, Jiang B, Dietz MJ, Smith ES, Clovis NB, Rao KM. Evaluation of local MCP-1 and IL-12 nanocoatings for infection prevention in open fractures. J Orthop Res. 2010;28(1):48–54.
83. Hazer DB, Sakar M, Dere Y, Altinkanat G, Ziyal MI, Hazer B. Antimicrobial effect of polymer-based silver nanoparticle coated pedicle screws: experimental research on biofilm inhibition in rabbits. Spine (Phila Pa 1976). 2016;41(6):E323–9.
84. Polyzois I, Nikolopoulos D, Michos I, Patsouris E, Theocharis S. Local and systemic toxicity of nanoscale debris particles in total hip arthroplasty. J Appl Toxicol. 2012;32(4):255–69.
85. Sato M, Webster TJ. Nanobiotechnology: implications for the future of nanotechnology in orthopedic applications. Expert Rev Med Devices. 2004;1(1):105–14.
86. Nodzo SR, Hohman DW, Chakravarthy K. Nanotechnology: why should we care? Am J Orthop (Belle Mead NJ) 2015;44(3):E87–E88. PubMed PMID: 25750958.
87. Kelly MJ, Dean MC. A specific nanomanufacturing challenge. Nanotechnology. 2016;27(11):112501. https://doi.org/10.1088/0957-4484/27/11/112501.

14

Acceptability of a digital health intervention alongside physiotherapy to support patients following anterior cruciate ligament reconstruction

Emma Dunphy[1,2*], Fiona L. Hamilton[1], Irena Spasić[3] and Kate Button[4,5]

Abstract

Background: Physiotherapy rehabilitation following surgical reconstruction to the Anterior Cruciate Ligament (ACL) can take up to 12 months to complete. Given the lengthy rehabilitation process, a blended intervention can be used to compliment face-to-face physiotherapy with a digital exercise intervention. In this study, we used TRAK, a web–based tool that has been developed to support knee rehabilitation, which provides individually tailored exercise programs with videos, instructions and progress logs for each exercise, relevant health information and a contact option that allows a patient to email a physiotherapist for additional support. The aim of this study was to evaluate the acceptability of TRAK–based blended intervention in post ACL reconstruction rehabilitation.

Methods: A qualitative research design using semi-structured interviews was used on a convenience sample of participants following an ACL reconstruction, and their treating physiotherapists, in a London NHS hospital. Participants were asked to use TRAK alongside face-to-face physiotherapy for 16 weeks. Interviews were carried out, audio recorded, transcribed verbatim and coded by two researchers independently. Data were analyzed using thematic analysis.

Results: Of the 25 individuals that were approached to be part of the study, 24 consented, comprising 8 females and 16 males, mean age 30 years. 17 individuals used TRAK for 16 weeks and were available for interview. Four physiotherapists were also interviewed. The six main themes identified from patients were: the experience of TRAK rehabilitation, personal characteristics for engagement, strengths and weaknesses of the intervention, TRAK in the future and attitudes to digital healthcare. The main themes from the physiotherapist interviews were: potential benefits, availability of resources and service organization to support use of TRAK.

Conclusions: TRAK was found to be an acceptable method of delivering ACL rehabilitation alongside face-to-face physiotherapy. Patients reported that TRAK, specifically the videos, increased their confidence and motivation with their rehabilitation. They identified ways in which TRAK could be developed in the future to meet technological expectations and further support rehabilitation. For Physiotherapists time and availability of computers affected acceptability. Organization of care to support integration of digital exercise interventions such as TRAK into a blended approach to rehabilitation is required.

Keywords: Anterior cruciate ligament, Physiotherapy, Surgery, Rehabilitation, E-health, Internet

* Correspondence: emma.dunphy@ucl.ac.uk
[1]E-Health Unit, Research Department of Primary Care and Population Health, Upper Third Floor UCL Medical School (Royal Free Campus), Rowland Hill Street, NW3 2PF, London, UK
[2]Homerton University Hospital NHS Trust, Homerton Row E96SR, London, UK
Full list of author information is available at the end of the article

Background

Anterior cruciate ligament (ACL) injury represents a significant burden of serious knee injuries. An American study estimates that 100,000 ACL reconstructions are performed per year [1]. A UK based study estimates that in a 'catchment area of 400,000 population, accident and emergency departments can expect to see two acute ACL injuries per week [2]. There is a significant commitment to rehabilitation required for patients who wish to return to an active, athletic life [3–5].

There are many protocols for ACL rehabilitation available and evidence for both physical and psychological recovery continues to inform best practice in optimizing function [5–10]. Still, a high percentage of individuals never return to their pre-injury level of function [3, 6, 11–14]. Potential reasons for this are loss of confidence and self-efficacy [6, 11, 15] combined with poor engagement with the rehabilitation process [16], which is known to be lengthy in nature, often requiring commitment for a year or more [14]. Patients struggle with motivation, compliance and a clear understanding of what is recommended at each stage of their recovery [5, 16]. Patient knowledge and engagement are key to successful rehabilitation [17]. There is evidence to suggest that digital tools can support engagement with healthcare [18–22]. Patients can use the Internet to gain access to correct information and utilize digital tools such as progress logs and personalized prompts in order to be informed, motivated and encouraged [21, 23, 24]. One such tool is TRAK, a digital intervention developed to support self-management of knee conditions [24, 25]. TRAK, provides a platform for individually tailored exercise programs with videos, detailed instructions and progress logs for individual exercises, a health information section, and a contact option that allows a patient to email a physiotherapist for additional support. TRAK has recently been modified with specific content for ACL rehabilitation based on the best available evidence [4, 5, 9, 10, 16, 26]. The ACL-specific version of TRAK includes over 200 new exercise videos, mostly to support advanced stages of physiotherapy including return to sport activities. These exercises (see Fig. 1 for an example), target modifiable factors such as strength, neuromuscular control, motor learning, sport specific skills and fatigue resistance, and are specifically tailored to an ACL population of patients, who tend to be younger and more active, and therefore have higher expectations regarding knee function [27]. ACL-related health information focuses on managing expectations given a lengthy recovery process by providing detailed information, milestones and common problems associated with each stage of rehabilitation.

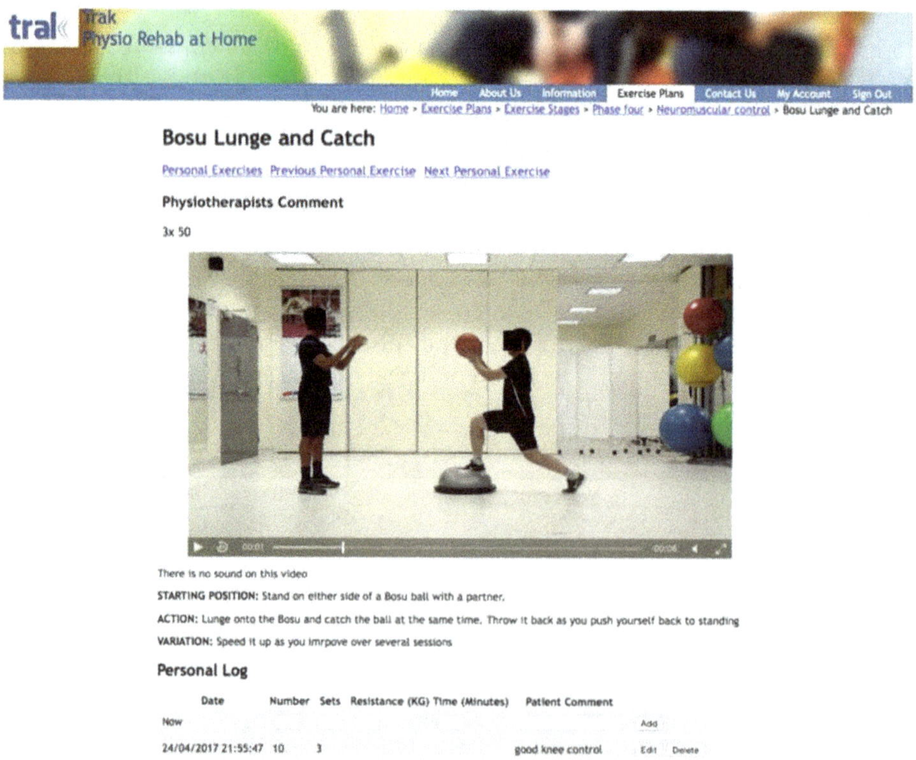

Fig. 1 A description of a neuromuscular control exercise in Phase 4 of rehabilitation where the goal is return to sport activities. (From TRAK website with permission)

As part of the development and testing of digital interventions, we need to understand the relationship between individuals' initial reactions to newly developed online interventions, the intention to use it and their actual use [28]. The usability study conducted for the initial version of TRAK, which was implemented originally as a Facebook app, suggested that a digital exercise intervention would facilitate communication, provide information, help recall information, improve understanding, enable exercise progression, and support self-management in general [24]. These finding were subsequently confirmed when a new version of TRAK re–implemented as web–based app (which is also the version discussed in this study) was integrated into routine healthcare and evaluated for its impact on the patient, clinician and organization [25, 29]. The aim of the current study, however, was to evaluate the acceptability of TRAK to a specific patient population – those following ACL reconstruction, whose rehabilitation on average takes 12 months to complete and, therefore, may struggle with long–term engagement. In addition to patients themselves, we also evaluated the acceptability of TRAK to physiotherapists. These findings will be used to inform more effective integration of TRAK into a blended exercise intervention, which should capture patients' needs over an extended duration of recovery pathway.

Methods

Patient public involvement

Patients and the public were involved in the early development of this study by suggesting exercise content appropriate to their rehabilitation goals. They participated in the filming of videos and gave consent for public use of these videos. They informed the study methodology by suggesting that a trial period of usage who be suitable to assess the website acceptability. This was not the group of patients who were the recruited to the study.

Study design

This research was done with qualitative methods using semi-structured interviews to ascertain the acceptability of TRAK to a population receiving rehabilitation following ACL reconstruction as well as their treating physiotherapists, who were based at one London NHS hospital. Five physiotherapists were trained on how to use TRAK and integrate it into patient care alongside face-to-face physiotherapy. They then used TRAK for four months with a group of patients who were at varying stages following ACL reconstruction. After four months semi-structured interviews were conducted by lead researcher ED, at a location convenient to both types of participants. The interviews focused on the overall experience of ACL rehabilitation and in particular experience of using TRAK. In relation to the latter, we examined the influence of contextual factors related to acceptability of new digital tools including performance expectancy, effort expectancy, social influence, facilitating conditions, self-efficacy, anxiety and behavioral intentions [28].

Standard ACL rehabilitation pathway

All patients who undergo ACL reconstruction are invited to follow a standard ACL rehabilitation pathway, which has been designed around published evidence and is delivered in a group format. [5, 7–10, 16, 26, 30]. This pathway consists of four rehabilitation stages (Table 1.). Progression through the stages is based on pre-set functional criteria. Treatment is delivered within a group environment. Individual consultations are provided for within that structure. Exercise prescription is individually tailored and in line with American College of Sports Medicine guidance [31].

There is a significant variety in patients' individual experiences and goals. TRAK rehabilitation is designed so that it can reflect any individual's pathway within these stages. It is designed to facilitate improved engagement, confidence, motivation and self-efficacy away from the class. The personalized exercise plans with videos, exercise log, information and remote e-mail support for any questions or concerns are in addition to the standard care ACL program.

Sample selection and recruitment

This study took place in a London hospital with an NHS caseload of predominantly recreational athletes. All patients were recruited from the physiotherapy department, where they were receiving treatment following ACL reconstructive surgery. Between two and four new ACL patients are referred weekly from orthopedics. A convenience sample method was used: patients were recruited from all stages of the physiotherapy post-operative ACL pathway (see Fig. 2). The inclusion criteria were: all patients on the ACL pathway who could freely consent, were over 18 years old, who spoke English fluently and had access to a smartphone. The

Table 1 Stages of ACL rehabilitation in standard care

Stage 1, 0–6 weeks approximately, depending on milestones achieved: focuses on restoration of active range of motion, muscle activation, gait and the management of swelling, pain and wound healing.
Stage 2, 6 weeks to 3 months approximately, depending on milestones achieved: weekly classes which initiate strength training and neuromuscular control.
Stage 3, from 3 months approximately, depending on milestones achieved: strength gains are consolidated and motor control is challenged with increasing dynamic activity. Some participants will complete care and return to sport in this stage where goals do not include cutting and pivoting activities such football, hockey, dancing etc.
Stage 4, from 6 months approximately, depending on milestones achieved: advanced sports specific skills and movement patterns are trained toward patient goals.

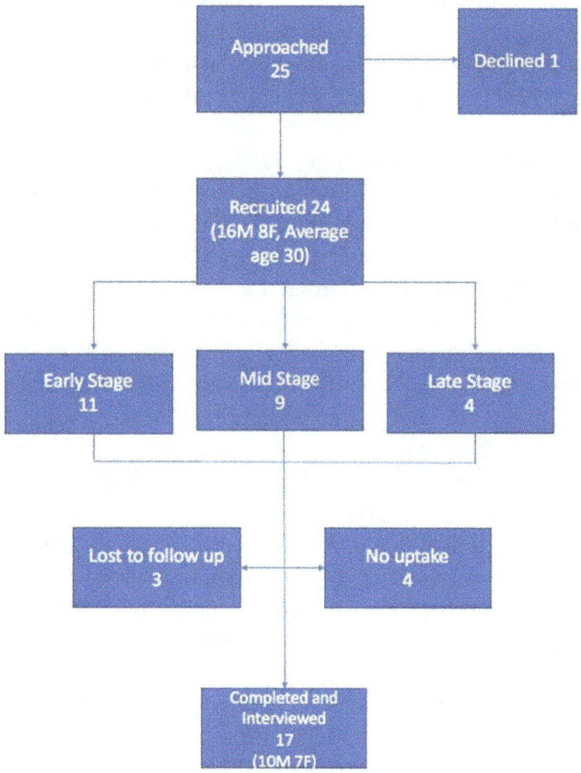

Fig. 2 Sample and Recruitment

exclusion criteria were: patients with multi-ligament reconstruction, revision ACL surgery or fractures, or patients with a poor command of English. Twenty-five patients were asked to take part in the study. One patient declined participation because of time concerns. A sample of 24 patients was recruited. Four patients withdrew from the study due to time constraints. Seventeen patients completed the study and were interviewed. Following provision of an information leaflet and obtaining written informed consent, participants were trained on how to use TRAK by their treating physiotherapist who provided them with a personalized exercise plan. This was delivered in a one-to-one session and patients were offered informal user guidance as needed.

The Principal Investigator (PI) was one of 5 treating physiotherapists in the ACL group from Band 5, 6 and 7 level of experience. Thirteen participants knew the PI before being recruited but were unaware of any role or motivation in the study. Physiotherapist training on how to use TRAK as part of the standard care took place over a 30 min period in a group session led by the lead researcher. The TRAK exercise programs were maintained and updated by all physiotherapists involved in the group.

Data collection

Semi-structured interviews took place at a convenient time and place for the participants, at the hospital, over the phone and in two cases at an agreed, appropriate public place. All physiotherapists were interviewed in the physiotherapy department. All interviews were digitally audio recorded and transcribed verbatim by the lead researcher. All interviews were participant and PI only.

The interview questions were guided by topics that arose in previous related studies and from ongoing informed discussion within the research team [20, 24, 25]. The topic guide was minimally refined throughout the process to responds to emerging data.

Data analysis

Data from the interviews were analyzed using pragmatic thematic analysis to inform factors that relate to acceptability of new digital tools like TRAK. This sees the data itself rather than the theory driving the process. The themes emerging from the interviews are grouped stringently so all the interview data relating to a particular theme are recorded. Data are weighted and reported secondary to frequency of occurrence or explanatory value [32]. The data were analyzed and coded by the principal investigator and separately coded by another team member. Saturation of data was agreed upon. A dialectic process followed until agreement was reached. Data are presented in the results as a descriptive narrative to reflect the patient and physiotherapist experience [32].

Results

Ten male and seven female patients with an average age of 30 were interviewed. Four Physiotherapists were also interviewed. The patient and physiotherapists interviews have been reported separately to illustrate with clarity how using TRAK alongside face-to-face physiotherapy was experienced by patients and physiotherapists. Key quotes from the interviews are included to express the specific words of the participants. The results show how and why users accept or do not accept TRAK. They explore in particular, performance and effort expectancy, social conditions and environment, self-efficacy, anxiety and behavioral intentions relating to the combination of TRAK with standard care [28].

Patient interviews

Theme 1 – Experiences of the blended approach of standard ACL rehabilitation with TRAK

Using TRAK blended with standard physiotherapy enhanced the patient experience for most participants. The blended combination of their face-to-face care and the use of the website to support self-management gave patients access to the resources they needed at all times.

P13: There are certain things that I couldn't remember from week to week but it was good to be able to go back and look at it again.

P8: Oh definitely, I couldn't imagine it (rehab) without it. It is such a lot of work ... it's been 6 months since my surgery. You have to put in so much work. You need that support to keep.

P10: I mean...I do refer to internet anyway because of the accessibility issue. It's so easy. So I think there are positives for that reason alone. It's so easy to get to. If there is detailed information on there, I want to use it. I think it's a good thing.

Patients found that the group structure was a positive experience. They discussed the learning environment and the support they felt from one another. They also described replacing something of the loss of their usual activities while they rehabilitated.

P2: I wasn't sure how it would be to be part of a class but I really like it. I know it helps with volume control but actually it's really nice to be around other people who have gone through the same thing and see the different stages before and ahead and how far you have come. How people are doing. And ... I also think it's a pretty good job of providing one to one during those classes too.

P9: One thing I really like was to come here and see the guys who had the same injury I had and you ask them, hey mate, what happened to you and they say football. Me too!

P6: Motivation and comparing yourself. It's important to review other people and their training and it tells you a lot about what you should be doing. Why are you so good at that and why are you doing that so much better than what I do? You know it drives you. I had a very joyful moment of three times ten at 80 kg and others from my level couldn't do it. I felt proud.

Eight patients mentioned that they felt lucky to have been in an area where ACL injury and surgery are commonplace and so an evidence-based rehabilitation group is provided with high levels of support. Their perception was that NHS care was varied and they felt lucky to be in this particular hospital.

P14: I felt very lucky to have happened to live in the right area.

P5: I think it's really good because I have heard that other hospitals ...doesn't have a programme that is as good as yours and physios that look after you.

P6: I feel like I am one of those who won the postcode lottery.

P7: I think it has been pretty brilliant, the support I have received in comparison to other people I know who have gone to other hospitals.

Theme 2 - Personal characteristics and rehabilitation engagement

Patients broadly seemed to find the ACL rehabilitation experience exceeded their expectations, but the commitment to rehabilitation was undoubtedly a burden for many patients and marked their lives in a significant way. Key concepts that recurred for patients were, commitment, motivation and confidence in physical ability.

Commitment

P7: There is a lot to do ...you have work and your life and then this rehab is a whole other thing.

Motivation

P2: I think the toughest thing now is to keep the motivation to go to the gym three or four times a week. ... you need to think of it as a lifestyle change, to keep fit.... Just trying to fit it with work and commuting and everything is hard.

Confidence in physical ability

P7: I felt like I couldn't do (things) and was letting people down. A lot of those jobs were hinging on me being able to do physical things. ... so yes it has really affected me quite a lot.

Many patients described a loss of function and participation after ACL injury. There was a sense of being changed and often a feeling that the extent of their loss of function was not understood.

P6: I tried skiing without my ACL, I tried and tried but it felt awful. The more I thought about it, I needed the surgery. It would have ended up being injured more if I continued on that knee.

P9: I was in pain... I had 1 or 2 times ...where I took a step and my knee just collapsed.

Some people reflected on how their pre-existing personality traits affected the way they engaged with both traditional physiotherapy and TRAK. Those who were disposed to improve self-care with the use of technology did so, whereas those who saw themselves as being differently motivated or skilled, engaged differently.

P14: In terms of tracking on the website I haven't done it that well and I have been trying to work out why ... and I am not very good at being consistent with my methods in anything in life and it includes that.

P1: I am lazy with the internet and it's easier to watch a video and just do it but I'll not report or log.

Theme 3 – Attitudes to the internet and healthcare

As there are so many websites providing healthcare advice and services, patients expressed concern about knowing with confidence what information is 'safe' when it comes to digital resources. They worried about self-diagnosis, poor exercise technique and inappropriate advice exercise apps or websites where their personal injury and abilities were not fully understood and taken into account. Patients were very clear that they go online for information despite the risks and that they feel the

NHS should be providing them with approved digital rehabilitation tools and information sources.

P5: it's overwhelming too. You might think there is something wrong with you and you might do the wrong thing. You need to check with a real professional.

P14: Even if you think of putting that on YouTube with every other videos people will all go to the one that is NHS approved. Obviously that's the one people would pick.

P6: If I don't know how to do an exercise or something and I will go on YouTube or whatever but you get a varied standard and some may be downright dangerous. It is not good, for obvious reasons. So I think opt have a site that I know my physios or the hospital I am with, the NHS, has approved that these are the good stuff to do or links to the right stuff. That is kind of important.

Theme 4 – Benefits of using TRAK for rehabilitation

The patient participants gave positive patient feedback on the key functions of TRAK. They felt that all the key functions (video-based personal plans, information, exercise logs and email support) impacted directly on their knowledge, motivation and confidence, but to differing degrees.

Patients felt that they went to the videos to inform their technique and give them confidence that they were doing the exercises correctly. They also reported that the videos reminded them of what exercises they should be doing.

P10: You can't rate it highly enough really. It's somewhere to go and check on what you're supposed to be doing and make sure to do it right.

There was a mixed response to the exercise log, it was popular as a method to monitor progress but it was reported to be somewhat user-unfriendly and did not provide an option of a general progress report.

P6: It really makes me because I think, oh god I haven't filled anything in to my log this week and it looks so bad. It really drags me to the gym, I look at it and think, I have to do something. I have to do something ... even when I feel yuk.

P8: Again at the beginning I was inputting few things but it was adding half an hour onto my gym session. Trying to get a connection and all that.

The information section was popular immediately post-operatively and at phase-to-phase transitional points. Several patients suggested that the information was too wordy and would be improved by presenting it in video format and linking it with the exercise phases, i.e. a more seamless transition between the personal plans and information.

P6: In the beginning when you have more issues and you are fresh out of surgery and a bit ahhhhh. Then it's very useful.

The 'contact us' section was not as popular as expected. Patients reported that they wanted the face-to-face reassurance when they had concerns. This identified a challenge for new technology to find effective ways of reassuring patients through a digital medium.

P10: I thought before I started using it that I would use the contact us more but didn't because I waited until the session and asked my questions there. Maybe I didn't come into such huge problems where I had to contact you urgently.

Some individuals emphasized the importance of TRAK to support rehabilitation when they were unable to attend physiotherapy due to work commitments or because of personal circumstances.

P14: I think the videos are like a revolution! It's amazing ...but it's not like what you see on YouTube because you trust it. ... it doesn't exist anywhere else as far as I can see.

P3: There are lots of exercises that people can do. And if it's too easy for you, you can move up different stages. Some harder ones and some easier ones... I think it gives you a focus and a way to approach it. It's like a weekly target to do it and not think of the long road.

It also acted as a motivator to comply with their rehabilitation:

P6: Well TRAK works very well for me. Firstly, it makes me go to the gym. It really makes me because I think, oh god I haven't filled anything in to my log this week and it looks so bad. I love the videos; I look at them every time before I do my exercise. Because I am paranoid about bad technique and sometimes so paranoid about it that I stay away from doing things.

Theme 5 – Limitations of TRAK for rehabilitation

Patients were asked about their user experience of TRAK as a tool to support self-management. The answers were broadly divided into extrinsic and intrinsic factors. Patients discussed extrinsic problems they experienced, which could have been addressed by better physiotherapist management of the personal plans or e-mail links.

P4: in terms of communication. Right from the off, I write a couple of messages in the contact us section and I never received anything back. It kind of killed the point of the website for me... to a degree.

P10: I refer back to the paper in the class sometimes as that is more up to date than my plan....

Other extrinsic factors such as access to and the speed of Internet connection also affected usability. Without exception, every patient mentioned this as a limitation.

P15: The problem is the internet connection, in the gym it's impossible to navigate between pages so I just gave up. Some apps you can use offline, that is what is needed.

P8: Again at the beginning I was inputting few things but it was adding half an hour onto my gym session. Trying to get a connection and all that.

Intrinsic factors referred to the website function itself. Patients discussed functional limitations of TRAK in comparison to other apps they were exposed to through the commercial market.

P9: (I used it) out of commitment (to the study). If it was more designy (sic) or there was an app easy to use then definitely.... If it was done like the Nike one, you can bet there would have been so many downloads.... There is nothing on there to say 'come on'. Like the Nike app, if you run there is this voice saying 'great job, you did 5 K today'.

P14: I found it difficult, well, clunky to add it add the bottom of every page. To put that in each time. It's the kind of ins and out of the techy stuff ... it wasn't smooth.

Theme 6 – TRAK in the future: How to increase the impact on positive behaviors

Patients saw the use of TRAK blended together with face-to-face physiotherapy as the future of ACL rehabilitation. They agreed universally that a digital exercise intervention was needed and they used their own experience with new technology to provide more information about their user needs. They would like to see the usability of existing functions improved, e.g. the ways of providing health-related information (educational videos alongside written information), easier identification of exercises (thumbnails alongside their descriptions), easier logging of exercise progression (slider scales and speech notes as an alternative to text input). New functionality that TRAK could benefit from mainly focused on personalization aspects such as prompts and cues that could be set individually, summary of overall progress, web chat, etc. The majority of patients felt that the web site needed to be converted into an app accessible on handheld devices such as tablets and smartphones and in particular with functions that are accessible offline.

P4: I would very much like to stress that it should be an app. It's just that it would really help because it is really tricky on the phone. It's hard in the gym I want to look at the examples really quick and remind myself ... an app would be better. You can use it offline.

P9: I want it to prompt me, I want it to give me a weekly record, I want it to shout at me through the phone that I need to be doing my single leg squats today, that kind of thing. Something that comes up saying 'don't forget this, do this today'.

They requested further prompts to emphasize exercises they may be missing, prompt a help link, a chat log that you could refer back to, a dashboard of completed sessions and milestones that can generate a weekly report, a set of different workouts that the can be automatically generated such as A, B & C, per week, a body map to show where they should feel the exercises, further links to relevant resources such as evidence or sport-specific information and pop ups that remind them where they are relative to milestones.

P6: I wish I could reflect all the exercise that I am doing. Even stuff that's not on TRAK, so I can keep a complete record of my exercise and progress. Drills, squats that aren't on TRAK. Sounds banal but there is a pride in showing all that I have done to myself and the physio. It's what I do to get better.

P7: the kind of comparison I have is when I was going to do a half marathon and I used this app and it told me every day. Go and run this far, now do a strength and conditioning class and now go do some yoga.

Patients were very clear that they did not think TRAK was a replacement for physiotherapy, but should be used to complement face-to-face treatment in a 'blended approach'. They were very keen to explain that it was an aid to their self-care when they were not in physiotherapy. Interestingly several patients who were in the middle stage of their rehabilitation did say that when they became too busy at times they were happy to manage through the website and attend physiotherapy less often.

P16: I would like to have both but I wouldn't have it instead.

Physiotherapist interviews

Physiotherapist discussed the benefit of having a website to enhance their patients' self-management during rehabilitation. Physiotherapists explained that they want to improve their patients' confidence, quality of exercise technique and compliance with exercise as the evidence suggests this would ensure better outcomes. The website provides a more evolved way of influencing these factors than traditional exercise handouts. They also noted that digital health options do not interest all patients and that patients' self-selection is key to acceptability of digital interventions.

Theme 1 - Benefits to physiotherapists

Physiotherapists expressed enthusiasm for TRAK on behalf of themselves and their patients, however they also seemed to acknowledge that not all patients would be suitable for this digital tool.

PHY1: We are giving back that locus of control to the patient .... You pick a patient who is appropriate for it. I mean there are so many patients who you may have say 6 appointments with, the middle three might just be exercise progressions. Some patients would be more than happy with email review... well, you could save the patient time too.

PHY4: Anyone that wants. Self-selecting group and definitely. I am refusing to be ageist because I have 80-year-old patients who email me and who are very engaged with technology. Equally I have 30 years olds that don't care or don't get it.

Rotational physiotherapists particularly felt that they used the website to educate themselves. That it was a go to summary of the education for each stage and a library of exercise ideas that they could use to help patients.

PHY3: As a junior physio I found it really useful in terms of information and a quick go to resource for reviewing milestones and do's and don'ts.... I quite relied on it and it fed me information. Especially band 5 physios who come into a trust new and it's a great learning tool to help you.

PHY1: If we had much more digital contact with patients I would be very happy with that. We could be emailing patients and caring a lot remotely. Simple progressions and checking on exercises could save contact time, patients' own time and money I guess.

Theme 2 - Suggestions to improve the usability of TRAK for physiotherapists

Of particular concern to physiotherapists was the time it took to build personal exercise programs and maintain them as patients progressed. Practical suggestions that recurred in interviews included the use of tablets in class to update programs quickly, thumbnail images alongside the names of exercises so they could quickly see what each one was without having to click on it and load new pages. Another suggestion was an inbuilt spelling checker, as one dyslexic physiotherapist felt they were slow in adding instructions because this functionality was not available. Physiotherapists would also like to see the exercise section have several 'bolted' key exercises for each stage.

PHY1: It would be good to build a smoother understanding of how we use the TRAK in the sessions. Some patients expect to be updated, some don't and then we don't know... in the sessions, having TRAK open on iPad or something would work. So patients could almost go through it with you as you upgrade it.

One physiotherapist was concerned about the use of patients in the videos because their exercise technique may not be perfect, e.g. a hop that showed inadequate valgus control of the knee. This emphasized the need to upgrade some of the videos. Another physiotherapist was concerned that not enough variations of exercises were available, which meant some exercise videos differed from what the patients were taught in the group.

Importantly, they would like to see a weekly dashboard or a report generated on what the patients have done. This could be printed as a notes record and can be added to paper or digital notes kept in the department instead of duplicating an exercise compliance and progression record.

Physiotherapists discussed the risks associated with TRAK training and management for physiotherapists. They were concerned about delays in picking up patient contacts and felt an emphasis on red flags in the information or red flag pop up reminders might help to identify potentially vulnerable patients.

PHY4: I have a disclaimer about slow contacts on my email and the phone number of the department in case of problems ...It needs to have an out of office function or a re-routing function for when therapists are off. The information section, it should have ...a clear red flag lists, when to stop and exercise, FAQ's etc. again to reduce anxiety and reassure.

Further suggestions for improvement included providing information on using videos in addition to written material. One physiotherapist suggested that in line with commercial apps, perhaps a celebrity or famous athlete who had a similar injury would be involved in the production of information videos. Patient-experience videos were also suggested as well as voiceover instructions to some of the videos to highlight key guidance on technique. Similar to the patients, the physiotherapists wanted to see prompts and pop ups that engaged patients and directed to different sections of information. They also felt that a group or board should be reviewing the content on an ongoing basis so that the evidence is up to date and exercises or information can be added as appropriate. Opinions were mixed about how much information about physiology or advanced rehabilitation knowledge patients would benefit from. However, it was agreed that links to approved information or research were a good addition.

Discussion

This study found that patients generally accepted a TRAK, a digital self-management support tool that was personalized with their own ACL rehabilitation plan and saw it as a positive addition to be blended with standard care. Physiotherapists likewise engaged well with the website as a support tool for patients and found it helpful to work with patients through this interface. Of the 17 interviewed patients and 4 physiotherapists, all thought that the blended approach of standard care and the website, notwithstanding its ongoing technical improvement, was an improvement on standard care alone. Every interviewed patient thought that the website should be a choice available to all ACL rehabilitated patients on the NHS.

In the interviews, the emergence of social influence, expectations and anxieties regarding TRAK usage reflect the established paradigm for acceptability of new digital technology discussed by Venkatesh et al. [28]. Performance expectancy (the degree to which an individual believes that using the system will help them attain goals), effort expectancy (the degree of ease associated with using the technology), social influence (the degree to which an individual perceives that important others believe they should use) and facilitating conditions (the degree to which an individual believes the organizational and technical infrastructure exist to support use) are considered the key factors in determining acceptability. As well as self-efficacy, anxiety and behavioral intentions.

Social influences in the group were evident where patients described their engagement with one another as an incentive for using the TRAK website. More importantly, individuals reported that interest in TRAK was dependent on the engagement of their physiotherapist. They reported less use if their physiotherapists were slow to respond to e-mails or because personal plans were not updated in a timely manner. This establishes the physiotherapist as the necessary agent behind the blending of standard care with TRAK. Physiotherapists expressed awareness of this and highlighted a number of facilitating conditions that influenced their ability to deliver this. Clinical time was the main challenge for TRAK management, but they felt that through use of better hardware such as tablet devices and improved organization of TRAK data, they could improve efficiency and maintenance of personalized programs.

Performance and effort expectancy of TRAK found a gap in functionality between this prototype and participants' experience of commercial health apps such as 'the Nike App'. In particular, they wished to see TRAK as an app with offline functions. Physiotherapists wanted a function for prompts and reminders that could be set by patients depending on patient goals in order to facilitate further engagement, and incentives such as, 'if you achieve these target, you may begin the running program' [33]. Patients and physiotherapists reported that TRAK was easy to use and did not frustrate their effort expectancy, with the exception of maintaining the log, though this was also discussed as having a positive effect on behavior.

The Behavior Change Wheel model outlines the importance of understanding the patients' physical, social and psychological sources of behavior in order to understand developing interventions for changing behavior [34]. This group of patients described their sense of loss, their goals and the burden of a long and physically challenging rehabilitation program. These contextual factors inform their feelings about the target behavior, the rehabilitation program. The patients discussed how the website informed, motivated and improved confidence in carrying out the desired behaviors. Specifically the website functions provided clear plans, videos and instructions as well as persuading them with targeted information and an opportunity to record and monitor progress [34]. Overall, individuals indicated that TRAK helped them as part of a blended approach to physiotherapy (face-to-face and digital) as opposed to exclusive face-to-face or digital options.

Some patients who participated highlighted that they would not have chosen ordinarily to use a digital health intervention as they were not sure they would like it or it would be beneficial. Interestingly they worried about how their lack of usage would impact on the physiotherapists' opinion of them. They described themselves as 'lazy' and 'sorry' [23]. This raises questions about how organizational changes to incorporate digital tools may affect patients who choose not to use these tools [28, 35]. Morden et al. found that "care must be taken to balance the needs of clinicians and patients whilst avoiding the scenario where patient information becomes a substitute rather than a supplement" [36]. Every patient that was interviewed without exception said that they did not see TRAK as an alternative to their face-to-face physiotherapy appointments but it should be used in a blended approach combining the digital tool with face-to-face. This is an approach taken by Bossen et al. with knee OA [20]. While some patients will continue to prefer standard care, this blended approach facilitates patients who wish to work more independently to do so safely. Some patients did say they would accept TRAK instead of appointments in stage 3 of their rehabilitation where exercise goals were clear and they felt confident to work independently with longer gaps between appointments. This can be explored further in a planned feasibility trial of TRAK for ACL patients [37] . Given the established psychological factors in determining return to function and sport the role of patient confidence in the blended approach is key to its usefulness [15]. As such TRAK is a unique digital tool for ACL reconstructed patients to facilitate the self-care component of their rehabilitation.

Conclusion

Exploring patients' opinions showed an evolved understanding of the potential benefits of a blended approach. TRAK aims to influence patient engagement and behavior change in line with established theory by motivating patients, giving them the capability to perform well and creating opportunities to record development toward well-defined goals. The study results suggest that TRAK, subject to technical improvement, was acceptable to patients in effort and performance expectancy. The value of TRAK was understood by participants to be a personalized reflection of their rehabilitation program with interactive components that aimed to inform, motivate and engage. However, physiotherapists highlighted organizational changes are needed to better integrate its use into standard physiotherapy practice.

Abbreviations
ACL: Anterior Cruciate Ligament; NHS: National Health Service; PI: Principal Investigator; TRAK: Taxonomy for the Rehabilitation of Knee Conditions

Acknowledgements
Emma Dunphy was supported in part by the National Institute for Health Research (NIHR) Collaboration for Leadership in Applied Health Research and Care North Thames at Bart's Health NHS Trust. The views expressed are those of the authors and not necessarily those of the NHS, NIHR, or the Department of Health.

Funding
ED was supported in part by National Institute for Health Research (NIHR) Collaboration for Leadership in Applied Health Research and Care North Thames at Bart's Health NHS Trust.

Authors' contributions
ED was the PI on this study and worked with supervision from KB and FH. KB and IS designed TRAK and ED made content changes to reflect the needs of ACL patients. ED and KB separately analyzed data and prepared the final manuscript for publication. All authors read and approved the final manuscript.

Consent for publication
Given in written form by all study participants.

Competing interests
The authors declare that they have no competing interests.

Author details
[1]E-Health Unit, Research Department of Primary Care and Population Health, Upper Third Floor UCL Medical School (Royal Free Campus), Rowland Hill Street, NW3 2PF, London, UK. [2]Homerton University Hospital NHS Trust, Homerton Row E96SR, London, UK. [3]School of Computer Science & Informatics, Cardiff University, Queens Building, 5 The Parade, Cardiff CF24 3AA, UK. [4]School of Healthcare Sciences, Cardiff University, Eastgate House, Newport Road, Cardiff CF24 0AB, UK. [5]Cardiff & Vale University Health Board, Health Park, Cardiff CF14 4XW, UK.

References

1. Bollen S. Advances in the management of anterior cruciate ligament injury. Curr Orthop. 2000;14(5):325–8.
2. Kapoor B, et al. Current practice in the management of anterior cruciate ligament injuries in the United Kingdom. Br J Sports Med. 2004;38(5):542–4.
3. Ardern CL, et al. Fifty-five per cent return to competitive sport following anterior cruciate ligament reconstruction surgery: an updated systematic review and meta-analysis including aspects of physical functioning and contextual factors. Br J Sports Med. 2014:bjsports-2013-093398.
4. Adams D, et al. Current concepts for anterior cruciate ligament reconstruction: a criterion-based rehabilitation progression. J Orthop Sports Physic Ther. 2012;42(7):601–14.
5. Risberg MA, Lewek M, Snyder-Mackler L. A systematic review of evidence for anterior cruciate ligament rehabilitation: how much and what type? Physical Therapy in Sport. 2004;5(3):125–45.
6. Ardern CL, et al. A systematic review of the psychological factors associated with returning to sport following injury. Br J Sports Med. 2013;47(17):1120–6.
7. Herrington L, Myer G, Horsley I. Task based rehabilitation protocol for elite athletes following anterior cruciate ligament reconstruction: a clinical commentary. Physical Therapy in Sport. 2013;14(4):188–98.
8. Risberg MA, Ekeland A. Assessment of functional tests after anterior cruciate ligament surgery. J Orthop Sports Phys Ther. 1994;19(4):212–7.
9. Risberg MA, et al. Design and implementation of a neuromuscular training program following anterior cruciate ligament reconstruction. J Orthop Sports Phys Ther. 2001;31(11):620–31.
10. EltzEn I, et al. A progressive 5-week exercise therapy program leads to significant improvement in knee function early after anterior cruciate ligament injury. J Orthop Sports Physic Ther. 2010;40(11):705–21.
11. Ardern CL, et al. The impact of psychological readiness to return to sport and recreational activities after anterior cruciate ligament reconstruction. Br J Sports Med. 2014;48(22):1613–9.
12. Ardern CL, et al. Return-to-sport outcomes at 2 to 7 years after anterior cruciate ligament reconstruction surgery. Am J Sports Med. 2012;40(1):41–8.
13. Ardern CL, et al. Return to sport following anterior cruciate ligament reconstruction surgery: a systematic review and meta-analysis of the state of play. Br J Sports Med. 2011:bjsports76364.
14. Ardern CL, et al. Return to the preinjury level of competitive sport after anterior cruciate ligament reconstruction surgery two-thirds of patients have not returned by 12 months after surgery. Am J Sports Med. 2011;39(3):538–43.
15. Ardern CL, et al. Psychological responses matter in returning to preinjury level of sport after anterior cruciate ligament reconstruction surgery. Am J Sports Med. 2013;41(7):1549–58.
16. Lynch AD, et al. Consensus criteria for defining 'successful outcome'after ACL injury and reconstruction: a Delaware-Oslo ACL cohort investigation. Br J Sports Med. 2013:bjsports-2013-092299.
17. Croft P, Porcheret M, Peat G. Managing osteoarthritis in primary care: the GP as public health physician and surgical gatekeeper. Br J Gen Pract. 2011;61.
18. Grindem H, et al. Online registration of monthly sports participation after anterior cruciate ligament injury: a reliability and validity study. Br J Sports Med. 2013:bjsports-2012-092075.
19. van Mechelen DM, Van Mechelen W, Verhagen EA. Sports injury prevention in your pocket?! Prevention apps assessed against the available scientific evidence: a review. Br J Sports Med. 2014;48(11):878–82.
20. Bossen D, et al. Effectiveness of a web-based physical activity intervention in patients with knee and/or hip osteoarthritis: randomized controlled trial. J Med Internet Res. 2013;15(11):e257.
21. Alkhaldi G, et al. The effectiveness of prompts to promote engagement with digital interventions: a systematic review. J Med Internet Res. 2016;18(1)
22. Semple JL, et al. Using a mobile app for monitoring post-operative quality of recovery of patients at home: a feasibility study. JMIR mHealth and uHealth. 2015;3(1):e18.
23. Moore GC, Benbasat I. Development of an instrument to measure the perceptions of adopting an information technology innovation. Inf Syst Res. 1991;2(3):192–222.
24. Spasić I, et al. TRAK app suite: a web-based intervention for delivering standard care for the rehabilitation of knee conditions. JMIR research protocols. 2015;4(4)
25. Button K, et al. TRAK ontology: defining standard care for the rehabilitation of knee conditions. J Biomed Inform. 2013;46(4):615–25.
26. Risberg MA, et al. Neuromuscular training versus strength training during first 6 months after anterior cruciate ligament reconstruction: a randomized clinical trial. Phys Ther. 2007;87(6):737–50.
27. Magnussen RA, et al. Cross-cultural comparison of patients undergoing ACL reconstruction in the United States and Norway. Knee Surgery Sports Traumatology Arthroscopy. 2010;18(1):98.
28. Venkatesh V, et al. User acceptance of information technology: toward a unified view. MIS Q. 2003:425–78.
29. Button KSI. Implementation of the TRAK intervention to enable e-rehab for knee conditions: a web-based intervention suite to support self-management in. Rehabilitation. 2017.
30. Myer GD, et al. Rehabilitation after anterior cruciate ligament reconstruction: criteria-based progression through the return-to-sport phase. J Orthop Sports Phys Ther. 2006;36(6):385–402.

31. Garber CE, et al. American College of Sports Medicine position stand. Quantity and quality of exercise for developing and maintaining cardiorespiratory, musculoskeletal, and neuromotor fitness in apparently healthy adults: guidance for prescribing exercise. Med Sci Sports Exerc. 2011;43(7):1334–59.
32. Pope C, Ziebland S, Mays N. Analysing qualitative data. Br Med J. 2000; 320(7227):114.
33. Knight E, et al. Public health guidelines for physical activity: is there an app for that? A review of android and apple app stores. JMIR mHealth and uHealth. 2015;3(2):e43.
34. Michie S, van Stralen MM, West R. The behaviour change wheel: a new method for characterising and designing behaviour change interventions. Implement Sci. 2011;6(1):42.
35. Bossen D, et al. Adherence to a web-based physical activity intervention for patients with knee and/or hip osteoarthritis: a mixed method study. J Med Internet Res. 2013;15(10):e223.
36. Morden A, et al. Acceptability of a 'guidebook' for the management of osteoarthritis: a qualitative study of patient and clinician's perspectives. BMC Musculoskelet Disord. 2014;15(1):427.
37. Dunphy E, Hamilton FL, Button K. Taxonomy for the rehabilitation of knee conditions (TRAK), a digital intervention to support the self-care components of anterior cruciate ligament rehabilitation: protocol of a feasibility study. JMIR Research Protocols. 2016;5(4)

15

Efficacy of standardized training on a virtual reality simulator to advance knee and shoulder arthroscopic motor skills

Stefan Rahm*, Karl Wieser, David E. Bauer, Felix WA Waibel, Dominik C. Meyer, Christian Gerber and Sandro F. Fucentese

Abstract

Background: Most studies demonstrated, that training on a virtual reality based arthroscopy simulator leads to an improvement of technical skills in orthopaedic surgery. However, how long and what kind of training is optimal for young residents is unknown. In this study we tested the efficacy of a standardized, competency based training protocol on a validated virtual reality based knee- and shoulder arthroscopy simulator.

Methods: Twenty residents and five experts in arthroscopy were included. All participants performed a test including knee -and shoulder arthroscopy tasks on a virtual reality knee- and shoulder arthroscopy simulator. The residents had to complete a competency based training program. Thereafter, the previously completed test was retaken. We evaluated the metric data of the simulator using a z-score and the Arthroscopic Surgery Skill Evaluation Tool (ASSET) to assess training effects in residents and performance levels in experts.

Results: The residents significantly improved from pre- to post training in the overall z-score: − 9.82 (range, − 20.35 to − 1.64) to − 2.61 (range, − 6.25 to 1.5); $p < 0.001$. The overall ASSET score improved from 55 (27 to 84) percent to 75 (48 to 92) percent; $p < 0.001$. The experts, however, achieved a significantly higher z-score in the shoulder tasks ($p < 0.001$ and a statistically insignificantly higher z-score in the knee tasks with a $p = 0.921$. The experts mean overall ASSET score (knee and shoulder) was significantly higher in the therapeutic tasks ($p < 0.001$) compared to the residents post training result.

Conclusions: The use of a competency based simulator training with this specific device for 3-5 h is an effective tool to advance basic arthroscopic skills of resident in training from 0 to 5 years based on simulator measures and simulator based ASSET testing. Therefore, we conclude that this sort of training method appears useful to learn the handling of the camera, basic anatomy and the triangulation with instruments.

Keywords: Education, Simulation, Arthroscopy, Orthopaedic surgery, Virtual reality simulation, Training

Background

Training of residents is a very important, but demanding and time consuming job in teaching hospitals. Arthroscopic surgery in particular is difficult to learn since it cannot be acquired by observation and assisting alone [1, 2]. Virtual-reality based training has become more popular in the past, but there is still a lack of a standardized integration of virtual reality based simulator training in orthopaedic post-graduate programs [3–10]. The benefit of virtual-reality based teaching is proven to be at least of equal value as direct observation, animal and/or cadaver models or videotape learning tools [11–13].

The potential 24/7 availability of a training tool is increasingly important since the hands-on operation time gets less for residents. The initial high investment of such a simulator as well as the service expenses are recognized downsides. In a previous study [14] it was shown that medical students have a steep learning curve in the first 2 hours of training on a virtual reality based knee arthroscopy simulator but there were no

* Correspondence: stefan_rahm@yahoo.com
Orthopaedic Department, Balgrist University Hospital, University of Zurich, Forchstrasse 340, CH-8008 Zurich, Switzerland

identifiable predictors of talent or magnitude of improvement of skills.

It is not known which type of training on a virtual-reality based arthroscopy simulator is the most efficient and beneficial for residents. Further, there are different types of measuring the quality of an arthroscopic procedure and there is still a lack of validated outcome score for the evaluation of an arthroscopic performance [10]. Metric data such as task time or instrument movements can be measured and the skill level of an arthroscopist can be evaluated with scores such as the Arthroscopic Surgery Skill Evaluation Tool (ASSET) [5, 15].

It was the purpose of this study to determine whether a standardized, competency based training advances arthroscopic skills of residents. Two hypotheses were tested: First, arthroscopic novices (residents) improve their skills significantly through a standardized competency based training program on a virtual reality simulator. Second, the residents can reach an arthroscopic proficiency skill level based on the metric data and the ASSET score compared to fellowship trained arthroscopists after the training program.

Methods

Prior to the study all participants gave their written, informed consent. Our local IRB waived the need for ethical approval; BASEC Nr: Req-2016-00442.

Twenty residents (16 males and 4 females) with a mean age of 31 (27 to 37) years and a mean of 2.5 (0 to 5.5) years experience in the orthopaedic field were included in this study. Furthermore, there were five fellowship trained experts (all males) with a mean age of 45 (34 to 63) years and a mean of 17 (8 to 35) years experience in the orthopaedic field also included in this study as a reference group. Three of them were shoulder specialists and two of them knee specialists, of which all had a very long experience in arthroscopic surgery. Detailed information on demographic data and previous experience in real and simulated arthroscopy are depicted in Table 1.

Protocol

All participants (residents and experts) performed a test on the validated VirtaMed AG (Schlieren, Switzerland) virtual reality based knee- and shoulder arthroscopy simulator [3, 16]. The residents had to pass a competency based training program, which included several knee- and shoulder arthroscopy tasks. Thereafter, the previously completed test was redone.

Test description

To start all participants, who did not know the simulator ($n = 9$) got a standardized introduction, explaining the hard- and software. A 2 minutes hands on time trying out the test tasks was allowed to all these participants. Further, all participants could get familar with the system using the camera and the tools for exactly 60 s.

Knee

Three knee arthroscopy tasks needed to be performed. One standard diagnostic knee arthroscopy task including the visualisation of the complete intraarticular anatomic structures. One foreign body removal task including fishing of six rings with the hook (three in the lateral and three in the medial compartment) and one guided task of removal of a flaptear of the lateral meniscus using the punch to achieve a stable meniscus. The time was stopped when the participants judged their job to be completed.

Shoulder

Twice, the same two shoulder arthroscopy tasks were performed, once in beach chair and once in lateral decubitus position. First, a standard diagnostic shoulder arthroscopy using the camera through the posterior

Table 1 Overview of the demographic information of the residents and the experts

Total arthroscopies performed	0	1 to 20	21 to 50	51 to 100	> 100	> 200
Residents	6	1	5	0	0	0
Experts	0	0	0	0	0	5
Total hours on knee / shoulder virtual reality based	0	1 to 5	6 to 20			
Residents	3	10	7			
Experts	1	3	1			
Total hours of playing video games per week	0	1 to 5	6 to 20			
Residents	19	1	0			
Experts	4	1	0			
Handedness	right	left				
Residents	16	4				
Experts	5	0				

The distribution of the demographic data and previous real arthroscopy- and simulator experience are depicted of the 20 residents and the five experts portal visualizing the intraarticular and the subacromial (coracoacromial ligament and the acromioclavicular joint) structures was performed. Second, a therapeutic task consisting in touching five balls by the probe for 3 seconds. Either the anterior or anterolateral portal could be used.

Training protocol

The training protocol was, as mentioned before, competency based, which means, that residents with a certain level of performance regarding operation time and overall camera and instrument pathway were allowed to proceed to the next task and therefore have a shorter overall training period. Less experienced residents, which did not achieve a certain benchmark, had to repeat the tasks until it was completed in the required level. The training program was chosen to be at least 3 hours and maximum 5 hours if all tasks were repeated to the maximum. All participants began with training of knee arthroscopy. Overall 32 tasks including diagnostic and therapeutic arthroscopy were completed. The tasks comprised diagnostics, guided diagnostics, diagnostics and palpation with the probe, catching rings with the hook, foreign body removal with the grasper/hook (stars) and partial meniscectomy.

Afterwards the training continued with shoulder arthroscopy, first in beach chair and then in lateral decubitus position. Twenty tasks each including diagnostic and therapeutic arthroscopy were completed. The tasks comprised diagnostics, guided diagnostics, diagnostics and palpation with the probe, catching rings with the hook, foreign body removal with the grasp.

Outcome parameters

Metrics All the metric data (time in seconds, camera, hook/probe and punch pathway in centimeters) were recorded by the simulator system. We evaluated these metric data of the simulator itself and additionally used z-scores for comparison of the tests [14].

Arthroscopic surgery skill evaluation tool (ASSET) Furthermore, of two particular knee (one diagnostic arthroscopy/one therapeutic arthroscopy catching six rings) and two shoulder (one diagnostic arthroscopy in beach chair/one therapeutic arthroscopy palpating five balls with the probe in lateral decubitus) arthroscopy tasks, the ASSET was evaluated to measure the performance. The ASSET score is based on these following domains; safety, field of view, camera dexterity, instrument dexterity, bimanual dexterity, flow of procedure, quality of procedure, which had to be scored from one to five (one being a novice level and five an expert level). The additional domains, autonomy and added complexity of procedure were not evaluated in this study. This scoring was performed by two experienced knee and shoulder surgeons (S.R. and K.W.) in a fully blinded (pre- or post training/resident or expert) consensus read-out. As instrument and bimanual dexterity in diagnostic arthroscopies could not be evaluated, the maximum ASSET score was 25 points for the diagnostic tasks and 35 points for the therapeutic tasks, respectively.

The metric data were correlated to the ASSET score. The learning curve of the residents using the metric data and the ASSET scores were analyzed. The final post training test results of the residents were compared with the basic test results of the experts. Furthermore, the demographic data from the questionnaire were correlated with the metric data and the ASSET score of the final basic test.

Statistical analysis

Data are presented as mean and standard deviation (SD) for continuous variables and as proportion (%) for categorical variables, if not stated otherwise. A two-tailed Kolmogorov–Smirnov test was used for testing normal distribution, if $p \leq 0.05$, the data were considered as normally distributed. The Wilcoxon signed-rank Test was used for testing differences between means of pre- to post training results for each participant. The Mann-Whitney U Test was used for testing differences between the expert and non-expert subpopulations.

The Pearson's Chi-squared test was applied for testing differences of distribution of categorical variables. A p-value of < 0.05 was considered to be statistically significant.

For comparison of metric data of different dimensions, variables were normalized to the expert population by subtracting the individual score of each participant from the expert populations mean and dividing the difference by the expert populations standard deviation. The thereby calculated z-scores of each variable were then summed up and an arithmetic mean was calculated to obtain a single score for each task. The statistical analysis was performed by a professional bio-statistician.

Results

Metrics

The overall mean z-score of the basic test improved significantly pre- to post training from − 9.82 (range, − 20.35 to − 1.64; SD 5.05) to − 2.61 (range, − 6.25 to 1.5; 1.63); $p < 0.001$. A statistically significant improvement was found in all pre- to post training metric shoulder tasks and all except two metric knee tasks. Only the hook pathway in the removal of six rings and the punch pathway in the partial meniscectomy task showed no significant difference from pre-to post training. (see Table 2).

The experts reached an overall mean z-score of 0.0 (range, − 0.55 to 0.52; SD 0.47) which was significantly better than the post training result of the residents ($p < 0.001$). The experts reached a higher mean *knee z-score* with 0.00 (range, − 0.69 to 0.83; SD 0.61) than the post training residents result with − 0.87 (range, − 4.48 to 0.66; SD 1.50) not reaching statistical significance; $p = 0.192$.

Table 2 Overview of the metric pre- to posttraining results and the expert results

Test; Task	Metric Parameter	Residents Pretraining Test (mean)	min	max	SD	Residents Posttraining Test (mean)	min	max	SD	Wilcoxon: pre-to-posttraining	Experts Test (mean)	min	max	SD	Mann-Whitney-U: Residents posttraining to experts
Knee: Diagnostic Arthroscopy	Time (sec)	254	77	571	133	121	79	219	39	< 0.001	118	71	174	50	0.621
	Camera pathway (cm)	145	39	621	127	74	40	191	36	0.001	75	42	113	30	0.767
Knee: Removal of 6 rings	Time (sec)	159	77	367	83	97	55	203	40	0.001	65	53	73	8	0.029
	Camera pathway (cm)	50	18	174	42	32	12	79	19	0.048	20	14	27	5	0.169
	Hook pathway (cm)	107	38	343	76	82	27	350	74	0.067	53	39	84	19	0.243
Knee: Lateral partial meniscectomy	Time (sec)	332	128	952	235	149	109	231	35	< 0.001	134	87	191	50	0.408
	Camera pathway (cm)	147	53	665	159	70	35	200	35	0.001	87	47	135	35	0.243
	Punch pathway (cm)	42	20	77	16	33	17	60	12	0.057	46	22	77	25	0.447
Shoulder (BC): Diagnostic Arthroscopy	Time (sec)	439	201	728	189	186	91	425	79	< 0.001	60	31	95	25	< 0.001
	Camera pathway (cm)	627	152	3291	694	201	67	385	90	< 0.001	73	25	107	33	0.001
Shoulder (BC): Touching of 5 balls	Time (sec)	271	108	704	171	121	58	244	43	< 0.001	66	43	82	16	< 0.001
	Camera pathway (cm)	103	21	272	74	48	14	118	25	0.004	28	17	33	7	0.071
	Hook pathway (cm)	282	96	1018	233	101	55	286	54	< 0.001	59	33	80	21	0.035
Shoulder (LAT): Diagnostic Arthroscopy	Time (sec)	296	96	1026	213	151	77	399	72	0.005	70	51	99	18	< 0.001
	Camera pathway (cm)	288	79	1152	237	145	62	385	74	0.004	73	57	81	9	0.003
Shoulder (LAT): Touching of 5 balls	Time (sec)	155	50	693	156	61	30	117	21	0.003	42	31	57	11	0.042
	Camera pathway (cm)	93	20	444	116	38	16	66	15	0.023	21	15	27	5	0.015
	Hook pathway (cm)	182	53	505	122	72	27	144	36	0.005	33	28	38	5	0.003

Complete overview of the results. The metric data are all seperately depicted using the mean, maximum, minimum and standard deviation. The p-value was calculated using the Wilcoxon signed rank test

In the the experts scored a significantly higher score with 0.00 (range, − 0.47 to 0.63; SD 0.46) compared to the post training z-score of the residents − 4.35 (range, − 8.56 to − 0.36; SD 2.28); $p < 0.001$. The results between the lateral decubitus and the beach chair position did not significantly differ.

All except one parameter in the knee tasks (time in the knee removal of six rings) showed no significant difference between the post training result and the expert result. However, in the shoulder tasks the experts were significantly better in all but one parameter (camera pathway in beach chair position of shoulder touching five balls). A complete overview of the pre- to post training results and the expert results of every parameter is depicted in Table 2.

Asset

The mean overall ASSET score improved significantly in all four tasks from pre- to post training; from 55% (range, 27 to 84) to 75% (range, 48 to 92); $p = 0.001$. In all four tasks the residents reached a higher (or close to reference) score in the post training assessment, although the experts ASSET score was still significantly better in two tasks (knee triangulation (rings) and shoulder triangulation (balls)). In Fig. 1 the complete results of the ASSET score are summarized.

Correlations

There was a good correlation (correlation coefficient = 0.688; $p = 0.013$) between the overall z-score and the overall ASSET score. There were no positive or negative correlations of the data regarding previous real or simulated experience, the handedness, the sports activity and the video games experience to the improvement of the scores or the final score.

Discussion

The most important finding in this study is that a standardized, competency based training leads to significant improvements of arthroscopic skills measured by both, metric data as well as structured assessment of performance and safety using the ASSET score. The difference between experts performance and residents post training remains significantly bigger for shoulder arthroscopy than for knee arthroscopy (see Fig. 1). Therefore, we could confirm our hypothesis that a significant improvement is achieved for residents, but had to reject the second hypothesis that a proficiency level, similar to the one of a fellowship trained arthroscopist, based on the metric data and the ASSET score can be reached by simulator training alone.

The significant improvement from pre- to post training was shown in the objective metric simulator data (overall z-score, $p < 0.001$, overall ASSET score $p < 0.001$). However, the residents improved their knee arthroscopy skills to a level almost as good as the experts, not showing a significant difference in the z-scores; $p = 0.192$. There was no correlation between the previous experience in arthroscopy and/or simulator training (especially knee arthroscopy) to the tests. On the other hand 50% of the residents already had knee arthroscopy simulator experience compared to only 30% having had shoulder. The tests in the simulated shoulder arthroscopy might have been less anatomically defined, favouring actual surgical experience and therefore explaining the somewhat smaller effect.

The clear correlation of the metric data and the ASSET score, used to measure the arthroscopic skill level including aspects such as the flow of the camera and instruments, as well as the safety aspect, such as not

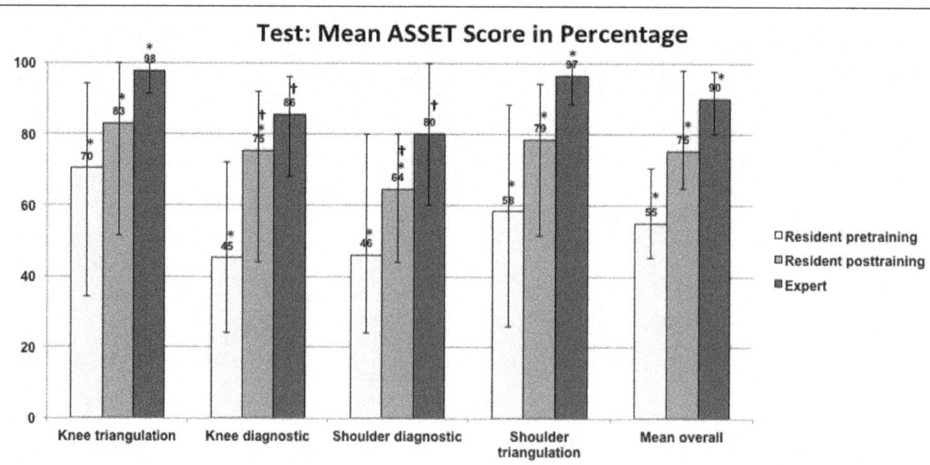

Fig. 1 Shows the percentage of the mean ASSET score of the four tested tasks. It shows a significant improvement in all four tasks from pre- to post training in the residents. Additionally there was again an improvement from the expert group with a better result in the diagnostic tasks and a significantly better result in the therapeutic tasks of knee- and shoulder arthroscopy

scratching the intraarticular cartilage, is another important finding in this study. Good final ASSET scores of the residents in the diagnostic tasks (shoulder and knee), which were not significantly inferior to the experts, was a confirmation of our tested training program. Also, for therapeutic arthroscopy, where an additional instrument was used and triangulation required, a strong increase for the residents was seen particularly in the knee. It seems that this competency based approach works and all participants improved relevantly with a variable time, which has been spent on the simulator (fast learners vs slow learners).

We see the main value of the method in improved camera handling relative to the anatomy to be identified, as well as in the improvement of triangulation skills. For this purpose we intend to use this training program on a regular basis in the future. In addition a relevant advantage of this type of training is the independency from additional medical staff. Other practical arthroscopic issues, such as swelling of the tissue and bleeding can of course not be fully simulated with the current technology. Nevertheless, from a handling standpoint, we feel that residents with a completed simulator training have a competent skill basis for a step-wise initiation of their OR surgical training and confirm similar investigational results for the shoulder (Waterman et al. [17]) or for laparoscopic surgery (Aggarwal et al. [1]) To define a benchmark (Angelo et al. [18]) at what level real expert level is reached, remains difficult, particularly considering that the best results of the trained residents exceeded those of some experts. When looking at maximally reached values however, the best expert was usually still approximately twice as fast as the best resident, indicating an actual correlation with practical experience. Our findings are in line with a finding of Ferguson et al. who stated that basic arthroscopic skills can not immediately be transferred to an unfamiliar anatomical environment within a simulated setting [19]. In a study of Jackson et al. there is evidence, that residents can retain their skills over a time period of 6 months [20]. Our study did not test this important point in skill retaining.

As a limitation, the study group showed a natural, but large heterogeneity for the residents in all different stages with different levels and experience in real arthroscopy and on the simulator, which may explain the poor correlations with the demographic data. Still there were significant improvements found regardless the previous experience. The intensity of the training was not standardized by number of hours spend on the simulator, but we have designed a proficiency based curriculum consisting of 32 knee arthroscopy and 2×20 shoulder arthroscopy cases (to be completed in both, beach chair and lateral position). Participants had to repeat the cases until they passed a pre-defined performance level. Using this approach, we were able to have shorten the training for fast learners and for participants with higher baseline performance. On average, training time was in the range of 3-5 h (which is in accord with reports) [14]. A limitation of the current study is the fact, that the training frequency was not standardized: some of the participants completed baseline assessment, training and post-assessment on 1 day. We observed that in some of these participants, the learning effects were covered by fatigue effects resulting in "negative learning effects", i.e. some participants showed lower performance after training than at baseline. As we know that more training would add some further skill improvement [21], the average training effects reported in this study are smaller than they would be in reality. Reppenhagen et al. systematically analysed optimal training frequency for arthroscopic skill acquisition and concluded that a training frequency of two sessions per week leads to best skill acquisition and retention [22].

The important question remains whether these results can be transferred in the operating room. Considering the improvement in basic arthroscopic triangulation skills, reaching for some residents the level of experts in the simulator, our results seem to support earlier findings regarding the positive transfer validity in orthopaedic surgery [21, 23]. To lay a basis for the handling of the camera and instruments we conclude that this sort of training makes sense and should be integrated in residents training programs since the hands on time in the operating room decreases for current residents in training [24].

Conclusions

The use of programmed simulator training with this specific device for 3-5 h is an effective tool to advance basic motor skills of residents in training from 0 to 5 years based on simulator measures and simulator based ASSET testing. Therefore, we conclude that this sort of training method appears useful to learn the handling of the camera, basic anatomy and the triangulation with instruments.

Authors' contributions

All (SR, KW, DEB, FW, DCM, CG, SFF) authors have made substantial contributions to this study; SR was involved in conception and design, analysis and interpretation of data and in drafting the manuscript. KW was involved in conception and design and interpretation of data. DB was involved in conception, analysis and statistics. FW was involved in the acquisition of data, analysis and interpretation of data. DCM, CG AND SFF were involved in conception, analysis and interpretation of data and revising the manuscript critically for important intellectual content. All authors read and approved the final manuscript.

Competing interests

The authors declare that they have no competing interests.

References

1. Aggarwal R, Grantcharov T, Moorthy K, Hance J, Darzi A. A competency-based virtual reality training curriculum for the acquisition of laparoscopic psychomotor skill. Am J Surg. 2006;191:128–33.
2. Rosenthal R, Gantert WA, Scheidegger D, Oertli D. Can skills assessment on a virtual reality trainer predict a surgical trainee's talent in laparoscopic surgery? Surg Endosc. 2006;20:1286–90.
3. Fucentese SF, Rahm S, Wieser K, Spillmann J, Harders M, Koch PP. Evaluation of a virtual-reality-based simulator using passive haptic feedback for knee arthroscopy. Knee Surg Sports Traumatol Arthrosc. 2015;23:1077–85.
4. Haque S, Srinivasan S. A meta-analysis of the training effectiveness of virtual reality surgical simulators. IEEE Trans Inf Technol Biomed. 2006;10:51–8.
5. Koehler RJ, Nicandri GT. Using the arthroscopic surgery skill evaluation tool as a pass-fail examination. J Bone Joint Surg Am. 2013;95:e1871.
6. Modi CS, Morris G, Mukherjee R. Computer-simulation training for knee and shoulder arthroscopic surgery. ArthroscopyYJARS. Elsevier Inc. 2010;26:832–40.
7. Pedowitz RA, Marsh JL. Motor skills training in orthopaedic surgery: a paradigm shift toward a simulation-based educational curriculum. J Am Acad Orthop Surg [Internet]. 2012;20:407–9. Available from: http://eutils.ncbi.nlm.nih.gov/entrez/eutils/elink.fcgi?dbfrom=pubmed&id=22751159&retmode=ref&cmd=prlinks
8. Sutherland LM, Middleton PF, Anthony A, Hamdorf J, Cregan P, Scott D, et al. Surgical Simulation. Ann Surg. 2006;243:291–300.
9. Tuijthof GJM, Visser P, Sierevelt IN, Dijk CN, Kerkhoffs GMMJ. Does perception of usefulness of arthroscopic simulators differ with levels of experience? Clin Orthop Relat Res. 2011;469:1701–8.
10. Slade Shantz JA, Leiter JRS, Gottschalk T, MacDonald PB. The internal validity of arthroscopic simulators and their effectiveness in arthroscopic education. Knee Surg Sports Traumatol Arthrosc. 2012;22:33–40.
11. Henn RF III, Shah N, Warner JJP, Gomoll AH. Shoulder arthroscopy simulator training improves shoulder arthroscopy performance in a cadaveric model. Arthroscopy. 2013;29:982–5. YJARS [Internet]. Arthroscopy Association of North America Available from: http://linkinghub.elsevier.com/retrieve/pii/S074980631300159X
12. Basdogan C, Sedef M, Harders M, Wesarg S. VR-based simulators for training in minimally invasive surgery. IEEE Comput Graph Appl. 2007;27:54–66.
13. Moorthy K, Munz Y, Sarker SK, Darzi A. Objective assessment of technical skills in surgery. BMJ. 2003;327:1032–7.
14. Rahm S, Wieser K, Wicki I, Holenstein L, Fucentese SF, Gerber C. Performance of medical students on a virtual reality simulator for knee arthroscopy: an analysis of learning curves and predictors of performance. BMC Surg. 2016;16:14.
15. Koehler RJ, Amsdell S, Arendt EA, Bisson LJ, Bramen JP, Butler A, et al. The arthroscopic surgical skill evaluation tool (ASSET). Am J Sports Med. 2013;41:1229–37.
16. Rahm S, Germann M, Hingsammer A, Wieser K, Gerber C. Validation of a virtual reality-based simulator for shoulder arthroscopy. Knee Surg Sports Traumatol Arthrosc. 2016;24(5):1730-7.
17. Waterman BR, Martin KD, Cameron KL, Owens BD, Belmont PJ Jr. Simulation training improves surgical proficiency and safety during diagnostic shoulder arthroscopy performed by residents. Orthopedics. 2016;39:e479–85.
18. Angelo RL, Pedowitz RA, Ryu RKN, Gallagher AG. The Bankart Performance Metrics Combined With a Shoulder Model Simulator Create a Precise and Accurate Training Tool for Measuring Surgeon Skill. YJARS. Arthroscopy Association of North America; 2015;31(9):1639-54.
19. Ferguson J, Middleton R, Alvand A, Rees J. Newly acquired arthroscopic skills: Are they transferable during simulator training of other joints? Knee Surg Sports Traumatol Arthrosc. 2017;25(2):608-15.
20. Jackson WFM, Khan T, Alvand A, Al-Ali S, Gill HS, Price AJ, et al. Learning and retaining simulated arthroscopic meniscal repair skills. J Bone Joint Surg Am [Internet]. 2012;94:e1321. Available from: http://eutils.ncbi.nlm.nih.gov/entrez/eutils/elink.fcgi?dbfrom=pubmed&id=22992861&retmode=ref&cmd=prlinks
21. Cannon WD, Garrett WE, Hunter RE, Sweeney HJ, Eckhoff DG, Nicandri GT, et al. Improving residency training in arthroscopic knee surgery with use of a virtual-reality simulator. A randomized blinded study. J Bone Joint Surg Am. 2014;96:1798–806.
22. Reppenhagen S, Zimmermann L, Buerklein D, Rudert M, Barthel T. Effectivity of arthroscopic skill acquisition in virtual reality knee arthroscopy training. Barcelona: Posterpresentation ESSKA; 2016.
23. Howells NR, Gill HS, Carr AJ, Price AJ, Rees JL. Transferring simulated arthroscopic skills to the operating theatre: a randomised blinded study. J Bone Joint Surg Br. 2008;90:494–9.
24. Aïm F, Lonjon G, Hannouche D, Nizard R. Effectiveness of Virtual Reality Training in Orthopaedic Surgery. YJARS. Arthroscopy Association of North America; 2015;32(1):224-32.

16

Outcomes of arthroscopic debridement of isolated Ligamentum Teres tears using the iHOT-33

Nicholas Pergaminelis[1,2*], Jesse Renouf[1,2], Camdon Fary[1], Oren Tirosh[1] and Phong Tran[1,2,3]

Abstract

Background: Tears of the Ligamentum Teres are a common cause of groin pain. Tears of the ligament frequently co-exist alongside other bony or labral intra-articular hip lesions, which are also treated at the time of arthroscopy. For this reason, it is often difficult to assess the effect that debridement alone has on improving patient pain and function. This study aims to assess the short-term outcomes of arthroscopic debridement of isolated Ligamentum Teres tears using a validated patient-reported outcome score – the International Hip Outcome Tool (iHOT-33).

Methods: A retrospective review was performed of 35 patients (37 hips) who had an isolated Ligamentum Teres tear treated with arthroscopic radiofrequency debridement between September 2012 and September 2015. Patients with concomitant intra-articular hip pathology (femoroacetabular impingement, labral lesions, hip dysplasia) were excluded from the study. All patients completed the iHOT-33 questionnaire pre-operatively and post-operatively. The mean age was 37.7 years (range 16–67 years) and patients were followed up for a mean period of 17.7 months (range 6–42 months). Thirty-one patients were female and 4 were male.

Results: Thirty-seven isolated partial tears were managed with arthroscopic radiofrequency debridement. At follow up, the mean iHOT-33 score improved from 26.9 pre-operatively to 48.0 post-operatively, representing a mean improvement of 21.1 ($p < 0.001$). The minimum clinically important difference of the iHOT-33 is 6.1 points. Significant improvements were noted in all four sub-sections of the iHOT-33.

Conclusion: Arthroscopic radiofrequency debridement of isolated Ligamentum Teres tears provides short-term benefit in the majority of patients, including significant improvement in sporting function.

Keywords: Hip arthroscopy, Ligamentum Teres, Outcomes, International hip outcome tool

Background

Ligamentum Teres tears are being increasingly diagnosed during hip arthroscopy [1–3]. Having long been considered a vestigial structure of little significance, tears of the ligament are now recognised as a common cause of debilitating hip pain and mechanical hip symptoms [2–4]. They occur most frequently in young, active females, and are today routinely managed during hip arthroscopy with radiofrequency debridement [3, 4]. However, tears of the Ligamentum Teres are often diagnosed and managed arthroscopically at the same time as other co-existing bony or labral intra-articular hip pathology. It has therefore proved difficult to assess the effect that arthroscopic debridement of the ligament alone has on patient symptoms. Indeed, studies which solely evaluate the outcomes of arthroscopic debridement of isolated Ligamentum Teres tears remain limited [3, 4]. Previous studies have produced encouraging preliminary results but none have thus far utilised the International Hip Outcome Tool (iHOT-33) – a patient-reported outcome questionnaire that has been validated and recommended for use in hip arthroscopy and hip preservation surgery [5]. The aim of this study was to assess the short-term outcomes of arthroscopic debridement of isolated tears of the Ligamentum Teres using the iHOT-33.

* Correspondence: n.pergaminelis@gmail.com
[1]Orthopaedic Department, Western Health, Footscray, VIC 3011, Australia
[2]The University of Melbourne, Parkville, VIC, Australia
Full list of author information is available at the end of the article

Methods

A retrospective review of a hip arthroscopy database was carried out. The database included 2541 hip arthroscopies performed by two surgeons experienced in the procedure between September 2012 and September 2015. Of these, 557 (22.7%) involved debridement of a tear of the Ligamentum Teres. Patients who had concomitant intra-articular hip pathology (femoroacetabular impingement, labral lesions, hip dysplasia) also managed during arthroscopy were excluded from the study, as were patients who had previous hip surgery.

The study ultimately included 37 operations in 35 patients who had had an isolated Ligamentum Teres tear managed with arthroscopic debridement. There were two indications for surgery in these patients. 1) Evidence of an isolated Ligamentum Teres tear on pre-operative MRI. 2) Undifferentiated hip/groin pain refractory to conservative management, with no intra-articular hip pathology identified on pre-operative imaging. The patient population had a mean age of 37.7 years (range 16–67 years) and were followed up for a mean period of 17.7 months (median 16.6 months, range 6–42 months). The majority of the patients were female (31 females, 4 males). Twelve arthroscopies were performed on the left hip and 25 on the right hip. Patients were most commonly involved in amateur netball, gymnastics, dancing and running (Table 1).

Surgical technique

All arthroscopies were carried out by two surgeons experienced in the procedure. Surgeries were performed in the lateral decubitus position under general anaesthesia (without muscle relaxants), in a manner consistent with the method described by Glick [6]. Traction was applied to the operative leg using a McCarthy Hip Distractor (Innomed, Inc., Savannah, GA, USA), and two portals (direct lateral and anterolateral) were established using an image intensifier. Distension of the joint was maintained during the procedure using an arthroscopic pump, and pressure was kept constant at 40 mmHg. A 70^0 arthroscope was used throughout and an initial assessment of intra-articular pathology was performed. The Ligamentum Teres was routinely assessed in external rotation and internal rotation. Where tears of the Ligamentum Teres were present, they were classified as partial or complete in accordance with Gray and Villar's classification system [7]. The presence of associated chondropathy was also noted, and was graded according to the Outerbridge classification system [8]. In the setting of chondropathy, mild chondroplasty was performed in some cases. All tears of the Ligamentum Teres were debrided using a radiofrequency ablation probe (Vulcan Eflex Ablator Probe, Smith & Nephew, Andover, MA, USA). Where synovitis was present, a localised or generalised synovectomy was also performed, also using a radiofrequency ablation probe. Post-arthroscopy, the joint was injected with local anaesthetic (Ropivicaine 150 mg) and morphine (5 mg). All surgeries were performed as day-cases or overnight stays. Post-operatively, crutches were used as required in the days following surgery and patients were advised to fully weight-bear. A standard rehabilitation protocol was adhered to in all cases [9].

Table 1 Patient demographics

	Number
Number of patients	35
Mean age	37.7
Female: Male	31: 4
Number of hips	37
Left: Right	12: 25
Sport / Activity	
Netball	6
Gymnastics	2
Dancing	2
Running	2
Horse-riding	1
Rowing	1
Soccer	1
Basketball	1
Cycling	1
Swimming	1

Outcome score

Patients completed the iHOT-33 pre-operatively and post-operatively. The iHOT-33 is a self-administered patient-reported outcome questionnaire that was developed in 2012 for active patients between the ages of 18 and 60 with a variety of hip pathologies [10]. It has been recommended as the most appropriate tool for evaluating the outcomes of hip arthroscopy in young, active patients [11, 12]. The iHOT-33 contains 33 questions and is divided into four sub-sections, each of which assesses a distinct domain of a patient's daily life. It culminates in a total score from 0 to 100, where 100 represents an optimal score. Both the total iHOT-33 scores and the average scores for the questionnaire's four sub--sections were analysed.

Statistical analysis

Mean pre-operative and post-operative iHOT-33 scores were calculated. The difference between the mean pre-operative and mean post-operative iHOT-33 scores were investigated with a paired sample t Test. P was be considered statistically significant if it was less than 0.05.

Single-factor ANOVA was used to determine the effect of performing a synovectomy on patient outcomes.

Results

Of the 37 hips operated on, partial tears of the Ligamentum Teres were identified in all cases. No patients had complete tears of the Ligamentum Teres. All patients presented with hip or groin pain, and 7 reported additional mechanical symptoms such as catching, clicking or giving way. In 12 cases patients could recall an acute, traumatic event that precipitated their symptoms, while they could not in 25 cases. On examination, all patients were found to have hip irritability, with 29 of these recording a positive Flexion Adduction Internal Rotation (FADIR) Test and 3 recording a positive Flexion Abduction External Rotation (FABER) Test.

Before orthopaedic referral and review, all patients had been managed conservatively by their general practitioner or a sports physician with analgesia and in some cases physical therapy. The duration of symptoms before specialist referral was highly variable, with a median period of 16 months (range 3 months – 5 years). Following their initial orthopaedic review, all patients chose to pursue arthroscopic intervention. The mean waiting time between orthopaedic review and surgery was 13 weeks (95% CI 9–17 weeks), and during this period patients continued conservative management for their symptoms.

All patients had a degree of synovitis detected at arthroscopy. A localised synovectomy was performed in 19 cases and a generalised synovectomy was performed in 9 cases (Table 2). Performing a synovectomy did not significantly impact post-operative iHOT-33 scores (p = 0.72). Associated chondral damage was present in 22 hips (Table 2). Eleven had both acetabular and femoral chondral damage, 8 had femoral chondral damage alone and 3 had acetabular chondral damage alone. Six patients underwent mild chondroplasty in for chondral damage. Capsular tightening was performed in addition to arthroscopic debridement of the Ligamentum Teres in 2 operations, once by radiofrequency debridement and once by suture plication. One patient had a second operation to debride their Ligamentum Teres due to persistent symptoms following their initial arthroscopy.

Table 2 Operative findings and details

	Number	Percent
Synovectomy		
Localised	19	51.4
Generalised	9	24.3
Chondropathy (Outerbridge Classification)		
Femoral	*18*	*48.6*
Grade 1	2	5.4
Grade 2	8	21.6
Grade 3	8	21.6
Grade 4	0	0
Acetabular	*12*	*32.4*
Grade 1	3	8.1
Grade 2	4	10.8
Grade 3	1	2.7
Grade 4	4	10.8
Capsular Tightening	2	5.4

At follow up, the mean total iHOT-33 score improved from 26.9 pre-operatively (95% CI 22.1–31.7) to 48.0 post-operatively (95% CI 40.6–55.3), representing a mean improvement of 21.1 (95% CI 14.2–27.9, $p <$ 0.001). The minimum clinically important difference of the iHOT-33 is 6.1 points [10]. Significant improvements were noted in all four sub-sections of the iHOT-33 (Table 3). For the single patient who underwent a second arthroscopy, revision surgery led to an improvement of 26.7 points. Tears of the Ligamentum Teres were successfully diagnosed pre-operatively on MRI in only 9 cases (21.6%).

Discussion

Tears of Ligamentum Teres are being increasingly identified at the time of arthroscopy [13]. There is also a growing body of evidence regarding the Ligamentum Teres' role as a secondary stabiliser of the hip joint, as well as its potential nociceptive and proprioceptive function [14–16]. Debriding tears of the ligament (without resecting the ligament itself) potentially reduces inflammation around its torn fibres, which in turn relieves pain and improves its mechanical function.

This study demonstrated that arthroscopic debridement of isolated tears of the ligament leads to significant short-term improvements in both pain and function. After a mean follow up of 17.7 months, the mean iHOT-33 score improved from 26.9 pre-operatively to 48.0 post-operatively. These findings are consistent with positive results described elsewhere in the literature.

Byrd and Jones produced the first prospective case series that assessed the outcomes of arthroscopic debridement in 2004 [2]. Twenty-three patients (mean age 28.3) were followed for a mean period of 29.2 months. They noted a significant improvement in the mean Modified Harris Hip Score (MHHS) from 47 pre-operatively to 90 post-operatively. However, patients with concomitant intra-articular hip pathology were not excluded from their study.

Subsequently, two retrospective case series have evaluated the outcomes of arthroscopic debridement of the isolated Ligamentum Teres tear. Haviv and O'Donnell followed 29 patients (mean age 25) for a mean period of

Table 3 Pre-operative and post-operative iHOT-33 scores

	Mean Pre-Operative Score	Mean Post-Operative Score	Mean Change	*p*
Section 1: Symptoms & Functional Limitations	33.6	57.2	23.6	< 0.001
Section 2: Sports & Recreational Activities	15.0	31.9	16.9	< 0.001
Section 3: Job-Related Concerns	38.4	56.1	17.7	0.007
Section 4: Social, Emotional & Lifestyle Concerns	19.1	42.6	23.6	< 0.001
Total Score	26.9	48	21.1	< 0.001

30 months [3]. They observed significant improvements in both the mean MHHS (70 pre-operatively to 86 post-operatively) and Non-Arthritic Hip Score (NAHS) (65–86).

Similar improvements were noted in Amenabar and O'Donnell's 2013 study of 26 patients (mean age 24.4), who underwent both arthroscopic debridement and capsular tightening by either radiofrequency or suture plication [4]. At follow up (mean 32 months), significant improvements in both the MHHS (65–89) and NAHS (66–87) were noted.

Numerous patient-reported outcome scores have been utilised to assess hip arthroscopy outcomes [5]. The Modified Harris Hip Score is derived from the Harris Hip Score, which itself was created for older, arthritic patients undergoing total hip arthroplasty [17]. As such, it has been shown to have a ceiling effect in younger patients [12]. Furthermore, it has been demonstrated to have limited correlation with patient satisfaction in the setting of hip arthroscopy [18]. The Non-Arthritic Hip Score was developed in 2003 for younger patients between the ages of 20 and 40 with non-arthritic hip pathology. It has good reliability and validity but is not validated for monitoring post-operative changes [19]. It has also been shown to have a ceiling effect in younger patients [12].

The iHOT-33 is validated for use in hip arthroscopy, particularly in young, active patients. Although it has been found to be a valid tool to measure hip arthroscopy outcomes, few publications have utilised it to date [20, 21]. The iHOT-33 was formulated in 2012 for active patients between the ages of 18 and 60 with a variety of hip pathologies [10]. It has excellent validity, and has been recommended by two recent systematic reviews as the most appropriate questionnaire in appraising outcomes of arthroscopic hip surgery [11, 12].

In addition, the iHOT-33's four sub-sections further allow for further sub-analysis of surgical outcomes. Significant improvements were observed in all four sections of the iHOT-33 with the greatest improvements in the domains of 'Symptoms and Functional Limitations' and 'Social, Emotional and Lifestyle Concerns'. Lesser levels of improvement were observed in the domains of 'Job-Related Concerns' and 'Sports and Recreational Activities'.

Participation in sport is common amongst patients with tears of the Ligamentum Teres [2–4]. This study's population were young and athletic, with patients most commonly participating in netball, gymnastics, dancing and running. As such, the findings related to the 'Sports and Recreational Activities' sub-section provide useful insights. The sub-sections of the iHOT-33 have not been validated for individual use, but it has been suggested that individual analysis may in fact provide a more valuable assessment of a patient's functional limitations than their total iHOT-33 score [10, 22].

Clinical diagnosis of tears of the Ligamentum Teres is difficult, as findings on both history and examination are often non-specific for intra-articular hip pathology [2, 3, 23]. In this study, patients most commonly presented with hip or groin pain, with some experiencing mechanical symptoms such as clicking, catching and feelings of instability. A majority of patients could not recall an acute traumatic injury which preceded the onset of their symptoms. The natural history of these symptoms was heterogeneous, with patients being managed conservatively by general practitioners or sports physicians from 3 months to up to 5 years before being referred to an orthopaedic surgeon. Hip irritability and a positive FADIR sign were the most common findings on examination, reinforcing the non-specific nature of clinical findings. Like other intra-articular hip pathology, MRI is the preferred method of detecting tears pre-operatively, but multiple studies have found that it is neither sensitive nor specific [1, 24, 25]. Our study demonstrated improved detection rates. 21.6% of tears were successfully diagnosed pre-operatively on MRI, albeit in a relatively small population. This perhaps suggests that the ability to diagnose tears is improving as recognition of Ligamentum Teres pathology continues to increase. Nonetheless, MRI was still an unreliable diagnostic tool. Ultimately, all patients progressed to arthroscopy following their initial orthopaedic review, regardless of the nature of their symptoms, acuity of their presentation and initial radiological findings.

Although the use of the iHOT-33 and the exclusion of concomitant intra-articular hip pathology remain valuable aspects of this study, several limitations still exist. The most significant is that the study did not include a control group. Despite the fact that all patients had been unsuccessfully managed non-operatively before arthroscopic intervention, both the timeframe and nature of conservative management was highly variable. In addition, data collection was retrospective and there are inherent limitations of such a study design. While most of the study's participants were young females, there was still a relative level of heterogeneity in their age and level of physical activity. Furthermore, follow up only occurred over a short-term period. Nevertheless, initial results are promising and represent the largest population of patients in the current literature. Extended follow up is now required, and is currently being performed, to assess the long-term outcomes of arthroscopic debridement.

Conclusion

Arthroscopic debridement of isolated tears of the Ligamentum Teres leads to short-term improvements in pain and function, when using the iHOT-33 to measure outcomes. Improvements were most significant in the domains of symptoms and functional limitations, as well as social, emotional and lifestyle concerns. They were less marked in job-related and sporting activities. Despite this, significant improvement was observed in sporting function, providing positive and valuable prognostic information for the athletic patients who commonly suffer from tears of the ligament.

Abbreviations

FABER: Flexion abduction external rotation test; FADIR: Flexion adduction internal rotation test; iHOT-33: International hip outcome tool

Acknowledgements

Not applicable

Funding

Not applicable.

Authors contributions

NP: Involved in conception of study, acquisition of iHOT-33 score data, drafting of manuscript. JR: Involved in conception of study, acquisition of iHOT-33 score data, drafting of manuscript. CF: Performed surgeries, analysis of and interpretation of data, drafting of manuscript. OT: Involved in design of the study, assisted in acquisition of and collection of data electronically, analysis of data. PT: Performed surgeries, analysis and interpretation of data, drafting of manuscript. All authors read and approved the final manuscript.

Consent for publication

Not applicable.

Competing interests

The authors declare that they have no competing interests.

Author details

[1]Orthopaedic Department, Western Health, Footscray, VIC 3011, Australia. [2]The University of Melbourne, Parkville, VIC, Australia. [3]Australian Institute for Musculoskeletal Science (The University of Melbourne and Western Health), St. Albans, VIC, Australia.

References

1. Botser IB, Martin DE, Stout CE, Domb BG. Tears of the ligamentum teres: prevalence in hip arthroscopy using 2 classification systems. Am J Sports Med. 2011;39(Suppl):117S–25S. https://doi.org/10.1177/0363546511413865.
2. Byrd JWT, Jones K. Traumatic rupture of the ligamentum teres as a source of hip pain. Arthroscopy. 2004;4:385–91.
3. Haviv B, Donnell J. Arthroscopic debridement of the isolated Ligamentum Teres rupture. Knee Surgery, Sport Traumatol Arthrosc. 2011;19:1510–3. https://doi.org/10.1007/s00167-010-1318-7.
4. Amenabar T, O'Donnell J. Successful treatment of isolated, partial thickness ligamentum teres (LT) tears with debridement and capsulorrhaphy. HIP Int. 2013;6:576–82.
5. Ramisetty N, Kwon Y, Mohtadi N. Patient-reported outcome measures for hip preservation surgery-a systematic review of the literature. J hip Preserv Surg. 2015;2:15–27. https://doi.org/10.1302/2046-3758.47.2000380.
6. Glick J. Hip arthroscopy. The lateral approach. Clin Sports Med. 2001;20:733–47.
7. Gray AJR, Villar RN. The ligamentum teres of the hip: an arthroscopic classification of its pathology. Arthroscopy. 1997;13:575–8. https://doi.org/10.1016/S0749-8063(97)90182-1.
8. Outerbridge R. The aetiology of chondromalacia patellae. J Bone Jt Surg. 1961;43:752–7.
9. Takla A. The hip. Assessment, arthroscopy and TOP protocol. Sport Physio Aust. 2009;1:18–21.
10. Mohtadi NGH, Griffin DR, Pedersen ME, et al. The development and validation of a self-administered quality-of-life outcome measure for young, active patients with symptomatic hip disease: the international hip outcome tool (iHOT-33). Arthrosc. J Arthrosc Relat Surg. 2012;28:595–610. https://doi.org/10.1016/j.arthro.2012.03.013.
11. Kemp JL, Collins NJ, Roos EM, Crossley KM. Psychometric properties of patient-reported outcome measures for hip arthroscopic surgery. Am J Sports Med. 2013;41:2065–73. https://doi.org/10.1177/0363546513494173.
12. Thorborg K, Tijssen M, Habets B, et al (2015) Patient-Reported Outcome (PRO) questionnaires for young to middle-aged adults with hip and groin disability: a systematic review of the clinimetric evidence. Br J Sports Med. https://doi.org/10.1136/bjsports-2014-094224.
13. Domb BG, Martin DE, Botser IB. Risk factors for ligamentum teres tears. Arthrosc - J Arthrosc Relat Surg. 2013;29:64–73. https://doi.org/10.1016/j.arthro.2012.07.009.
14. Dehao BW, Bing TK, Young J. Understanding the ligamentum teres of the hip: a histological study. Acta Orthop Bras. 2015;23:29–33.
15. Leunig M, Beck M, Stauffer E, et al. Free nerve endings in the ligamentum capitis femoris. Acta Orthop Scand. 2000;71:452–4.
16. Martin RL, Palmer I, Martin HD. Ligamentum teres: a functional description and potential clinical relevance. Knee Surgery, Sport Traumatol Arthrosc. 2012;20:1209–14. https://doi.org/10.1007/s00167-011-1663-1.
17. Byrd JWT, Jones KS. Prospective analysis of hip arthroscopy with 2-year follow-up. Arthroscopy. 2000;16:578–87. https://doi.org/10.1053/jars.2000.7683.
18. Aprato A, Jayasekera N, Villar RN. Does the modified Harris hip score reflect patient satisfaction after hip arthroscopy? Am J Sports Med. 2012;40:2557–60. https://doi.org/10.1177/0363546512460650.
19. Christensen C, Althausen P, Mittleman M, et al. The nonarthritic hip score: reliable and validated. Clin Orthop Relat Res. 2003;406:75–83.
20. Hetaimish BM, Khan M, Crouch S, et al. Consistency of reported outcomes after arthroscopic management of femoroacetabular impingement. Arthrosc - J Arthrosc Relat Surg. 2013;29:780–7. https://doi.org/10.1016/j.arthro.2012.11.011.
21. Yeung M, Khan M, Schreiber VM, et al. Global discrepancies in the diagnosis, surgical management, and investigation of femoroacetabular impingement. Arthroscopy. 2014;30:1625–33. https://doi.org/10.1016/j.arthro.2014.06.008.
22. Dwyer MK, Green M, McCarthy JC. Assessing outcomes following arthroscopic labral debridement-what can the IHOT-33 reveal? J Hip Preserv Surg. 2015;0:1–6. https://doi.org/10.1093/jhps/hnv022.

17

Risk factors of perioperative complications for posterior spinal fusion in degenerative scoliosis patients

Hai Wang[1†], Zheping Zhang[2†], Guixing Qiu[1], Jianguo Zhang[1*] and Jianxiong Shen[1*]

Abstract

Backgrounds: Rare study has been conducted to detect risk factors of perioperative complications, which are closely related to preoperative status of the patients and surgical stress. The aim of this study is to detect these relationships in degenerative scoliosis (DS) patients.

Methods: Perioperative complications of 226 cases with DS (56 males and 170 females; 65.5 ± 8.1 years old), who accepted posterior fusion in our hospital from January, 2013 to July, 2017, were retrospectively reviewed. Potential risk factors were first compared between patients with or without perioperative complications using student t test or Chi-squared test. Then, the unevenly distributed variables between the two groups were analyzed with binary logistic regression model.

Results: All patients separately underwent decompression with short limited instrumentation (116, 51.3%) or with long instrumentation for correction (110, 48.7%). The mean operation duration (OD) was 216.9 ± 64.2 min and the average amount of bleeding was 587.4 ± 357.2 ml. 44 cases (19.5%)suffered from the complications during the perioperative phase, including incision complications (5.3%), urinary infection (3.5%), dura tears/cerebrospinal fluid (CSF) leakages (3.5%) and new neurological deficits (2.7%). Hospital stay was significantly extended for the complications ($p < 0.001$). Univariate analysis showed that OD ($p < 0.001$), bleeding ($p = 0.014$), American Standards Association (ASA) grade > 2 ($p = 0.011$) and RBC transfusion≥4 U($p = 0.028$) were associated with these complications. Multivariate logistic regressions revealed that only ASA grade > 2($p = 0.011$, Odds Ratio[OR] = 4.104, 95% Confidence Interval[CI] = 1.413~ 11.917) and OD ($p = 0.013$, OR = 2.697, 95% CI = 1.233~ 5.899) were the independent risk factors.

Conclusions: The high morbidity of perioperative complications for posterior spinal fusion would significantly extend hospital stay of DS patients. It was independently related to higher ASA grade and longer OD.

Keywords: Degenerative scoliosis, Perioperative complication, Risk factors, American standards association (ASA) classification, Operation duration (OD)

Background

Degenerative scoliosis (DS), firstly described as "de novo" scoliosis, is a scoliosis caused by progressive degeneration of the spine in individuals without preexisting spinal deformity [1]. Most patients suffered from severe low back pain, nerve root compression symptoms and/or neurogenic claudication. Surgery is the most common therapy for patients who have failed conservative treatment, which can significantly alleviate the pain and improve the quality of life [2]. With the population aging, there is an associated rise in the prevalence of degenerative spinal disorders, including DS [3]. The demand for surgical treatment for DS had increased, with an increase of 3.4 times in more than 60 years of age from 2004 to 2011 according to the Scoliosis Research Society (SRS) database [4].

Surgical management of DS in the elderly population represents a challenge for spinal surgeons in clinic with the postoperative complication rate of 49% [2]. Perioperative complications accounted for more than half of postoperative

* Correspondence: jgzhang_pumch@yahoo.com; sjxpumch@163.com
†Hai Wang and Zheping Zhang contributed equally to this work.
1 Department of Orthopaedic Surgery, Peking Union Medical College Hospital, Peking Union Medical College and Chinese Academy of Medical Sciences, No. 1 Shuaifuyuan, Beijing 100730, China
Full list of author information is available at the end of the article

complications [5], and were closely related to preoperative status of the patients and surgical stress [6]. Understanding risk factors of perioperative complications could help to optimize treatment plan and improve cost-effectiveness. Up to now, there are few reports about the relationship between the perioperative complications and their risk factors.

The aim of this study is to report and analyze the perioperative complications and the potential risk factors related to preoperative status of the patients and surgical stress in DS patients.

Methods

Patients

A total of 226 consecutive patients with DS, who underwent posterior spinal fusion in our medical center from January, 2013 to July, 2017, were retrospectively reviewed. The patients who received minimally invasive surgery or with malignant tumor were excluded. General Characteristics, including age, sex, body mass index (BMI), smoking history, medication history (especially for insulin), comorbidities, lumbar operation history, preoperative hemoglobin (Hgb) and hospital stay, were charted. American Society of Anesthesiologists (ASA) grade was evaluated by two anesthetists.

Surgical procedures

X-rays, computerized tomography, and magnetic resonance imaging were routinely performed before operation. The surgical method was decided by all spine experts in our department based on its symptoms, signs, and images according to Lenke-Silva's suggestions in combination with its age, medical comorbidities, and socioeconomic status [7, 8]. Surgical methods included decompression with limited short fusion and decompression with long fusion for correction. Fusion levels, iliac fixation, operation duration (OD), bleeding, and homologous red blood cells (RBC) transfusion were recorded after surgery. All perioperative complications occurring within 30 days after the operation were also collected in detail.

Statistic analysis

Means and proportions were used to describe the overall sample as well as the groups identified by the presence (Group A) or absence (Group B) of perioperative complications. The quantitative variates (age, BMI, preoperative Hgb, OD, bleeding, and hospital stay) were compared between the two groups (Groups A&B) using student t test. The qualitative variates (sex [male or female], smoking [yes or no], ASA grade [1~2 or > 2], medical comorbidities [with or without heart disease/ respiratory disease/ diabetes mellitus(DM)/ insulin-dependent DM/immune disease], allograft [yes or no], RBC transfusion [< 4 U or ≥ 4 U], surgical method [short fusion (≤3 levels) or long fusion (> 3 levels) with correction], interbody fusion [yes or no], iliac fixation [yes or no], osteotomy [yes or no] and lumbar operation history [yes or no]) were compared by using Chi-square tests (Fisher exact tests where appropriate). All unevenly distributed variates between these two groups (Groups A&B) were analyzed with binary logistic regression model. The selection method was ENTER. Statistical analysis was performed with SPSS version 19.0 software (IBM Company, Armonk, New York, USA). All the potential risk factors were also analyzed between the patients with one complication and with multiple complications. $P < 0.05$ was set as significant difference.

Results

General characteristics

A total of 226 patients with DS were enrolled in this study, including 56 males and 170 females. Their mean age was 65.5 ± 8.1 years old. The average hospital stay was 15.9 ± 7.6 days. There were 133 cases (58.8%) with medical comorbidities, including 116 cases (51.3%) with heart disease, 35 cases (15.5%) with DM (8 cases with insulin-dependent DM), 11 cases (4.9%) with respiratory disease, and 11 cases (4.7%) with immune disease. Among them, there were about 34 cases (15.0%) with more than two medical morbidities. 7 cases (3.1%) had the history of lumbar surgery.

Table 1 Perioperative complications of degenerative scoliosis within postoperative 30 days

Complications	Patients (n)
Incision complications	12 cases
Superficial infection/ fat liquefaction	7 cases
Deep infection	4 cases
Hematoma	1 case
Urinary infection	8 cases
Dura tear/cerebrospinal fluid leakage	8 cases
New neurological deficits	6 cases
Respiratory complications	4 cases
Pulmonary infection	3 cases
Pleural effusion	2 cases
Atelectasis	1 cases
Myocardial ischemia	2 cases
Venous thromboembolism	3 cases
Plexus venosus leg muscle thrombosis	2 cases
Pulmonary embolism	1 cases
Sepsis	2 cases
Delirium	1 cases
Abnormal glutamic-pyruvic transaminase	2 cases
Central nervous system infection	1 case
Cerebral infarction	1 case
Total	44 cases

Table 2 The results of Univariate analysis between the patients with or without perioperative complications

Variates	Perioperative complications		*P* value
	No (*n* = 182)	Yes (*n* = 44)	
Age(years)	65.6 ± 8.2	65.1 ± 7.9	0.729
Preoperative Hgb(g/L)	134.6 ± 13.9	131. 0 ± 14.2	0.130
BMI(kg/m^2)	25.6 ± 3.7	26.8 ± 3.6	0.065
Bleeding(ml)	558.8 ± 339.7	705.7 ± 405.1	0.014
OD(minutes)	208.6 ± 58.1	251.7 ± 77.2	0.000
Hospital stay(days)	14.3 ± 5.3	22.2 ± 11.6	0.000
Sex			
Female	135(79.4%)	35(20.6%)	0.459
Male	47(83.9%)	9(16.1%)	
ASA grade			
1~2	172(82.7%)	36(17.3%)	0.011*
> 2	10(55.6%)	8(44.4%)	
Heart disease			
No	91(82.7%)	19(17.3%)	0.417
Yes	91(78.4%)	25(21.6%)	
Respiratory disease			
No	173(80.5%)	42(19.5%)	1.000*
Yes	9(81.8%)	2(18.2%)	
DM			
No	151(79.1%)	40(20.9%)	0.191
Yes	31(88.6%)	4(11.4%)	
Insulin-dependent DM			
No	176(80.7%)	42(19.3%)	0.655*
Yes	6(75.0%)	2(25.0%)	
Immune disease			
No	174(80.9%)	41(19.1%)	0.451*
Yes	8(72.7%)	3(27.3%)	
Smoking			
No	161(82.1%)	35 (17.9%)	0.118
Yes	21(70.0%)	9(30.0%)	
Allograft			
No	54(79.4%)	14(20.6%)	0.780
Yes	128(81.0%)	30(19.0%)	
RBC transfusion			
< 4 U	167(82.7%)	35(17.3%)	0.028*
≥ 4 U	15(62.5%)	9(37.5%)	
Surgical method			
Short fusion	96(82.8%)	20(17.2%)	0.385
Long fusion	86(78.2%)	24(21.8%)	
Interbody fusion			
No	166(81.8%)	37(18.2%)	0.170*

Table 2 The results of Univariate analysis between the patients with or without perioperative complications *(Continued)*

Variates	Perioperative complications		*P* value
	No (*n* = 182)	Yes (*n* = 44)	
Yes	16(69.6%)	7(30.4%)	
Osteotomy			
No	176(80.4%)	43(19.6%)	1.000*
Yes	6(85.7%)	1(14.3%)	
Lumbar operation history			
No	175(80.3%)	43(19.7%)	1.000*
Yes	7(87.5%)	1(12.5%)	
Iliac fixation			
No	177(80.8%)	42(19.2%)	0.624*
Yes	5(71.4%)	2(28.6%)	

*Fisher exact test

Surgical characteristics

Decompression with limited short fusion was done in 116cases (51.3%), and decompression with long fusion and correction of deformity was done in 110 cases (48.7%). Osteotomy was performed in 7 cases (3.1%), including 4 Smith-Peterson osteotomies and 3 pedicle subtraction osteotomies. The mean OD was 216.9 ± 64.2 min and the average amount of bleeding was 587.4 ± 357.2 ml. 142 cases (62.8%) used autologous blood transfusion system and 79 cases (35.0% accepted allogeneic blood transfusion with RBC of 2.8 ± 1.3 U and plasma of 374.5 ± 122.4 ml.

Perioperative complications

Perioperative complications occurred in 44 patients (19.5%) within 30 days after operation, including 12 cases (5.3%) with incision complications, 8 cases (3.5%) with urinary infections, 8 cases (3.5%) with dura tears/cerebrospinal fluid (CSF) leakages, 6 cases (2.7%) with new neurological deficits and others (Table 1). The incision complications included 7 superficial infections/fat liquefactions, 4 deep infections and 1 hematoma. 5 patients (2.2%) suffered from more than 2 complications, including 1 case with superficial infection and urinary infection; 1 case with deep infection, urinary infection, CSF leakage, and central nervous system infection; 1 case with deep infection and sepsis; 1case with superficial infection, pleural effusion,atelectasis and pulmonary embolism and 1case with pleural effusion and pulmonary infection. 3 patients (1.3%) underwent unplanned second surgeries for their complications, including 2 deep infections and 1new neurological deficit because of poor screw position. One patient with incision hematoma accepted the interventional puncture therapy.

Statistic analysis

Hospital stay of the patients was significant prolonged by their perioperative complications (14.3 ± 5.3 vs 22.2 ± 11.6 days, $p < 0.001$). As shown in Table 2, the distributions of bleeding ($p = 0.014$), OD ($p < 0.001$), ASA grade ($p = 0.011$), and RBC transfusion ($p = 0.028$) were significantly different between the patients with and without perioperative complications. In order to eliminate influences of farraginous factors, a binary logistic regression model was used for multivariate analysis of unevenly distributed variates. The results showed that ASA grade > 2 ($p = 0.009$, Odds Ratio[OR] = 4.104, 95% Confidence Interval[CI] =1.413~ 11.917) and OD ($p = 0.013$, OR = 2.697, 95% CI = 1.233~ 5.899) were two independent risk factors (Table 3). Further, the risk factor of multiple complications was also evaluated. But there was no significant one to be associated with multiple complications (Table 4).

Discussion

There was a relative higher morbidity of perioperative complications for DS, similar to that of postoperative complications. The morbidities of perioperative complications were about 20.4% in this study and 29.8% in Cho's report [5]. They would significantly prolong the hospital stay ($p < 0.001$), and consequently increase the medical cost, and lower the postoperative satisfaction. Thence, it was a major challenge for spinal surgeons to deal with perioperative complications in DS patients.

Incision complications were the most common perioperative complications in DS patients (5.3%). Although some patients lack bacteriological evidence of infection after superficial fat liquefaction, we still considered that there was a high possibility of superficial infections. Therefore, superficial fat liquefaction and infections were put together, accounting for 58.3% of the total incision complications. Most of them could be healed by dressing and antibiotic therapy. The key points were close observation, early detection and treatment to prevent spreading to the deep structure. For deep infections, vacuum-assisted closure device was recommended, because it could significantly reduce the rate of reoperation of deep infection after spinal internal fixation, shorten the use of antibiotics, improve the retention rate of internal fixation [9]. In this study, 4 cases with deep infection were cured by the combination of vacuum-assisted closure device and systemic antibiotic therapy.

Table 3 The results of binary logistic regression analysis of unevenly distributed variates between the patients with or without perioperative complications. (method = "Enter")

Variates	P value	Odds Ratio (95% Confidence Interval)
Bleeding	0.694	1.000(0.999~ 1.001)
RBC transfusion	0.274	1.840(0.616~ 5.494)
ASA grade	0.009	4.104(1.413~ 11.917)
OD	0.013	2.697(1.233~ 5.899)

Urinary infection was another common complication of DS with the incidence of 3.5% in this study. It was one of the risk factors for incision infection after posterior spinal fusion [10]. There were 2 cases with incision infections following urinary infections in this study. Therefore, it was very important to prevent and early detect urinary infection. Most nosocomial urinary infections were associated with indwelling urinary catheters, and its incidence could be significantly reduced by shortening indwelling time [11]. It was suggested to remove urinary catheter as soon as possible.

Dural tear /CSF leak was one of the major complications of DS. The incidence was 3.5%, similar to 2.9% for adult scoliosis according to the SRS database [12]. It might lead to incision complications, pseudomeningocele, cerebrospinal fluid sinuses, arachnoiditis, meningitis, epidural abscess and psychiatric symptoms [13]. Once dural tear was found during operation, it was suggested to intraoperatively repair as far as possible [14]. The other recommended measures included suturing the para-spinal muscle to reduce the dead space, suturing the incision closely, and lying supine for 4–7 days after operation to reduce hydrostatic pressure.

New neurological deficits were common complications of concern in DS patients. The morbidity was 2.7% in this study, in accordance with 2.0% reported by SRS [12]. They were mostly associated with the performance of these extensive decompressions because DS patients often had significant spinal canal stenosis [15]. Most of them were transient nerve root complications and only needed conservative treatment [16]. But it was still necessary to be careful about the position of implants. There was one new neurological deficit for poor position of screw in this study. For these cases, it was very important to detect and address them to keep more neurological functions as early as possible.

Perioperative complications were associated with preoperative status of the patients and surgical stress [6]. Some variates about preoperative status and surgical stress were considered as potential risk factors of perioperative complications in this study, referring to the previous related studies [6, 17, 18]. Univariate analysis results showed that bleeding ($p = 0.014$), OD ($p < 0.001$), ASA grade ($p = 0.011$), and RBC transfusion ($p = 0.028$) unevenly distributed between patients with and without perioperative complications. Further, multivariate regression analysis results revealed that only ASA grade > 2 ($p = 0.009$) and OD ($p = 0.013$) were the independent risk factors.

Table 4 The results of Univariate analysis between the patients with one or multiple perioperative complications

Variates	Perioperative complications		*P* value
	< 2 (*n* = 39)	≥ 2 (*n* = 5)	
Age(years)	65.3 ± 7.9	64.0 ± 9.6	0.738
Preoperative Hgb(g/L)	130.7 ± 14.5	133.4 ± 13.3	0.694
BMI(kg/m^2)	26.7 ± 3.6	27.6 ± 3.8	0.586
Bleeding(ml)	718.0 ± 395.8	610.0 ± 512.8	0.581
OD(minutes)	250.3 ± 69.8	263.0 ± 132.2	0.732
Sex			
Female	31(88.6%)	4(11.4%)	1.000*
Male	8(88.9%)	1(11.1%)	
ASA grade			
1~2	32(88.9%)	4(11.1%)	1.000*
> 2	7(87.5%)	1(12.5%)	
Heart disease			
No	17(89.5%)	2(10.5%)	1.000*
Yes	22(88.0%)	3(12.0%)	
Respiratory disease			
No	37(88.1%)	5(11.9%)	1.000*
Yes	2(100.0%)	0(0.0%)	
DM			
No	36(75.0%)	1(10.0%)	0.394
Yes	3(88.6%)	4(25.0%)	
Insulin-dependent DM			
No	37(88.1%)	5(11.9%)	1.000*
Yes	2(100.0%)	0(0.0%)	
Immune disease			
No	36(87.8%)	5(12.2%)	1.000*
Yes	3(100.0%)	0(0.0%)	
Smoking			
No	30(85.7%)	5(14.3%)	0.566*
Yes	9(100.0%)	0(0.0%)	
Allograft			
No	12(85.7%)	2(14.3%)	0.647*
Yes	27(90.0%)	3(10.0%)	
RBC transfusion			
< 4 U	31(88.6%)	4(11.4%)	1.000*
≥ 4 U	8(88.9%)	1(11.1%)	
Surgical method			
Short fusion	18(90.0%)	2 (10.0%)	1.000*
Long fusion	21(87.5%)	3(12.5%)	
Interbody fusion			
No	32(86.5%)	5(13.5%)	0.574*
Yes	7(100.0%)	0(0.0%)	
Osteotomy			
No	38(88.4%)	5(11.6%)	1.000*
Yes	1(100.0%)	0(0.0%)	
Lumbar operation history			
No	38(88.4%)	5(11.6%)	1.000*
Yes	1(100.0%)	0(0.0%)	
Iliac fixation			
No	38(90.5%)	4(9.5%)	0.217*
Yes	1(50.0%)	1(50.0%)	

*Fisher exact test

The ASA classification system was first proposed in 1963, on behalf of the patient's preoperative physical status [19]. Compared to other grading system (such as Acute Physiology and Chronic Health Evaluation II score, Physiological and Operative Severity Score for the Enumeration of Mortality and Morbidity, et al.), it was simple and easy to obtain [20]. The ASA grade had been confirmed to be associated with the morbidity and mortality in spinal surgery before [21, 22]. Its close relationship with the occurrence of postoperative complications in DS had also been reported [17]. In this study, the higher ASA grade (p = 0.009) was further founded to be related to the morbidity of perioperative complications in DS. It would be helpful in counseling individuals on risks of morbidity for perioperative complications.

Operative duration (p = 0.013) was the other independent risk factor for the development of perioperative complications in DS patients. First, it would likely result in higher incision infection rates. Because the surgical site exposed longer to the operating room surroundings with OD increasing. There was a significant correlation between the length of time that the sterile tray is exposed to the air and the contamination rate of the instruments [23]. Second, the duration of bleeding in the wound site would lead excessive intraoperative blood loss, which increased allogeneic blood transfusion. That's why bleeding (p = 0.694) and RBC transfusion (p = 0.274) were confounding factors of perioperative complications in this study. Third, it was also associated with overall complications, medical complications, and surgical complications as reported before [24]. Furthermore, OD was prone to be extended by the complexity of the type of procedure or patient health, level of training and expertise, and multilevel fusions [25].

As the results revealed that ASA > 2 and long OD were two independently risk factors of perioperative complications in this study. Thence, the surgical strategies should be optimized to shorten OD for those patients with ASA > 2 after preoperative evaluation, such as decompression without fusion or with short fusion, or minimally invasive surgery. In this study, the surgical method had been optimized according to its age, medical comorbidities, and socioeconomic status based on Lenke-Silva's suggestions. For some high-risk patients, short fusion was selected. That might be why long fusion was not related to perioperative complications.

There were several limitations for this study. The major limitation was the small sample size from one medical center. Some reported risk factors were not significant because the sample was relatively small such as insulin dependent DM [17]. For the same reason, we couldn't reveal any risk factors of multiple complications, and the association between the application of iliac fixation and complications ($n = 5$ for multiple complications; $n = 7$ for application of iliac fixation). Otherwise, it was a retrospective cohort study, and there was lack of standardized comparison groups.

Conclusion

The high morbidity of perioperative complications for posterior spinal fusion should draw more attention when planning operations in DS patients. It was independently associated with higher ASA grade and longer OD, respectively. For those high risk patients, such as ASA grade > 2, the optimized surgical strategies to shorten OD should be suggested to improve the patient outcomes.

Abbreviations

95%CI: 95% Confidence Interval; Alb: Albumin; ASA: American Society of Anesthesiologists; BMI: Body Mass Index; CSF: Cerebrospinal Fluid; DM: Diabetes Mellitus; DS: Degenerative Scoliosis; Hgb: Hemoglobin; OD: Operation Duration; OR: Odds Ratio; RBC: Red Blood Cells; SRS: Scoliosis Research Society

Authors' contributions

All authors made substantive intellectual contributions to this study to qualify as authors. HW and ZZ contributed to acquisition of data, analysis of data, statistical analysis, and interpretation of results. GQ contributed to study design and study coordination. JZ and JS contributed to study design, study coordination, and manuscript preparation. All authors read and approved the final manuscript.

Consent for publication

Not applicable.

Competing interests

The authors declare that they have no competing interests.

Author details

[1]Department of Orthopaedic Surgery, Peking Union Medical College Hospital, Peking Union Medical College and Chinese Academy of Medical Sciences, No. 1 Shuaifuyuan, Beijing 100730, China. [2]Department of Orthopaedic Surgery, Beijing Puren Hospital, Beijing, China.

References

1. Ailon T, Smith JS, Shaffrey CI, Lenke LG, Brodke D, Harrop JS, Fehlings M, Ames CP. Degenerative spinal deformity. Neurosurgery. 2015;77(Suppl 4): S75–91.
2. Liang CZ, Li FC, Li H, Tao Y, Zhou X, Chen QX. Surgery is an effective and reasonable treatment for degenerative scoliosis: a systematic review. J Int Med Res. 2012;40(2):399–405.
3. O'Lynnger TM, Zuckerman SL, Morone PJ, Dewan MC, Vasquez-Castellanos RA, Cheng JS. Trends for spine surgery for the elderly: implications for access to healthcare in North America. Neurosurgery. 2015;77(Suppl 4):S136–41.
4. Sing DC, Berven SH, Burch S, Metz LN. Increase in spinal deformity surgery in patients age 60 and older is not associated with increased complications. Spine J. 2017;17(5):627–35.
5. Cho KJ, Suk SI, Park SR, Kim JH, Kim SS, Choi WK, Lee KY, Lee SR. Complications in posterior fusion and instrumentation for degenerative lumbar scoliosis. Spine (Phila Pa 1976). 2007;32(20):2232–7.
6. Hirose J, Taniwaki T, Fujimoto T, Okada T, Nakamura T, Usuku K, Mizuta H. Validity of E-PASS system for postoperative morbidity of spinal surgery. J Spinal Disord Tech. 2015;28(10):E595–600.
7. Silva FE, Lenke LG. Adult degenerative scoliosis: evaluation and management. Neurosurg Focus. 2010;28(3):E1.
8. Kotwal S, Pumberger M, Hughes A, Girardi F. Degenerative scoliosis: a review. HSS J. 2011;7(3):257–64.
9. Kale M, Padalkar P, Mehta V. Vacuum-assisted closure in patients with post-operative infections after instrumented spine surgery: a series of 12 cases. J Orthop Case Rep. 2017;7(1):95–100.
10. Nunez-Pereira S, Rodriguez-Pardo D, Pellise F, Pigrau C, Bago J, Villanueva C, Caceres E. Postoperative urinary tract infection and surgical site infection in instrumented spinal surgery: is there a link? Clin Microbiol Infect. 2014;20(8): 768–73.
11. Lobao MJ, Sousa P. Hospital-acquired urinary tract infections: results of a cohort study performed in an internal medicine department. Acta Medica Port. 2017;30(9):608–14.
12. Sansur CA, Smith JS, Coe JD, Glassman SD, Berven SH, Polly DW Jr, Perra JH, Boachie-Adjei O, Shaffrey CI. Scoliosis research society morbidity and mortality of adult scoliosis surgery. Spine (Phila Pa 1976). 2011;36(9):E593–7.
13. Tosun B, Ilbay K, Kim MS, Selek O. Management of Persistent Cerebrospinal Fluid Leakage Following Thoraco-lumbar Surgery. Asian Spine J. 2012;6(3): 157–62.
14. Khan MH, Rihn J, Steele G, Davis R, Donaldson WF 3rd, Kang JD, Lee JY. Postoperative management protocol for incidental dural tears during degenerative lumbar spine surgery: a review of 3,183 consecutive degenerative lumbar cases. Spine (Phila Pa 1976). 2006;31(22):2609–13.
15. Fu KM, Smith JS, Polly DW Jr, Perra JH, Sansur CA, Berven SH, Broadstone PA, Choma TJ, Goytan MJ, Noordeen HH, et al. Morbidity and mortality in the surgical treatment of 10,329 adults with degenerative lumbar stenosis. J Neurosurg Spine. 2010;12(5):443–6.
16. Pateder DB, Kostuik JP. Lumbar nerve root palsy after adult spinal deformity surgery. Spine (Phila Pa 1976). 2005;30(14):1632–6.
17. Tang H, Zhu J, Ji F, Wang S, Xie Y, Fei H. Risk factors for postoperative complication after spinal fusion and instrumentation in degenerative lumbar scoliosis patients. J Orthop Surg Res. 2014;9(1):15.
18. Yang YH, Zheng J, Lou SL. Causes and managements of postoperative complications after degenerative scoliosis treatments with internal fixation. Int J Clin Exp Med. 2014;7(11):4300–7.
19. Yang KE. A new classification of tubal conditions in hysterosalpingography for prognosing and treating sterility: a study of 1,041 cases. Chin Med J. 1963;82:263–70.
20. de Cassia Braga Ribeiro K, Kowalski LP. APACHE II, POSSUM, and ASA scores and the risk of perioperative complications in patients with oral or oropharyngeal cancer. Arch Otolaryngol Head Neck Surg. 2003;129(7):739–45.

21. Pateder DB, Gonzales RA, Kebaish KM, Cohen DB, Chang JY, Kostuik JP. Short-term mortality and its association with independent risk factors in adult spinal deformity surgery. Spine (Phila Pa 1976). 2008;33(11):1224–8.
22. Fu KM, Smith JS, Polly DW Jr, Ames CP, Berven SH, Perra JH, McCarthy RE, Knapp DR Jr, Shaffrey CI, Scoliosis Research Society M, et al. Correlation of higher preoperative American Society of Anesthesiology grade and increased morbidity and mortality rates in patients undergoing spine surgery. J Neurosurg Spine. 2011;14(4):470–4.
23. Dalstrom DJ, Venkatarayappa I, Manternach AL, Palcic MS, Heyse BA, Prayson MJ. Time-dependent contamination of opened sterile operating-room trays. J Bone Joint Surg Am. 2008;90(5):1022–5.
24. Kim BD, Hsu WK, De Oliveira GS Jr, Saha S, Kim JY. Operative duration as an independent risk factor for postoperative complications in single-level lumbar fusion: an analysis of 4588 surgical cases. Spine (Phila Pa 1976). 2014;39(6):510–20.
25. Phan K, Kim JS, Capua JD, Lee NJ, Kothari P, Dowdell J, Overley SC, Guzman JZ, Cho SK. Impact of operation time on 30-day complications after adult spinal deformity surgery. Global Spine J. 2017;7(7):664–71.

18

Improving accuracy of opening-wedge osteotomies of distal radius using a patient-specific ramp-guide technique

Simon Roner[1*], Fabio Carrillo[1], Lazaros Vlachopoulos[2], Andreas Schweizer[2], Ladislav Nagy[2] and Philipp Fuernstahl[1]

Abstract

Background: Opening-wedge osteotomies of the distal radius, performed with three-dimensional printed patient-specific instruments, are a promising technique for accurate correction of malunions. Nevertheless, reports of residual malalignments and discrepancies in the plate and screw position from the planned fixation exist. Consequently, we developed a patient-specific ramp-guide technique, combining navigation of plate positioning, osteotomy cutting, and reduction. The aim of this study is to compare the accuracy of navigation of three-dimensional planned opening-wedge osteotomies, using a ramp-guide, over state-of-the-art guide techniques relying solely on pre-drilled holes.

Methods: A retrospective analysis was carried out on opening-wedge osteotomies of the distal radius, performed between May 2016 and April 2017, with patient-specific instruments. Eight patients were identified in which a ramp-guide for the distal plate fixation was used. We compared the reduction accuracy with a control group of seven patients, where the reduction was performed with pre-drilled screw holes placed with the patient-specific instruments. The navigation accuracy was assessed by comparing the preoperative plans with the postoperative segmented, computed tomography scans. The accuracy was expressed using a 3D angle and in measurements of all six degrees of freedom (3 translations, 3 rotations), with respect to an anatomical coordinate system.

Results: The duration of the surgery of the ramp-guide group was significantly shorter compared to the control group. Significantly less rotational and translational residual malalignment error was observed in the open-wedged osteotomies, where patient-specific instruments with ramp-guides were used. On average, a residual rotational malalignment error of 2.0° (± 2.2°) and a translational malalignment error of 0.6 mm (± 0. 2 mm) was observed in the ramp-guide group, as compared to the 4.2° (± 15.0°) and 1.0 mm (± 0.4 mm) error in the control group. The used plate was not significantly positioned more accurately, but significantly fewer screws (15.6%) were misaligned in the distal fragment compared to the control group (51.9%).

Conclusion: The use of the presented ramp-guide technique in opening-wedge osteotomies is improving reduction accuracy, screw position, and surgical duration, compared to the existing patient-specific instrument based navigation methods.

Keywords: Osteotomy, Distal radius, Extra-articular, Patient specific-instruments, Computer-assisted planning, Ramp-guide, Malunion

* Correspondence: simon.roner@balgrist.ch
[1]Computer Assisted Research and Development Group, Balgrist University Hospital, University of Zurich, Forchstrasse 340, 8008 Zurich, Switzerland
Full list of author information is available at the end of the article

Background

Malunions are one of the most common complications following fractures of the distal radius. As a consequence of alterations in the alignment, patients may have a limited range of motion (ROM) in the wrist and forearm or a painful or unstable distal radioulnar joint [1]. Typically, malunions of the distal radius fractures include a shortening and, especially after a Colles' type fracture, a dorsal angulation of the distal fragment [2]. Therefore, malunited distal radius fractures are often corrected through opening-wedge osteotomies.

Several studies have demonstrated the accurate restoration of radiological indices using corrective opening-wedge osteotomies to relieve the pain, and to improve the range of motion in symptomatic patients [3–5]. Nevertheless, three-dimensional (3D) deformities, especially with rotational malalignment, are not assessed accurately in two-dimensional (2D) plain radiographs [6]. A more reliable method is using 3D bone models, extracted from computed tomography (CT) for a precise deformity analysis, and preoperative planning for the corrective osteotomy [7–9]. Patient-specific instruments (PSI) for navigation can be designed based on the 3D-simulated postoperative bone models to accurately execute the surgical plan. A study in 2015 by Vlachopoulos [10] demonstrated a high reduction in the accuracy of closing-wedge and single-cut osteotomies, with a residual rotational malalignment error of 3.5° (± 1.1°), when using patient-specific instruments. Opening-wedge osteotomies were significantly less accurate at 8.30° (± 5.35°). The authors mention high soft-tissue tension as one of the reasons for difficulties when performing the reduction of opening-wedge osteotomies with only pre-drilled screw holes as reference.

Due to the weakness of the current PSI systems, we have developed a new patient-specific guide technique, for optimal plate and screw positioning in opening-wedge osteotomies. In 2016, the method was presented as a case of corrective osteotomy of a complex, malunited humeral fracture. With the aid of a ramp-guide, the reduction was performed indirectly using the predefined fixation of the plate on the humeral head [11]. The main feature is to create a guide for the navigation of the plate position using a ramp-like surface, on which the implant can be mounted, hereinafter called a ramp-guide. The goal of this study is to retrospectively compare the accuracy of the 3D planned opening-wedge osteotomies of the distal radius, using a ramp-guide for distal plate fixation, to that of the state-of-the-art patient-specific guides.

Methods

Nine patients were identified who underwent osteotomies of the distal radius, using patient-specific ramp-guides, between May 2016 and April 2017. The criteria for inclusion were the performance of an extra-articular opening-wedge osteotomy, and the presence of a postoperative CT scan. The control group was operated on between January and September 2013 in our department and consisted of seven patients who had been treated with open-wedge osteotomies, using commercial, state-of-the-art, patient-specific instruments (MyOsteotomy; Medacta SA, Castel San Pietro, Switzerland). The reduction accuracy of the control group was published in 2015 by Vlachopoulos [10]. Demographics of both groups are listed in Table 1.

Preoperative planning

Segmentations of pathological and contralateral healthy bone models from the CT data (Philips Brilliance 40 T, Amsterdam, Netherlands) were generated using commercial software, as discussed in a previous publication [10]. In-house preoperative planning software (CASPA; Balgrist CARD AG, Zurich, Switzerland) was used to create the 3D preoperative surgical plan. The mirror model of the contralateral bone was used as a template representing the physiological anatomy. The basic principle of 3D planning of opening-wedge osteotomies has been described previously [10].

Guide design

The plate is positioned exactly as desired on the simulated postoperative result (Fig. 1a). The position and direction of the screws in the proximal fragment are used to first design a pre-reduction guide on the surface of the pathological bone (Fig. 1b), used to pre-drill the proximal screws into the shaft fragment. This guide is also comprised of a cutting slot for partially navigating the osteotomy. In a second step, the plate is back-transformed on the pathological bone by applying the reduction to the plate and the distal fragment (Fig. 1c). Note that the position of the distal plate part relative to the distal fragment, did not change. Therefore, the back-transformation defines how the plate must be fixed on the distal fragment, before completing the corrective osteotomy. The ramp-guide is designed upon the pathological bone (Fig. 1d), defining the position of the plate, with respect to the distal fragment. Accuracy is guaranteed by a negative footprint of the plate on the slope, with a hole for the possibility of temporarily fixating the planned plate with a screw.

Patient-specific instruments of the control group were designed, as published in 2015 by Vlachopoulos [10]. In general, pre-reduction guides were used to define the

Table 1 Demographic data, clinical data, and type of corrective osteotomy is given to each patient

Group	Patient	Age ranges (years)	Side	Injury to surgery (months)	Previous treatment
Ramp Guide	1	60–69	right	12	cast
	2	50–59	right	7	cast
	3	40–49	left	274	cast following surgery
	4	50–59	left	7	cast
	5	50–59	left	11	cast
	6	40–49	left	218	surgery
	7	50–59	right	10	cast
	8	60–69	right	14	cast
Control	9	30–35	right	9	cast
	10	10–19	left	33	cast
	11	10–19	left	9	cast
	12	10–19	right	40	cast
	13	10–19	left	no trauma	none
	14	10–19	left	5	surgery
	15	40–49	right	13	cast

proximal and distal holes of the plate and the position of the cutting plane. A senior surgeon (A.S or L.N.) verified the 3D preoperative plan for both groups. Consequently, the patient-specific guides were designed by the same in-house planning software and produced externally by Medacta SA (Castel San Pietro, Switzerland).

Surgical technique

A standard modified Henry approach was performed to expose the malunion of the distal radius. After careful surface preparation of the malunited bone, the pre-reduction guide was applied, with K-wires defining the proximal screw hole positions. Subsequently, less than the half of

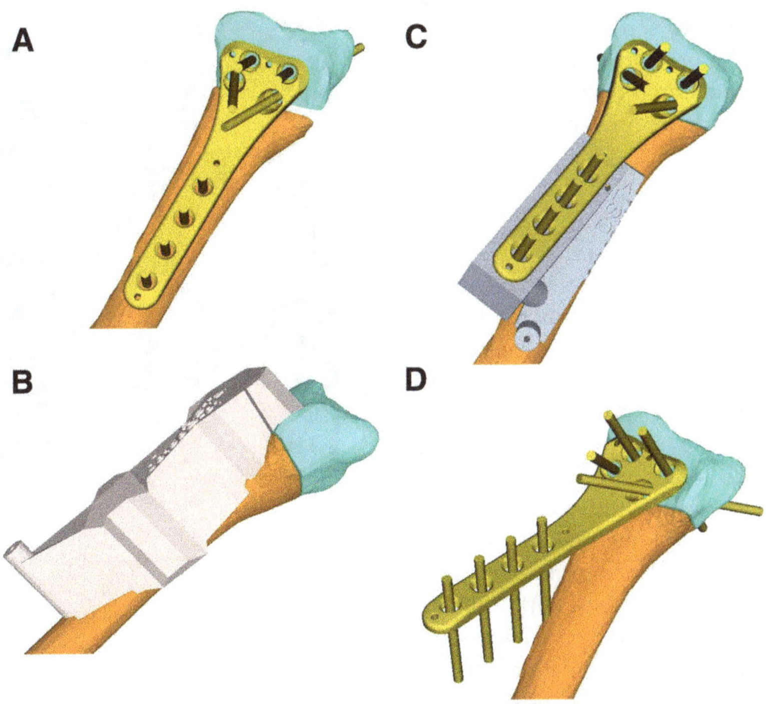

Fig. 1 a Planned opening-wedge osteotomy with shaft (orange) and distal fragment (cyan) with optimal plate position (yellow). **b** Pre-reduction guide (pink) with optimal fit on the malunited distal radius with cutting slit. **c** Ramp guide (gray) attached to malunited distal radius with fixated plate (yellow) on the slope. **d** Fixated plate (yellow) on the distal fragment before completing the osteotomy planned osteotomy was performed without losing the connection and position of the distal fragment. Optionally, this step of partially navigate the planned osteotomy can be included in the ramp-guide itself. After removing the pre-reduction guide, the described ramp-guide was fixed proximally, using the same K-wires to guarantee accurate guide position. The plate was latched on the ramp in the negative footprint and temporarily fixated with a cortical screw. Subsequently, drilling using conventional angular-stable sleeves (Intercus AG, Aarau, Switzerland), the plate was attached to the distal fragment with locking screws (Fig. 2a). To complete the osteotomy, the ramp-guide was detached from the plate after losing the ramp-screw and removal in the proximal direction. The final step is performing the reduction of the plate, with the fixated distal fragment in the pre-defined proximal screw holes on the shaft (Fig. 2b). After a fluoroscopy verification of the reduction and the screw lengths, a volar splint was applied on the wrist post wound closure. A two-week postoperative, clinical control was scheduled with suture removal. Aftercare was conducted with immobilization in a splint, and with functional treatment provided by a hand therapist for the first eight weeks.

Similar to the ramp-guide technique, pre-reduction guides were used to position and perform the osteotomy in the control group. After removing the guide, the planned plate involving locking screws was fixated on the distal fragment using the predefined direction of the drilled screw holes. Subsequently, reduction of the plate with the fixed distal fragment, as previously described was performed.

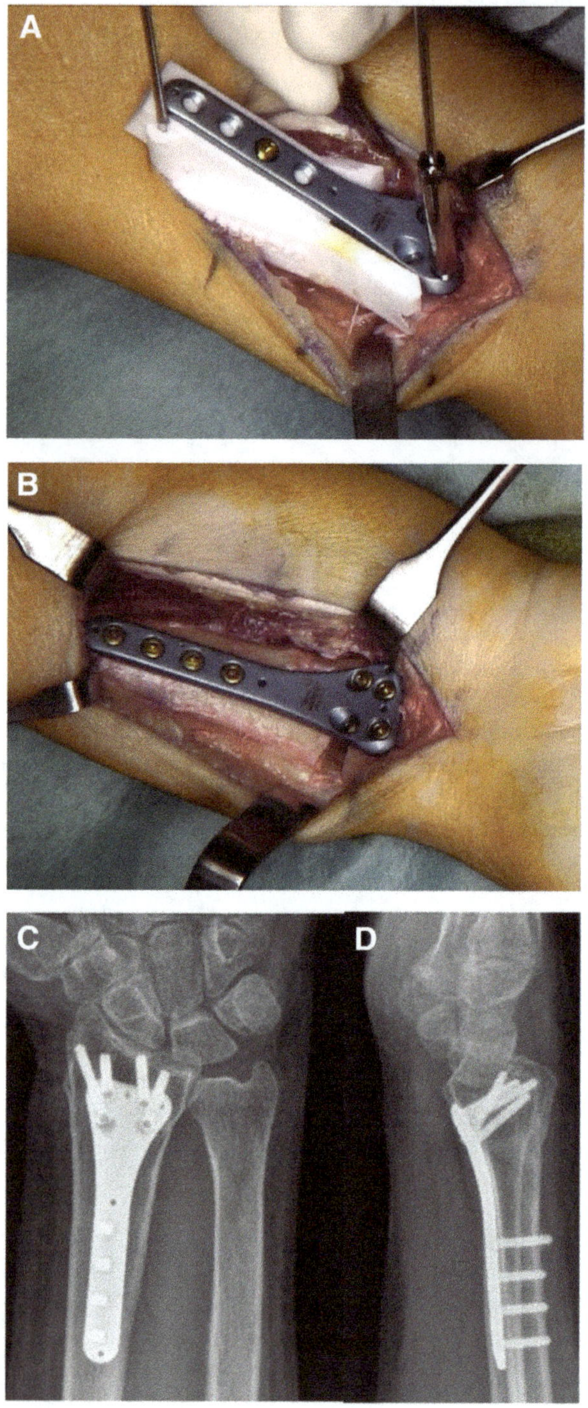

Fig. 2 a Ramp-guide (white) with temporal fixation by K-wires on the most proximal drilling-hole. **b** Plate reduction with fixated distal fragment after guide removal. **c** and **d** Posteroanterior and lateral radiographs after corrective osteotomy

Evaluation method

After eight weeks of postoperative care, a CT scan of the operated forearm was acquired to verify consolidation. As described in a previous publication [10], the residual malalignment error was measured by comparing the planned model with the postoperative result in 3D. Additionally, the postoperative plate and screw position was compared to the position in the 3D planning. Only if the distal part of the postoperative radius was present in the postoperative CT scan, axial alignment of the postoperative bone model with the model of the malunion was performed as follows: After superimposing, using the Iterative Closest Point (ICP) surface registration algorithm [9], the exact visual alignment of the cortical cross-section, on the proximal end of both models, was conducted by displaying the postoperative bone model in transparency mode (Fig. 3). The residual malalignment error was measured by calculating the relative transformation between the distal radius parts in planned and postoperative positions. The resulting 4×4 transformation matrix was decomposed in a rotational and translational part. The residual angulation was expressed with an axis-angle representation; additionally,

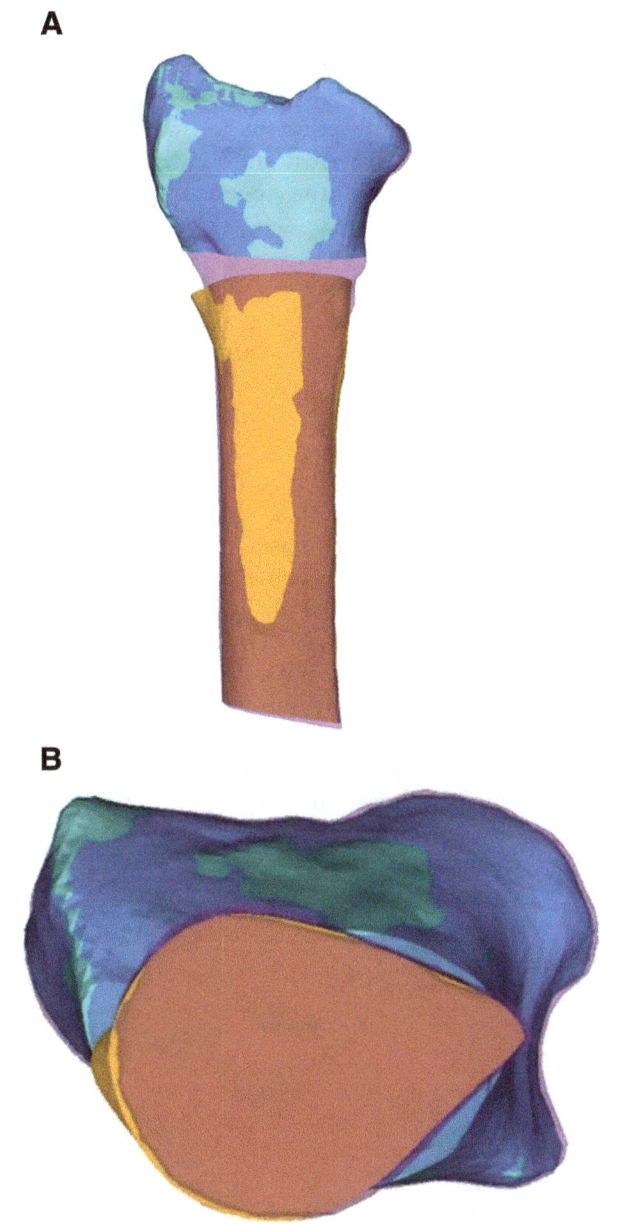

Fig. 3 a and **b** A Case with superimposition of the postoperative result in transparency mode (purple) with the surgical plan (orange and magenta). This demonstrates the alignment of the corticalis (**b**) when only the distal part of the radius is available

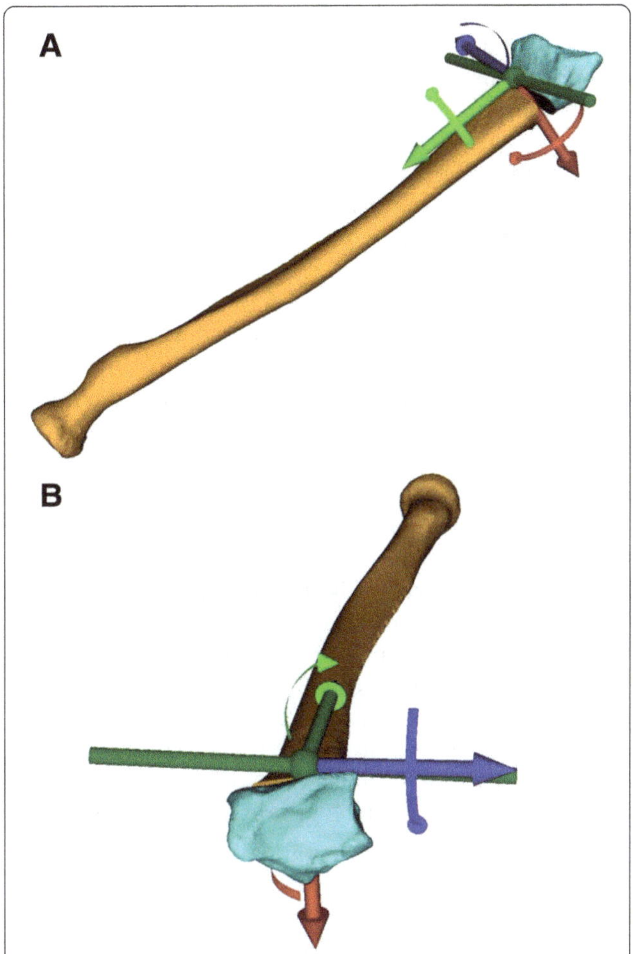

Fig. 4 a and **b** Center of the coordinate system, defined on the rotation axis (dark green) of the fragment transformation

as three consecutive rotations (i.e., Euler rotations) [12] around a standardized coordinate system, as depicted in Fig. 4. An anatomic coordinate system was set, with the x-axis pointing from dorsal to volar, defining the ulnar -/radial rotation axis. The y-axis was defined as perpendicular to the x-axis, pointing in the direction of the anatomical axis of the radius in the proximal direction. The z-axis was defined to be orthogonal to the x- and y-axes in the ulnar direction.

Statistical analysis

After the graphical verification of normal distribution, an unpaired t-test was performed to compare the residual rotational and translational error in absolute values, separately between both groups; the level of significance was established at $p < 0.05$. Likewise, the residual error of the postoperative plate position was compared to the plan, using an unpaired t-test between both groups. Comparison of age and operation time between the two groups was conducted using the Mann-Whitney U Test; the level of significance was established at $p < 0.05$. The software R (Version 3.4.3; R Foundation, Vienna, Austria) was used for statistical evaluation.

Results

The demographic data is summarized in Table 1. The ramp-guide group (mean age 42; range 30–66) was significantly older, compared to the control group (mean age 15; range 12–45). Consolidation of the osteotomy was observed in all patients between weeks 8 and 10 on the CT scans. No postoperative complications were reported in either of the two groups. In all ramp-guide cases, a correctus plate (Intercus AG, Aarau, Switzerland) was used; an implant with an uniaxial locking screw system. In the control group, angular-stable plate systems from two different companies (Intercus AG, Aarau, Switzerland; Synthes, West Chester, USA) were used.

The measurements of the planned correction and the residual malalignment error, with a calculated 3D axis-angle around the coordinate system, are summarized in Fig. 5. The interventional group showed a significantly lower residual rotational error of 2.0° (± 2.2°), and translational error of 0.6 mm (± 0.2 mm) than the control group, where the rotational and translation error were 4.2° (± 15.0°) and 1.0 mm (± 0.4 mm), respectively (Fig. 6). Instances of plate and screw position of each group are depicted in Fig. 7. Compared to the planned plate position, a mean, residual rotational error of 1.3° (± 2.3°), and a translational error of 0.6 mm (± 0.2 mm) of the plate was measured in the ramp-guide group. No significant differences in the residual plate error was observed compared to the control group, where a rotational error of 2.0° (± 5.8°) and translational error of 0.7 mm (± 0.2 mm) was measured. Significantly, in the ramp-guide group, 5 of the total 32 (15.6%) screws in the distal fragment were misaligned (> 10°), compared to the 14 of a total of 27 (51.9%) in the control group. The duration of the surgery for the ramp-guide group (86–161 min) was significantly shorter compared to the control group (140–240 min).

Discussion

Performing open-wedge osteotomies planned in 3D, and using patient-specific instruments, is a promising method to accurately restore bone anatomy of malunited distal radius. Several navigation techniques have been described to precisely achieve the desired reduction after performing the osteotomy. In laboratory studies, comparable results were reported between K-wire based specific reduction guides [13], and patient-specific drill guides with reduction based on the pre-drilled screw directions [14]. In 2013, Kunz et al. performed distal radius osteotomies on nine patients, with patient-specific drill guides based on the implant screw directions [15]. Similarly, Vlachopolous et al. reported a high reduction accuracy in 3D-planned closing-wedge and single-cut osteotomies of the forearm, performed with PSI [10]. A significantly higher residual

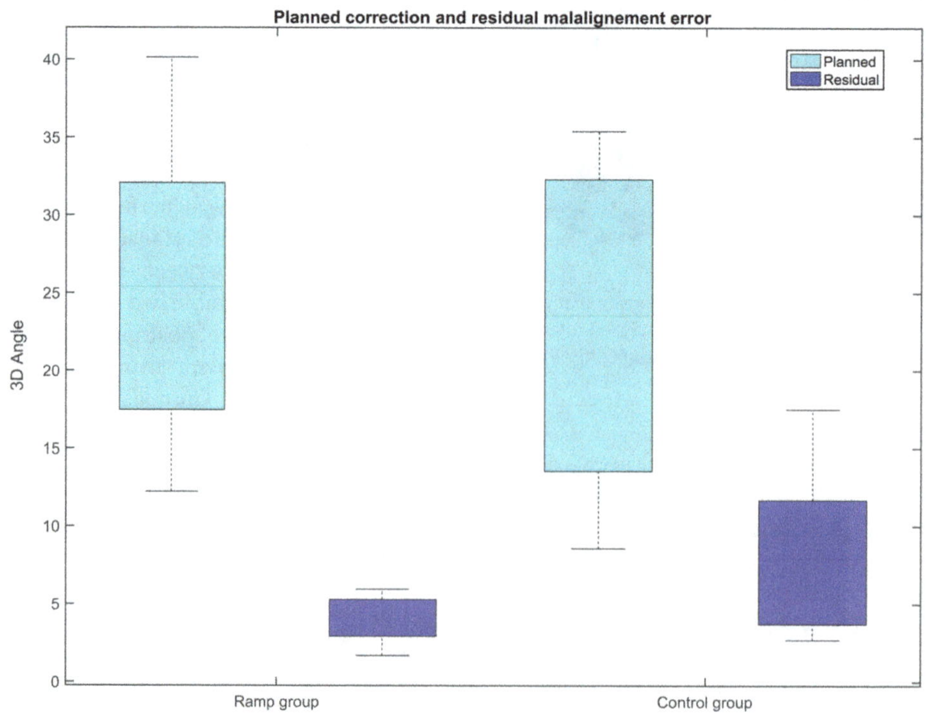

Fig. 5 Planned correction and residual malalignment error of both groups expressed as 3D angle

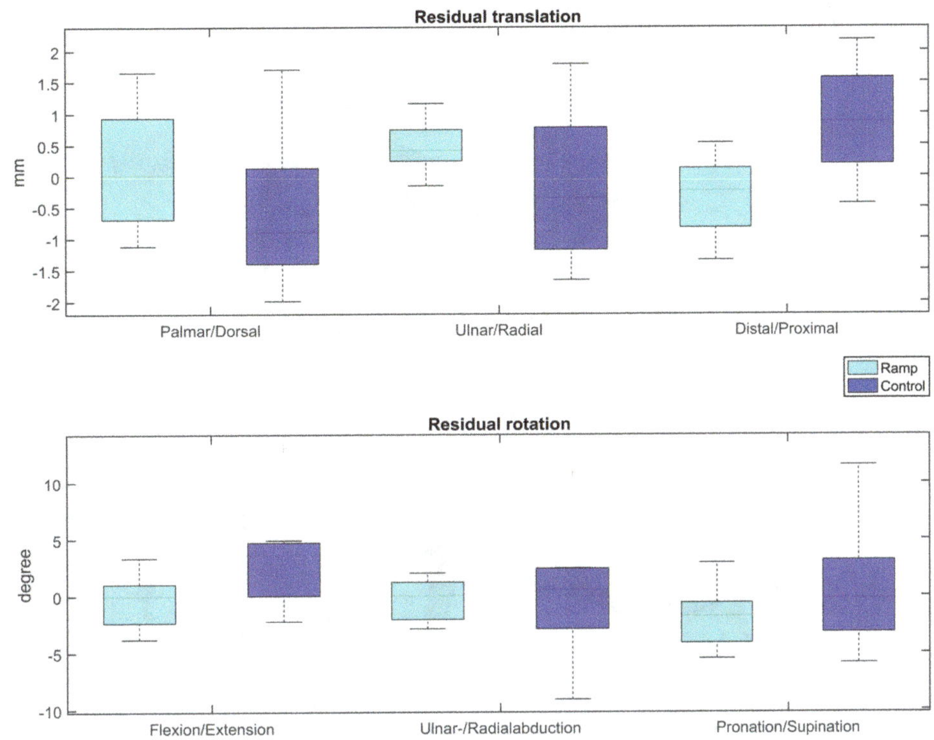

Fig. 6 Residual malalignment error measured in all six degrees of freedom (3 translations, 3 rotations) with respect to the anatomical coordinate system

rotational error was observed in opening-wedge osteotomies (8.30° ± 5.35°). In two cases a residual deformity of above 10° was reported. Excessive lengthening of the bone, additional to the rotational component, was required in both cases to achieve the planned reduction, resulting in very high soft tissue tensioning. They reported difficulties performing the reduction, solely based on the pre-drilled screw holes, and suggested that the stress between the fragments might additionally cause the screws to lock into the plate somewhat differently from the planned direction. Miyake et al. performed opening-wedge osteotomies of the distal radius on 10 patients, using a patient-specific guide technique, with prior plate-fixation to the distal radius fragment [16]. In contrast to the hereby described ramp-guide technique, the plate was fixated freehand by pre-drilling the screw holes on the distal fragment. The average deviation between the achieved and planned radial inclination was 1.8° (± 0.8°), for volar tilt, the average deviation between planned and achieved angle was 1.9° (± 1.5°).

In this study, we compared the accuracy of a new guide technique, where additionally the plate positioning was navigated with a patient-specific ramp-guide. Compared to state-of-the-art PSI techniques, using the pre-drilled screw holes, the hereby presented ramp-guide technique facilitates plate positioning on the distal fragment, and ensures a more accurate placement of the screws in the desired direction. Performing the reduction of the plate on the radius shaft, with a fixed and stable distal fragment, is technically less demanding in our opinion. Plate positioning on the distal radius prior to osteotomizing the radius can be performed more accurately, and therefore reduce misalignments. Postoperative 3D evaluation confirms this assumption by demonstrating a higher reduction accuracy in the ramp-guide group, compared to the control group. Rotational and translational residual malalignment error was significantly less, in each of the anatomical planes, in the ramp-guide group.

Comparison of the plate position between a 3D planned and performed surgery, did not support our assumption of significantly better implant positioning. Tough no outliners were detected in the ramp-guide group, contrasted by two outliners in the control group. Furthermore, in the control group 14 out of 27 (51.9%) of the screws in the distal fragment were misaligned compared to 5 out of 32 (15.6%) in the ramp-guide group. However, accurate screw placement is still an issue in corrective osteotomies, as incorrectly placed screws can compromise the planned reduction. In our

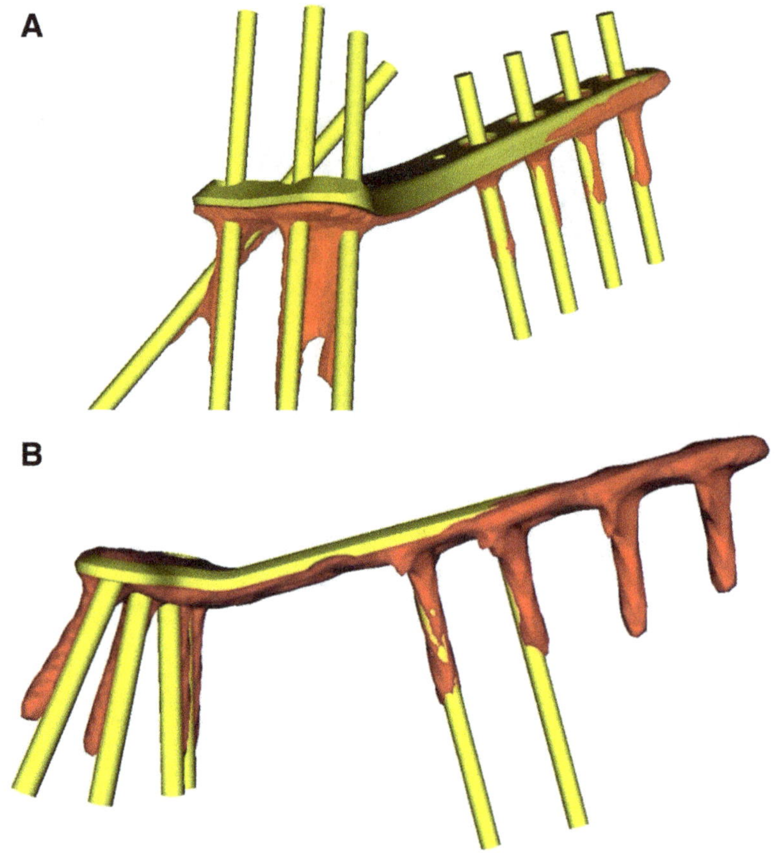

Fig. 7 Example of plate and screws of 3D planned (yellow) and obtained (orange) position of each group. **a** A case of the ramp-guide group with corresponding screws directions. **b** A case of the control group with mismatch of screw directions

opinion a larger thread on the plate, as used in the ramp-guide group, can support the correct direction of screws. Further investigation should be conducted on how to navigate screw placement more precisely, including the verification of cannulated screw application.

Despite the promising results and shorter surgery duration, the technique is only suitable for a subset of malunions. Application of a ramp-guide from palmar is only possible for malunions needing correction towards a palmar direction. The application of a ramp-guide from the opposite side may be an option to overcome this limitation. Application areas for a ramp-guide technique could be extended in the future, particularly in corrections desiring high accuracies. Further investigations are required to address PSI expansions in various anatomical regions.

Drawbacks of this technique could be the more challenging and time-consuming design of the ramp-guide, compared to state-of-the-art PSI. Furthermore, by using a ramp-guide the partially performed osteotomy must be completed freehand. The weakness of this study is the retrospective character and the small sample size. No clinical outcome was reported, since the aim of this study was to analyze the accuracy of different guide techniques. Nevertheless, the above mentioned studies demonstrated good clinical outcome in accurate restoration of forearm malunions, with PSI, without disadvantages. Finally, comparison of the outcome, with a long-standing follow-up of different techniques and accuracy results is necessary.

Conclusion

This study demonstrates the further development of patient-specific instruments in performing corrective osteotomies. The use of the presented ramp-guide technique in opening-wedge osteotomies of the distal radius is improving accuracy and reducing surgery duration, compared to existing state-of-the-art methods using PSI. Moreover, screw positioning is more accurate with the guide-ramp design.

Appendix

Table 2 Preoperatively planned correction and residual malalignment error after surgery are given for each patient

Group		Planned Correction							Residual error						
		Rotation (°)				Translation (mm)			Rotation (°)				Translation (mm)		
	Patient	3D angle	Flexion / Extension	Ulnar / Radial	Pronation Supination	Palmar / Dorsal	Ulnar / Radial	Distal / Proximal	3D angle	Flexion / Extension	Ulnar / Radial	Pronation Supination	Palmar / Dorsal	Ulnar / Radial	Distal / Proximal
Ramp guide	1	26.82	26.58	3.15	−2.63	0.00	−0.05	0.01	4.45	3.34	−2.86	−0.61	0.25	0.77	−0.18
	2	27.83	19.93	10.02	−18.63	0.47	−1.29	1.43	5.71	1.01	1.12	−5.52	1.65	0.27	0.06
	3	14.64	5.35	3.74	−12.94	0.95	1.26	2.80	2.24	−1.21	0.09	−1.99	1.28	0.31	−0.58
	4	12.24	11.28	2.71	−4.20	− 0.06	0.29	− 0.12	5.95	−3.84	− 0.06	− 4.55	−0.95	0.72	−1.35
	5	23.98	23.57	3.14	−3.91	2.58	−2.07	−8.74	4.88	1.06	−2.92	−3.80	−0.21	0.22	0.19
	6	36.31	34.33	4.49	−12.62	0.00	−0.26	0.11	1.69	−0.89	1.31	−0.61	−0.44	− 0.15	−0.29
	7	20.29	19.55	4.94	−3.33	0.45	2.03	−0.43	4.08	−3.57	−1.26	−1.56	−1.12	0.51	−1.08
	8	40.13	40.03	−2.54	−0.93	− 0.80	1.15	0.00	3.66	0.85	2.02	2.91	0.58	1.16	0.53
Control	9	22.79	19.33	10.98	−7.39	−1.66	1.16	5.31	7.94	4.90	2.33	−5.90	0.10	1.79	0.86
	10	10.49	5.78	8.76	−0.71	0.55	0.36	7.66	4.76	3.63	0.56	−3.05	−1.99	−0.31	1.60
	11	28.26	24.34	−9.81	12.96	−0.54	0.81	9.08	17.51	13.08	−3.74	11.50	−0.92	−1.66	1.44
	12	35.39	7.42	32.61	9.84	0.09	1.15	17.93	12.47	4.06	10.86	4.25	−1.56	−1.21	2.17
	13	23.58	−10.46	−19.88	5.70	0.09	0.72	5.81	9.38	−2.24	−9.11	−0.21	1.70	1.14	−0.44
	14	33.65	−12.59	−16.12	−28.73	1.13	1.50	1.93	3.36	−0.36	− 0.55	−3.29	−0.90	−1.08	0.08
	15	8.57	−2.51	0.48	8.19	4.43	4.57	1.83	2.70	1.14	2.44	−0.18	0.14	−0.35	0.53

Abbreviations
2D: Two-dimensional; 3D: Three-dimensional; CT: Computed tomography; PSI: Patient-specific Instruments; ROM: Range of motion

Funding
This work was partially funded by the Swiss Canton of Zurich through a Highly-Specialized Medicine grant.

Authors' contributions
SR and PF performed the measurements. AS and LN performed the osteotomies and were involved in the planning and supervising work. SR and PF performed the analysis, drafted the manuscript, and designed the Figs. LV and FC aided in interpreting the results and worked on the manuscript. All authors discussed the results and commented on the manuscript. All authors read and approved the final manuscript.

Consent for publication
Written informed consent for publication was obtained from all included patients. Informed consent of minors was obtained by the legally authorized representative.

Competing interests
A.S, L.N., and P.F. are shareholders of a computer-assisted surgical planning application. The authors declare that they have no competing interests.

Author details
[1]Computer Assisted Research and Development Group, Balgrist University Hospital, University of Zurich, Forchstrasse 340, 8008 Zurich, Switzerland. [2]Department of Orthopaedics, Balgrist University Hospital, University of Zurich, Zurich, Switzerland.

References
1. Fernandez DL. Reconstructive procedures for malunion and traumatic arthritis. Orthop. Clin. North am. [internet]. 1993;24:341–63. Available from. http://www.ncbi.nlm.nih.gov/pubmed/8479731.
2. Jenkins NH, Mintowt-Czyz WJ. Mal-union and dysfunction in Colles' fracture. J Hand Surg Am. 1988;13:291–3.
3. Fernandez DL. Correction of post-traumatic wrist deformity in adults by osteotomy, bone-grafting, and internal fixation. J. Bone Joint Surg. Am. The American Orthopedic Association; 1982 [cited 2015 Dec 21];64:1164–78. Available from: https://www.ncbi.nlm.nih.gov/pubmed/6752150
4. Jupiter JB, Ring D. A comparison of early and late reconstruction of malunited fractures of the distal end of the radius. J Bone Joint Surg Am. 1996;78:739–48.
5. Shea K, Fernandez DL, Jupiter JB, Martin C. Corrective osteotomy for malunited, volarly displaced fractures of the distal end of the radius. J Bone Joint Surg Am. 1997;79:1816–26 Available from: http://www.ncbi.nlm.nih.gov/pubmed/9409795.
6. Vroemen JC, Dobbe JGG, Strackee SD, Streekstra GJ. Positioning evaluation of corrective osteotomy for the malunited radius: 3-D CT versus 2-D radiographs. Orthopedics [Internet]. 2013;36:e193–9. Available from: http://www.ncbi.nlm.nih.gov/pubmed/23380014
7. Athwal GS, Ellis RE, Small CF, Pichora DR. Computer-assisted distal radius osteotomy. J. Hand Surg. Am. Elsevier; 2003 [cited 2015 Dec 21];28:951–8. Available from: http://www.jhandsurg.org/article/S0363502303003757/fulltext
8. Schweizer A, Fürnstahl P, Nagy L. Three-dimensional correction of distal radius intra-articular malunions using patient-specific drill guides. J. Hand Surg. Am. 2013;38:2339–47.
9. Murase T, Oka K, Moritomo H, Goto A, Yoshikawa H, Sugamoto K. Three-dimensional corrective osteotomy of malunited fractures of the upper extremity with use of a computer simulation system. J. Bone Joint Surg. Am. The American Orthopedic Association; 2008 [cited 2015 Dec 21];90:2375–89. Available from: https://www.ncbi.nlm.nih.gov/pubmed/18978406
10. Vlachopoulos L, Schweizer A, Graf M, Nagy L, Fürnstahl P. Three-dimensional postoperative accuracy of extra-articular forearm osteotomies using CT-scan based patient-specific surgical guides. BMC Musculoskelet Disord. 2015;16.
11. Vlachopoulos L, Schweizer A, Meyer DC, Gerber C, Fürnstahl P. Three-dimensional corrective osteotomies of complex malunited humeral fractures using patient-specific guides. J Shoulder Elb Surg [Internet]. Elsevier Inc.; 2016;25:2040–7. Available from: https://doi.org/10.1016/j.jse.2016.04.038
12. Schneider PJ. Eberly DH. Geometric tools for computer graphics. Geom. Tools Comput. In: Graph; 2002.
13. Oka K, Murase T, Moritomo H, Goto A, Nakao R, Sugamoto K, et al. Accuracy of corrective osteotomy using a custom-designed device based on a novel computer simulation system. J Orthop Sci [Internet]. 2011;16:85–92. Available from: http://www.ncbi.nlm.nih.gov/pubmed/21359511
14. Ma B, Kunz M, Gammon B, Ellis RE, Pichora DR. A laboratory comparison of computer navigation and individualized guides for distal radius osteotomy. Int. J. Comput. Assist. Radiol. Surg. 2014;9:713–24. Available from: http://www.ncbi.nlm.nih.gov/pubmed/24323402.
15. Kunz M, Ma B, Rudan JF, Ellis RE, Pichora DR. Image-guided distal radius osteotomy using patient-specific instrument guides. J Hand Surg Am. 2013. https://doi.org/10.1016/j.jhsa.2013.05.018.
16. Miyake J, Murase T, Moritomo H, Sugamoto K, Yoshikawa H. Distal radius osteotomy with volar locking plates based on computer simulation. Clin Orthop Relat Res [Internet]. 2011;469:1766–73. Available from: https://www.ncbi.nlm.nih.gov/pmc/articles/PMC3094613/.

19

Outcomes after bone grafting in patients with and without ACL revision surgery

Theresa Diermeier, Elmar Herbst, Sepp Braun, Emine Saracuz, Andreas Voss, Andreas B. Imhoff*
and Andrea Achtnich

Abstract

Background: Current literature is lacking of data regarding functional outcomes in patients following bone tunnel grafting with or without revision anterior cruciate ligament (ACL) reconstruction. Therefore, the aim of the present study was to evaluate the clinical outcome in patients with (RACL) or without revision ACL reconstruction (OBG) following bone grafting.

Methods: Fifty-nine patients (18 female, 41 male) who underwent bone grafting due to recurrent, symptomatic ACL deficiency following ACL reconstruction between 2011 and 2014 were retrospectively analyzed. In 44 patients (mean age: 30,5 ± 8,5 years) a staged revision ACL reconstruction (RACL) was performed after bone grafting. 10 patients (mean age: 33.2 ± 10.3 years) refused to have ACL revision surgery after bone grafting (OBG). Outcome measures included instrumented laxity testing, the International Knee Documentation Committee (IKDC) score, the Knee Injury and Osteoarthritis Outcome Score (KOOS), Lysholm score and Tegner activity scale.

Results: After mean period of 33,9 ± 17.0 months, 54 patients were available for follow up examination. In the RACL group, the Lysholm score was 77,2 ± 15,5 (range 35–100), the mean IKDC subjective knee score was 69,0 ± 13,4 (range 39,1–97,7) and the mean Tegner activity score was 4,1 ± 1,5 (range, 1–9). Similarly, in the OBG group the mean Lysholm score was 72,90 ± 18,7 (range 50–100), the mean IKDC subjective score was 69,3 ± 20,0 (range 44,1–100) and the mean Tegner activity score was 4,6 ± 1,2 (range, 3–6). No significant difference was observed between the two groups. Knee laxity measurements were elevated without revision ACL surgery, however the difference was not significant.

Conclusion: Bone tunnel grafting with or without second stage ACL revision surgery showed no significant difference in functional outcome score. Thus, in case of revision ACL instability careful patient selection is necessary and expectations should be discussed openly with the patients.

Keywords: ACL reconstruction, Autologous bone grafting, Revision ACL surgery, Recurrence

* Correspondence: imhoff@tum.de
Research performed at the Department for Orthopaedic Sports Medicine, Klinikum rechts der Isar, TU Munich, Germany
Department of Orthopaedic Sports Medicine, Klinikum rechts der Isar, TU Munich, Ismaninger Str. 22, 81675 Munich, Germany

Background

Revision anterior cruciate ligament (ACL) reconstruction is continuously increasing with a current incidence of up to 15% [1–3]. Younger age, secondary trauma, insufficient graft healing and technical factors such as graft fixation or position were associated with increased failure rate after primary ACL reconstruction [4].

In patients requiring revision ACL reconstruction, either a single-stage or a two-stage procedure is indicated based on tunnel position (especially partially anatomic tunnels) and width as well as other potential risk factors, such as lower limb malalignment and steep posterior tibial slope.

In contrast to a single-stage ACL revision, a two-stage procedure consists of 1) hardware removal and graft remnant debridement and bone tunnel grafting and 2) revision ACL reconstruction.

Although two-stage revision ACL reconstruction could achieve similar laxity measurement compared to primary ACL reconstruction, functional outcome parameters have generally been shown to be inferior [2, 5]. From the patient's perspective especially a two-stage surgery requires high commitment the expectations should be set properly. Clinically, a subset of patients refuses to have further ACL revision surgery despite an already performed bone grafting.

Current literature is lacking of studies evaluating the clinical outcome in patients with and without revision ACL reconstruction following bone grafting. Therefore, the purpose of this study was to evaluate the clinical outcome in patients with and without revision ACL surgery following bone grafting. It was hypothesized that patient reported outcomes are comparable, while knee laxity measures are inferior in patients without revision ACL surgery.

Methods

In this retrospective study, patients who underwent bone tunnel grafting with autologous bone from iliac crest due to ACL re-injury between January 2011 and December 2014 were included. The decision to perform a two-stage revision was based on computer tomography (CT) scan analysis. Partially anatomic tunnel position combined with tunnel widening > 12 mm, significant tunnel widening (> 12 mm), suboptimal bone stock or inability to place new tunnel properly were indications for a two-stage procedure. Additional inclusion criteria were available, including preoperative radiographs (a.p. and lateral), CT scans of the involved knee and age > 18 years. Patients with multiple ligament instability requiring surgical treatment or missing data from primary ACL reconstruction were excluded. Demographic data, date and type of primary ACL surgery were extracted from the medical reports.

Clinical examination

All patients underwent clinical examination after a mean follow-up period of 33,9 ± 17.0 months (range, 8,0 to 68 months). Clinical evaluation of the patient's knee joint was based on the International Knee Documentation Committee (IKDC) form. A goniometer was used to measure the range-of-motion (ROM). Knee stability testing included the medial collateral ligament (MCL) and lateral collateral ligament (LCL), as well as the ACL and posterior cruciate ligament (PCL). For the ACL, anterior laxity was evaluated using the KT-1000 at 30° of flexion and Pivot shift test, graded according to the IKDC grading system. Patient reported outcomes included the IKDC, Knee injury and Osteoarthrtitis Outcome Score (KOOS), Tegner and Lysholm Score.

Surgical technique

All surgical revision procedures were performed in one hospital. The patient was placed in a supine position and the surgery was performed with the patient under general anesthesia. First, a routine arthroscopy through a high anterolateral and an additional anteromedial portal was performed. A probe was used to examine the cruciate ligaments, menisci and the cartilage. Meniscus and cartilage lesions were treated as indicated.

Bone grafting technique

The remnants from the previous graft, scar tissue and previous fixation material (interference screws, staples, etc.) were removed. Furthermore, tunnel position and diameter were evaluated and the final decision of bone grafting the tunnels was made. To properly localize the center of the femoral tunnel a guide wire was inserted in the previous tunnel. Tunnels were reamed, curretaged and rasped until they were fully cleared from sclerotic bone. An incision was then made within the existing scar on the proximal tibia to clear the tibial tunnel as described above. Then, both tunnel diameters were estimated with the help of a specific guide system (Arthrex OATS system, Naples, FL, USA) and bone cylinders from the ipsilateral iliac crest were harvested and extracted. With a donor guide, the bone cylinders were placed arthroscopically and impacted in the cleared tunnels. Protrusion of the cylinders was excluded by direct visualization. If necessary, the procedure was performed for both tunnels, femoral and tibial. Postoperatively, only partial weight bearing was permitted for the first two weeks with immediate unrestricted ROM..

Revision ACL surgery

After confirming adequate bone healing on follow-up CT (minimum 3 months postoperatively) the second operation was planned. Graft choice depended on the initial graft used. Following routine arthroscopy, the femoral and tibial bone tunnels were then prepared in a standardized fashion. For tunnel placement, a specific drill guide was used (Arthrex, Naples, FL, USA). Graft fixation was depended of the chosen tendon type. Femorally, the graft was fixed with a resorbable interference screw (bone-to--bone fixation) or for tendon-to-bone fixation with an extra cortical button system (Arthrex TightRope, Naples, FL, USA). Tibial graft fixation was performed with a resorbable interference screw (Arthrex TightRope, Naples, FL, USA.).

Rehabilitation

Rehabilitation in revision ACL reconstruction comprised wearing a knee brace with unrestricted ROM for the first six weeks. Furthermore only partial weight bearing was permitted for the first for two weeks. Physical therapy with muscle strengthening and proprioceptive training was performed at least 3 months after the first operation.

The study was approved by the institutional review board of the Technical University of Munich (No. 353/15) and conducted according to the Declaration of Helsinki. All patients gave their written informed consent to participate in this investigation.

Statistical analysis

For statistical analysis the significance level was set at $p < 0{,}05$. Data distribution was evaluated using the Shapiro-Wilk test. As data were not normally distributed, the Mann-Whitney-U test was used to compare patient reported outcome scores between patients who underwent revision ACL surgery and those without revision ACL reconstruction following bone grafting. Laxity measurements were evaluated using the Pearson's chi-squared test.

Results

Fifty-nine patients with bone tunnel grafting were included. Five patients were excluded from the study, because they declined participating in the study. Of the remaining 54 patients, 9 declined to participate in follow-up examination, but all of them consented to complete the patient reported outcome scores. In 44 patients a two stage revision ACL reconstruction (RACL) was performed after bone grafting, whereas 10 patients did not undergo further operation after bone grafting (OBG). Primary ACL reconstructions were performed by several orthopedic surgeons and also at various hospitals. After ACL graft re-rupture all patients present with subjective instability and epsiodes of "giving way" in our outpatient clinic. ACL graft re-rupture was confirmed by clinical examination and magnetic resonance imaging (MRI).

In the RACL group consisting of 31 females and 13 males, the mean age at the time of bone grafting was 30,5 ± 8.5 years (range 16.7 to 49.4 years). For revision ACL reconstruction the contralateral hamstring tendons were used in 46.7% (21/45), ipsilateral hamstring tendons in 26.7% (12/45), ipsilateral quadriceps tendon in 22.2% (10/45) and ipsilateral BTB graft in 2.2% (1/45).

The group of patients without revision ACL reconstruction (OBG) after bone tunnel grafting included 7 females and 3 males with a mean patient age of 33.2 ± 10.3 years (range 18.2–47.7 years).

Meniscus status and cartilage injuries during bone grafting procedure

Concomitant meniscus and cartilage injuries were evaluated during arthroscopy, which was conducted at every patient before the bone grafting procedure (Table 1). Additional lesions were treated in 45% of the RACL group and in 60% of the subjects who remained without revision ACL reconstruction.

Clinical examination

Knee laxity measurements were elevated without revision ACL surgery, but the difference was not significant (NS). Laxity measurements for both groups (RACL and OBG) are summarized in Table 2. Postoperatively no complications were reported. None of the included patients had a flexion or extensions deficit.

Clinical outcome

At final follow up examination no significant differences were observed between both groups for IKDC ($p = 0.973$), Lysholm ($p = 0.525$) or Tegner activity scale ($p = 0.326$) (Table 3). Likewise, no significant difference was observed for the five KOOS subscales between the groups (Fig. 1).

Table 1 Concomitant meniscus and cartilage lesions which were evaluated during arthroscopy. Arthroscopy was always performed before bone grafting procedure

	Bone grafting without revision ACL (OBG)	Revision ACL Group (RACL)
Medical Meniscus lesion	1 (10.0%)	11 (25.0%)
Lateral Meniscus lesion	5 (50.0%)	8 (18.2%)
Medial cartilage defect	7 (70.0%)	27 (61.4%)
Lateral cartilage defect	3 (30.0%)	10 (22.7%)
Patellofemoral cartilage defect	4 (40.0%)	10 (22.7%)

Table 2 Laxity measurements, side -to-side difference in KT 1000 for group without revision ACL reconstruction (OBG) and patients with revision ACL reconstruction (RACL)

	Bone Grafting Without Revision ACL (OBG)	Revision ACL Reconstruction (RACL)
Side-to-Side Difference (SSD)		
0-2 mm	50,0%	79,5%
3–4 mm	33,3%	15,4%
≥ 5 mm	16,7%	5,1%
Pivot -Shift Test		
-	16,7%	74,4%
+	33,3%	25,6%
++	50,0%	–

Discussion

The main finding of the present study was that after bone tunnel grafting in case of ACL re-instability not every patient requires revision ACL reconstruction. However, there was also no significant difference in the objective clinical outcome between both groups.

Based on our results almost 20% refused a revision ACL reconstruction after bone tunnel grafting, although the initial plan was to perform a revision ACL reconstruction in all patients. Most of these patients have refused to a revision ACL reconstruction due to reduced symptoms after initial bone grafting. At final follow up, laxity measurements were clearly elevated when RACL reconstruction was not performed. However, no significant difference was observed in any of the other evaluated parameters.

The reasons why some patients refused a second ACL reconstruction might be multifactorial. Noyes et al. [6] divided patients with ACL injuries into three different groups depending on their behavior after the injury and the necessity of treatment. "Coper" could achieve recreational level of activity without reconstruction [7]. "Adapter" modified their level of activity until they could manage with the injury. "Non-coper" suffered from recurrent episodes of "giving-way" phenomena and subjective instability during activities of daily living. Therefore in non-coper ACL reconstruction is the treatment of choice [8]. On the other hand, conservative treatment in potential copers also leads to high rate of return to sport and significant reduced instability [9–11]. Interestingly, Moksnes et al. [12] also described non-copers, with the potential to be converted to real copers by non-operative treatment [12]. Although 70% of non-copers were converted to real copers, this proportion might be too high [12]. Nevertheless it demonstrated that non-coper could be changed in to true coper by conservative treatment [11]. In addition, Fitzgerald et al. [9] achieved after standard physical therapy with perturbation training a high return to high-level activity and significant reduced episodes of "giving- way".

After initial bone grafting, physical therapy with muscle strengthening and proprioceptive training was performed for at least 3 months. However, not only the improved muscle strength is the decisive factor, but the changed functional movement patterns after intensive physical therapy [11]. Therefore, one possible factor, why some patients in the current study rejected revision ACL reconstruction might be due to improved movement pattern. The comparable functional outcome score between both groups also confirm this.

Due to the retrospective character of the study a detailed interview, why the patients did not want to undergo the revision reconstruction right after bone grafting was not possible. But Feucht et al. [13] highlighted the inferior expectations concerning return to sport, pain and the overall condition in patients with revision ACL reconstruction or previous operations. Therefore, the reduced functional approach and the improved functional status after the bone grafting could be another explanation for the rejection.

Besides subjective instability, some patients also presented with deficits in motion or locking of the knee. Before the bone tunnel grafting a routine diagnostic arthroscopy and resection and debridement of the

Table 3 Functional outcome at final follow up for group without revision ACL reconstruction (OBG) and patients with revision ACL reconstruction (RACL)

	Bone Grafting Without Revision ACL (OBG) Mean ± SD (Range)	Revision ACL Reconstruction (RACL) Mean ± SD (Range)
IKDC ± SD	69.3 ± 20.0 (Range 44.8–100,0)	69.0 ± 13.4 (Range 39.1–97.7)
Lysholm ± SD	72.9 ± 18.7 (Range 50–100)	77.2 ± 15.5 (Range 35–100)
Tegner ± SD	4.6 ± 1.2 (Range 3–6)	4.1 ± 1.4 (range 1–9)

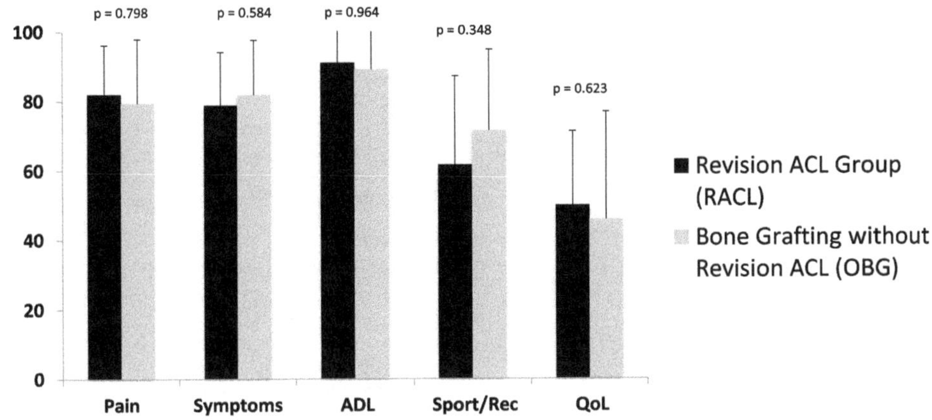

Fig. 1 KOOS Score at final follow up for group without revision ACL reconstruction (OBG) and patients with revision ACL reconstruction (RACL). No statistically significant difference was observed between the two groups

previous graft and scar tissue was performed. During this procedure additional pathologies, like meniscal tears or severe cartilage defects, were treated. Therefore, some of the complained symptoms might be reduced only by the first surgery. Nearly all of the patients (8 out of 10) without revision ACL reconstruction had additional treatment during the first stage of operation. Although these patients did not complain about subjective instability or recurrent episodes of "giving way" - phenomena, clinical instability was clearly evident without revision ACLR.

In case of revision surgery, a thorough analysis of already utilized tendons, muscle strength and preferred sports is necessary. A variety of possible grafts for revision ACL reconstruction are described [14, 15]. According to the results of the MARS group [16], autografts are favorable compared to allografts with regards to re-rupture rate, clinical outcome scores and sports function. Contralateral hamstrings were also the most common tendons for revision ACL reconstruction in our study population.

In general, ACL revision surgery is challenging and postoperative reported functional outcomes are reduced compared to primary reconstruction [2, 17]. Nevertheless, a recent meta-analysis demonstrated a significant improvement for Lysholm score by revision ACL reconstruction from average 61.5 to 87.5 points. Results for Lysholm scores in the present study are slightly below these values, but according to Briggs et al. [18] a normal to nearly normal overall knee function is associated with a Lysholm score of 73 ± 15 points. From previous literature, the minimum detectable difference for Lysholm score is reported to be between 8.9 and 10.1 points [18, 19]. However, in the current study, the difference between the two groups was 4.3 point. Therefore, no significant or clinically relevant difference was observed between the two study groups. Also, no significant difference between both groups for Tegner score was evident. After bone grafting patients with and without revision ACL reconstruction reached a mean Tegner activity score of 4. In case of revision a mean Tegner of 5 is reported in recent literature [20]. However, Tegner activity scale includes level of sport activity and occupational function [18]. A closer look what is included in a level 4 of Tegner score is necessary for a further interpretation. Patients with a score of 4 could do moderate heavy work and could at least run two times a week. Interestingly, the Tegner score in persons with a "normal knee function" is located at mean of 5.7 [21].

The present study has several limitations. First of all, it is a retrospective case series with known limitations. Furthermore, the number of included patients, especially in the group of patients without revision ACL surgery, is limited. In fact, the calculated power of the current study based on the Lysholm score was 0.33. As most of the patients regularly undergo revision ACL surgery following bone grafting, it is almost impossible to obtain sufficient statistical power. However, the current study highlights, that not every patient requires or is willing to undergo further ACL reconstruction without compromising patient reported outcomes. Follow- up in present study is short term and maybe difference between both groups only occur in mid and long term follow-up. On the other hand, to the authors' knowledge, this is one of the first studies to compare clinical outcome in patients with and without revision ACL reconstruction after bone grafting.

Conclusion

Bone tunnel grafting due to revision ACL instability with or without second stage ACL revision surgery showed similar clinical results. Thus, in case of revision ACL instability precise patient selection for a renewed operative treatment is necessary.

Abbrevations
ACL: Anterior cruciate ligament; CT: Computer tomography; IKDC: International Knee Documentation Committee Score; KOOS: Knee Injury and Osteoarthritis Outcome Score; LCL: Lateral collateral ligament; MCL: Medial collateral ligament; NS: Not significant; OBG: Only bone grafting; PCL: Posterior cruciate ligament; RACL: Revision anterior cruciate ligament; ROM: Range of motion

Acknowledgements
Not applicable.

Funding
This research received no specific grant from any funding agency in the public, commercial, or not-for-profit sectors.

Authors' contributions
AA, EH and ES made substantial contributions to conception and design, or acquisition of data, or analysis and interpretation of data; TD and AI have been involved in drafting the manuscript or revising it critically for important intellectual content; SB and AV made substantial contributions to conception and design of present study and give final approval to the version to be published. All authors have read and approved the manuscript.

Consent for publication
Not applicable.

Competing interests
The authors declare that they have no competing interests.

References
1. Taggart TF, Kumar A, Bickerstaff DR. Revision anterior cruciate ligament reconstruction: a midterm patient assessment. Knee. 2004;11(1):29–36. https://doi.org/10.1016/S0968-0160(02)00087-X.
2. Thomas NP, Kankate R, Wandless F, Pandit H. Revision anterior cruciate ligament reconstruction using a 2-stage technique with bone grafting of the tibial tunnel. Am J Sports Med. 2005;33(11):1701–9.
3. Yabroudi MA, Björnsson H, Lynch AD, Muller B, Samuelsson K, Tarabichi M, Karlsson J, Fu FH, Harner CD, Irrgang JJ. Predictors of Revision Surgery After Primary Anterior Cruciate Ligament Reconstruction. Orthop J Sports Med. 2016;4(9) https://doi.org/10.1177/2325967116666039.
4. Desai N, Andernord D, Sundemo D, Alentorn-Geli E, Musahl V, Fu F, Forssblad M, Samuelsson K. Revision surgery in anterior cruciate ligament reconstruction: a cohort study of 17,682 patients from the Swedish National Knee Ligament Register. Knee Surg Sports Traumatol Arthrosc. 2016; https://doi.org/10.1007/s00167-016-4399-0.
5. Weiler A, Schmeling A, Stöhr I, Kääb MJ, Wagner M. Primary versus single-stage revision anterior cruciate ligament reconstruction using autologous hamstring tendon grafts. Am J Sports Med. 2007;35(10):1643–52.
6. Noyes FR, Mooar P, Matthews D, Butler D. The symptomatic anterior cruciate-deficient knee. Part I: the long-term functional disability in athletically active individuals. JBJS. 1983;65(2):154–62.
7. Rudolph K, Axe M, Snyder-Mackler L. Dynamic stability after ACL injury: who can hop? Knee Surg Sports Traumatol Arthrosc. 2000;8(5):262–9.
8. Kaplan Y. Identifying individuals with an anterior cruciate ligament-deficient knee as copers and noncopers: a narrative literature review. J Orthop Sports Phys Ther. 2011;41(10):758–66.
9. Fitzgerald GK, Axe MJ, Snyder-Mackler L. The efficacy of perturbation training in nonoperative anterior cruciate ligament rehabilitation programs for physically active individuals. Phys Ther. 2000;80(2):128.
10. Fitzgerald GK, Axe MJ, Snyder-Mackler L. Proposed practice guidelines for nonoperative anterior cruciate ligament rehabilitation of physically active individuals. J Orthop Sports Phys Ther. 2000;30(4):194–203.
11. Chmielewski TL, Hurd WJ, Rudolph KS, Axe MJ, Snyder-Mackler L. Perturbation training improves knee kinematics and reduces muscle co-contraction after complete unilateral anterior cruciate ligament rupture. Phys Ther. 2005;85(8):740–9.
12. Moksnes H, Snyder-Mackler L, Risberg MA. Individuals with an anterior cruciate ligament-deficient knee classified as noncopers may be candidates for nonsurgical rehabilitation. J Orthop Sports Phys Ther. 2008;38(10):586–95.
13. Feucht MJ, Cotic M, Saier T, Minzlaff P, Plath JE, Imhoff AB, Hinterwimmer S. Patient expectations of primary and revision anterior cruciate ligament reconstruction. Knee Surg Sports Traumatol Arthrosc. 2016;24(1):201–7. https://doi.org/10.1007/s00167-014-3364-z.
14. Franceschi F, Papalia R, Del Buono A, Zampogna B, Diaz Balzani L, Maffulli N, Denaro V. Two-stage procedure in anterior cruciate ligament revision surgery: a five-year follow-up prospective study. Int Orthop. 2013;37(7): 1369–74. https://doi.org/10.1007/s00264-013-1886-5.
15. Garofalo R, Djahangiri A, Siegrist O. Revision anterior cruciate ligament reconstruction with quadriceps tendon-patellar bone autograft. Arthroscopy. 2006;22(2):205–14. https://doi.org/10.1016/j.arthro.2005.08.045.
16. Effect of graft choice on the outcome of revision anterior cruciate ligament reconstruction in the Multicenter ACL Revision Study (MARS) Cohort. Am J Sports Med. 2014;42(10):2301–10. https://doi.org/10.1177/0363546514549005.
17. Ahlden M, Samuelsson K, Sernert N, Forssblad M, Karlsson J, Kartus J. The Swedish National Anterior Cruciate Ligament Register: a report on baseline variables and outcomes of surgery for almost 18,000 patients. Am J Sports Med. 2012;40(10):2230–5. https://doi.org/10.1177/0363546512457348.
18. Briggs KK, Lysholm J, Tegner Y, Rodkey WG, Kocher MS, Steadman JR. The reliability, validity, and responsiveness of the Lysholm score and Tegner activity scale for anterior cruciate ligament injuries of the knee: 25 years later. Am J Sports Med. 2009;37(5):890–7. https://doi.org/10.1177/0363546508330143.
19. Briggs KK, Kocher MS, Rodkey WG, Steadman JR. Reliability, validity, and responsiveness of the Lysholm knee score and Tegner activity scale for patients with meniscal injury of the knee. J Bone Joint Surg Am. 2006;88(4): 698–705. https://doi.org/10.2106/jbjs.e.00339.
20. Andriolo L, Filardo G, Kon E, Ricci M, Della Villa F, Della Villa S, Zaffagnini S, Marcacci M. Revision anterior cruciate ligament reconstruction: clinical outcome and evidence for return to sport. Knee Surg Sports Traumatol Arthrosc. 2015;23(10):2825–45. https://doi.org/10.1007/s00167-015-3702-9.
21. Briggs KK, Steadman JR, Hay CJ, Hines SL. Lysholm score and Tegner activity level in individuals with normal knees. Am J Sports Med. 2009;37(5):898–901.

20

Should sagittal osteotomy line be parallel to tibial posterior slope in high tibial osteotomy?

Y. Akamatsu*, H. Kobayashi, M. Tsuji, S. Nejima, K. Kumagai and T. Saito

Abstract

Background: The reason why the osteotomy line in the sagittal view should be parallel to the medial tibial posterior slope in open wedge high tibial osteotomy (OWHTO) remains unclear. In addition, previous study reported that a posterolateral hinge position led to an increase in tibial posterior slope (TPS) after OWHTO. Our aims were to examine the relationships between angles among the tibial plateau and osteotomy planes or the hinge point and the change in TPS, and the location of the hinge position after OWHTO using three-dimensional computed tomography (3DCT). We hypothesized that the sagittal angle between the tibial plateau and osteotomy planes with an anterior-widening proximal tibial fragment resulted in increased TPS, and the hinge position located posterolaterally.

Methods: Preoperative planning anticipated a weight-bearing line ratio of 62% on the radiograph. The anterior gap was 67% of the posterior gap in OWHTO. We identified the tibial plateau and upper and lower osteotomy planes on 3DCT of 82 patients with symptomatic medial osteoarthritic knee after OWHTO. The osteotomy plane angles between the tibial plateau and upper osteotomy planes, and opening gap angles between both osteotomy planes in the coronal and sagittal views were measured. The anteroposterior (AP) and lateral hinge position was displayed as a percentage on the upper osteotomy plane. We assessed the relationships among them.

Results: The TPS significantly increased after OWHTO ($p = 0.002$). There was no significant difference between the sagittal osteotomy plane angle and the change in TPS. The sagittal opening gap angle and the AP hinge position ratio were significantly correlated with the change in the TPS ($r = 0.477$ $p < 0.001$ and $r = -0.342$, $p = 0.002$, respectively). The hinge position was located a mean of 16.0% from the lateral and 48.6% from the posterior tibial edge in the upper osteotomy plane.

Conclusions: Contrary to our expectation, the osteotomy plane did not need to be parallel to the tibial plateau plane in the sagittal view. However, the osteotomy gap should be rectangular in the sagittal view. The hinge position located nearly in the center of the sagittal view.

Keywords: Open wedge high tibial osteotomy, 3 dimensional computed tomography, Hinge position, Osteotomy plane, Tibial posterior slope

* Correspondence: akamatsu@yokohama-cu.ac.jp
Department of Orthopaedic Surgery, Yokohama City University, School of Medicine, 3-9, Fukuura, Kanazawa-ku, Yokohama 236-0004, Japan

Background

A surgical technique that the osteotomy line in the sagittal view should be parallel to the medial tibial posterior slope (TPS) in open wedge high tibial osteotomy (OWHTO) is recommended [1–4]. Lee et al. reported that the mean sagittal osteotomy plane angle, which is angle between the tibial plateau and upper osteotomy planes in the sagittal view, with an anterior-widening proximal tibial fragment on the radiograph was 15.1°, and 87.1% of knees had an anterior-widening proximal tibial fragment. They showed that the sagittal osteotomy plane angle was positively correlated with the change in TPS [4]. Regarding the control of TPS during surgery, two reports have suggested that the opening gap ratio, which was defined as the ratio of an anteromedial opening gap to a posteromedial opening gap, of 1/2 or 2/3 will minimize the change in TPS [2, 5]. The change in TPS may be controlled by intraoperatively measuring the TPS using two Kirschner wires [6, 7], lateral fluoroscopy projection, and a navigation system [2]. However, despite these techniques, the degree of change in TPS after OWHTO still varies [7].

Two previous studies have tried to investigate the relationship between the hinge position and the change in TPS after OWHTO, but have a small number of cases, which was one study to 12 knees using cadavers [8] and another to 19 knees using three-dimensional computed tomography (3DCT) [9]. They concluded that the hinge position affected the change in TPS, and a posterolateral hinge position led to an increase in TPS after OWHTO.

Our aims were to examine the relationships among the osteotomy plane, opening gap, and hinge position, and to determine the location of hinge position using 3DCT after OWHTO. We hypothesized that the sagittal osteotomy plane angle with an anterior-widening proximal tibial fragment resulted in increased TPS and the hinge position located posterolaterally.

Methods

Patients

This was a retrospective analysis of prospective collected data. One surgeon performed all OWHTO between April 2012 and March 2014. We retrospectively analyzed the radiographs and CT images. Inclusion criteria were patients with medial knee OA, an anatomical femorotibial angle (aFTA) of ≦185°, and a flexion contracture of ≦15°. Exclusion criteria were patients with a patellofemoral symptom, an anterior or posterior cruciate ligament insufficiency, and a lateral tibiofemoral joint space narrowing on radiograph. We collected data from 87 patients. Two cases had lateral tibial plateau fracture during OWHTO, and 3 cases did not have all of their radiographs and CT images examined until 2 years postoperatively. Therefore, 5 patients were totally excluded and the final total was 82 included patients. No patients had an extra-articular deformity, or an ipsilateral hip or ankle OA.

Radiography

The radiographs were projected using a Fuji computed radiography system, and the angles were measured using Fujifilm OP-A software (Fujifilm Co. Ltd., Tokyo, Japan). Anteroposterior (AP) and lateral whole leg radiographs were obtained with the patients in a standing position, as well as a skyline view of the knee; these radiographs were taken preoperatively and 24 months postoperatively. We took the radiographs 2 years after removal to exclude the influence of the fixation plate. The aFTA was defined as the lateral angle between the femoral and tibial anatomical shaft axes on an AP whole leg radiograph. The weight bearing line (WBL) ratio was defined as the ratio of the distance between the medial edge of the tibial plateau and the intersection point to the length of the tibial plateau. The WBL ratio of the medial tibial edge was considered to be 0% and the lateral tibial edge to be 100%. The medial TPS on the whole leg lateral radiograph was measured as the angle between the posterior slope and a line perpendicular to the tibial shaft axis [10]. We calculated the change in TPS by subtracting preoperative TPS from postoperative TPS. The anatomical lateral distal femoral angle (aLDFA) was defined as the lateral angle between the femoral anatomical axis and the tangent of the femoral condyles, and the anatomical medial proximal tibial angle (aMPTA) was defined as the medial angle between the tibial anatomical axis and the tibial plateau on the coronal view. The joint line convergence angle (JLCA) was defined as the angle between the tangents to the femoral condyles and the tibial plateau. JLCA with varus was represented as a "+" sign.

Computed tomography

Pre- and post-operative CT images of the whole lower extremity were obtained in 1.5-mm-thick slices using a SOMATOM Sensation 16 CT scanner (Siemens, Munich, Germany). The postoperative CT images were taken at 3 months after OWHTO. The analysis was performed using the CT images taken 3 months after OWHTO, because we could not confirm the borders between the osteotomy plane and artificial bones owing to bone union in later images. The data were incorporated into the Orthomap3D navigation software (Stryker, Kalamazoo, MI, USA), which enabled us to select anatomical landmarks and determine 3D linear and angular measurements by simultaneously referring to the sagittal, coronal, and axial planes [10, 11]. To measure each angle, the coronal and sagittal reference planes were set. The sagittal reference plane in the tibia was defined as the plane connecting the medial border of the patellar tendon at the level of the patellar tendon attachment, the middle of the posterior cruciate ligament at the level of the tibial plateau (connected to the Akagi line), and the ankle center [12]. The coronal reference plane in the tibia was defined as the plane perpendicular to the sagittal plane and passing through the middle point of the tibial eminences and the ankle center. The tibial plateau plane was defined as the plane connecting the anterior and posterior limits of the medial tibial plateau and the most lateral point on the line intersecting the lateral tibial plateau and the coronal plane. The upper osteotomy plane was defined as the plane connecting the following three cortical points: the anteromedial corner where the flange intersects with the upper osteotomy line, the posteromedial corner, and the center of the posterior cortex (Fig. 1a). The coronal and sagittal osteotomy plane angles were defined as the angles between the tibial plateau and the osteotomy planes in the coronal and sagittal views, respectively. The angle, which had an anterior-widening proximal tibial fragment, was showed as a positive value (Fig. 1b and c). The lower osteotomy plane, defined as the plane connecting the following three cortical points: the anteromedial corner where the flange intersected with lower osteotomy line, the posteromedial corner, and the center of the posterior osteotomy line (Fig. 2a). The coronal and sagittal opening gap angles were defined as the angles between the upper and lower osteotomy planes in the coronal and sagittal views, respectively. The angle, which is an anterior-opening gap, is showed as a positive value (Fig. 2b and c). When the opened upper and lower osteotomy planes was parallel in the tibial sagittal reference plane, the osteotomy gap in the sagittal view is rectangular. The hinge line was defined as the intersection line between the upper and lower osteotomy planes, as previously described (Fig. 2a) [9]. In the upper osteotomy plane, the midpoint of the line connecting the two points where the hinge line intersects the proximal tibial lateral cortex (hinge position) was displayed on the x-y coordinate system based on the mediolateral and anteroposterior width (Fig. 3). The percentage of the hinge position in the x-axis (lateral hinge position ratio) and y-axis (AP hinge position ratio) were defined. The AP and lateral hinge position ratio of the lateral tibial edge was considered to be 0%, the medial tibial edge to be 100%, the posterior tibial edge to be 0%, and the anterior tibial edge to be 100%. Two of the authors measured the osteotomy plane and opening gap angles in the coronal and sagittal views on CT images.

Clinical evaluation

Before and 2 years after OWHTO, arc of motion was measured, American Knee Society (AKS) knee and function scores were used to evaluate the degree of knee OA, and the Lysholm knee scoring scale was used to evaluate the conditions of the knee ligament [13, 14]. Clinical evaluations were measured by one of the authors preoperatively and at the 2 year after OWHTO.

Surgical technique

Preoperative planning anticipated a WBL ratio of 62% on the whole leg radiograph [15]. An arthroscopic examination was performed in all patients before OWHTO. After arthroscopic examination, a thigh tourniquet was applied while the patient was in the supine position. A 4–5-cm incision was made longitudinally at the 4–5-cm medial portion of the anterior ridge of the tibia. The superficial medial collateral ligament (MCL) was released subperiosteally from the medial proximal tibia. The osteotomy plane was obliquely directed from 35 mm distal to the medial

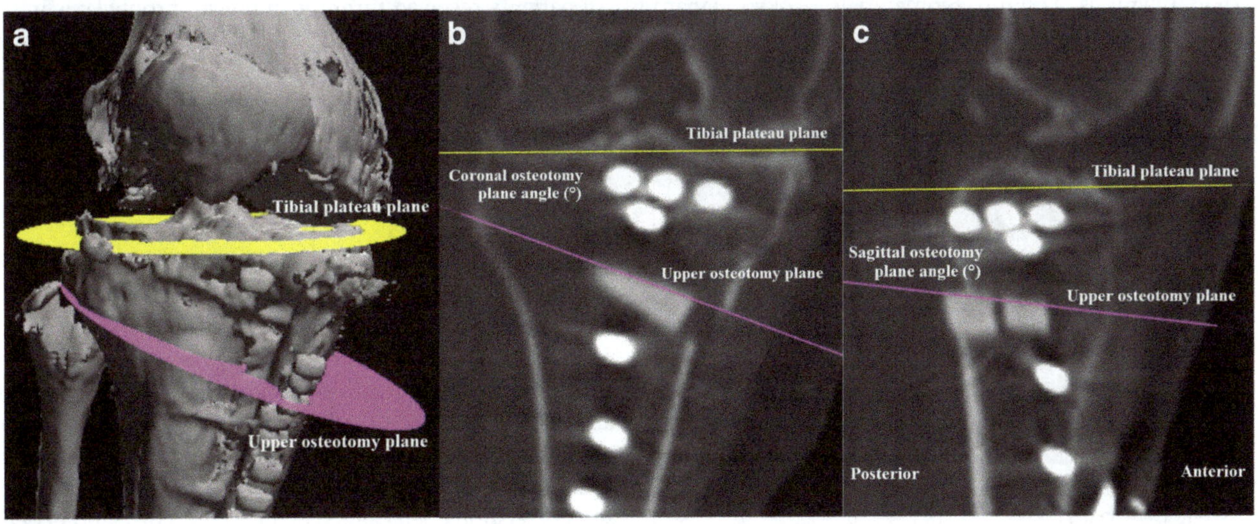

Fig. 1 **a** Three-dimensional computed tomography images of the knee joint. **b** The coronal osteotomy plane angle between the tibial plateau and the upper osteotomy planes in the coronal reference plane. **c** The sagittal osteotomy plane angle between the tibial plateau and the upper osteotomy plane in the sagittal reference plane

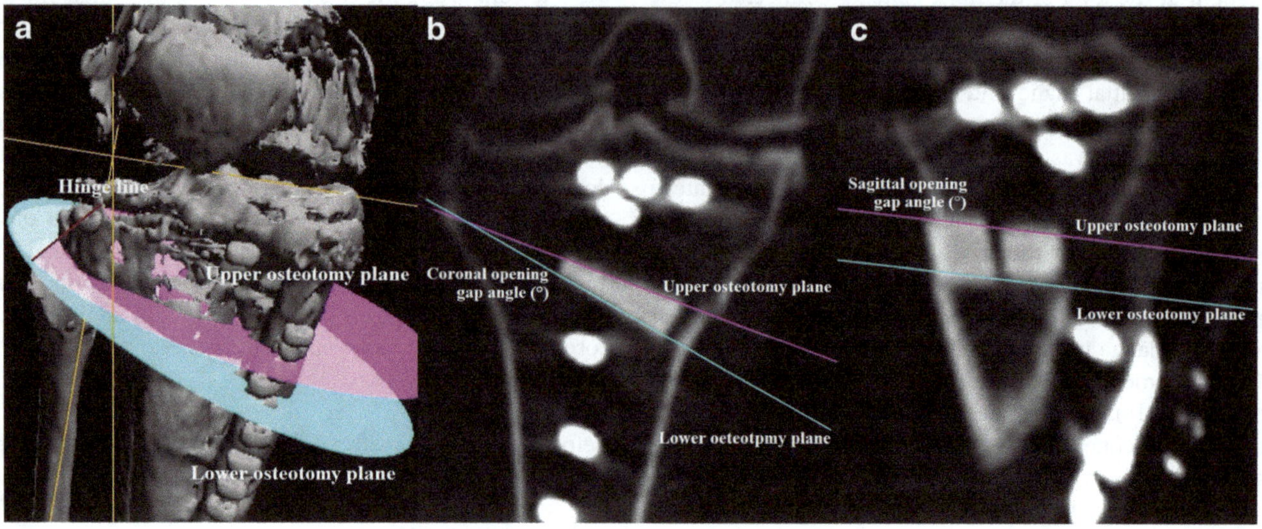

Fig. 2 **a** Three-dimensional computed tomography images of the knee joint. **b** The coronal opening gap angle between the upper and lower osteotomy planes in the coronal reference plane. **c** The sagittal opening gap angle between the upper and lower osteotomy planes in the sagittal reference plane

tibial plateau using two Kirschner wires parallel to the medial TPS [16, 17]. The osteotomy plane was planned to be parallel to the tibial plateau plane in the sagittal view. The anterior and posterior limits of the medial tibial plateau were superposed under fluoroscopy. Transverse osteotomy was performed from the medial tibia using a bone saw and chisels, while the lateral cortex was left intact of 10 mm as a hinge. The ascending osteotomy was performed under the tibial tuberosity at a 100–120° angle to the horizontal cut in the posterior 2/3 of the tibia in the sagittal view [2]. Under the image intensifier, the osteotomy site was gradually opened by stepwise insertion of 3–5 coupled chisels. The posterior beta-tricalcium phosphate (β-TCP; Olympus Terumo Biomaterials, Tokyo, Japan) was trimmed to a triangular shape the same width as the gap at the posteromedial corner, and the anterior β-TCP was trimmed to 2/3 of the width of the gap in the posteromedial corner. In cases of increased TPS, the posterior soft tissue was released. After the osteotomy and opening, two β-TCP wedges were inserted into the opened gap. The medial gap was filled by two formed β-TCP wedges and fixed with TomoFix and locking screws (DePuy-Synthes, Solothurn, Switzerland). The superficial MCL was not reattached. A drain was placed after closing the tissue layers.

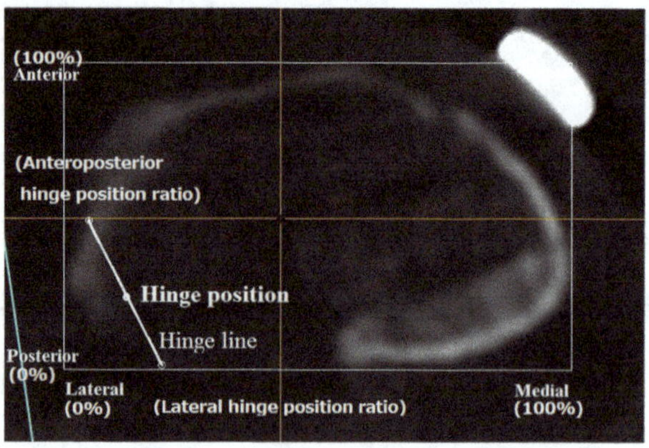

Fig. 3 Cross-sectional computed tomography image on the upper osteotomy plane. In the upper osteotomy plane, the midpoint of the line connecting the two points where the hinge line intersects the proximal tibial lateral cortex (hinge position) is displayed on the x-y coordinate system based on the mediolateral and anteroposterior width

Postoperative rehabilitation

All patients received thromboembolism prophylaxis in the form of low molecular weight heparin and venous impulse foot pumps. Patients began active and passive range of motion exercises and straight leg raising exercises on postoperative day 1. Full weightbearing was permitted to begin 1 week after surgery.

Statistical analysis

Data are expressed as means with 95% confidence intervals. To assess the intraobserver reproducibility and interobserver reliability, the measurements of each angle on postoperative CT were repeated twice by two observers in the first 40 knees. Preoperative and postoperative radiographic and clinical data were compared using t-test and Wilcoxon test. The relationships between the osteotomy plane or osteotomy gap and the TPS were calculated using the Pearson correlation coefficient. The interclass correlation coefficients (ICCs) for the intra- and inter-observer agreements were calculated. IBM SPSS Statistics Desktop for Windows version 21 software (SPSS Inc., Chicago, IL) was used for all statistical analyses. Values of $p < 0.05$ were considered statistically significant. Sample size calculation was performed using G*Power version 3.1.9 (Heinrich-Heine-Universität Düsseldorf, Germany). Priori power analysis (effect size = 0.3, $\alpha = 0.05$, power = 0.8) resulted in a sample size of 82.

Results

Patient characteristics are shown in Table 1. Table 2 shows the preoperative and postoperative radiographic and clinical data. The preoperative aFTA of 181.6° was significantly corrected to a postoperative aFTA of 168.5 ° ($p < 0.001$). The preoperative WBL ratio of 14.7% was significantly shifted to the postoperative WBL ratio of 69.8% ($p < 0.001$). The preoperative TPS of 11.9° significantly increased to the postoperative TPS of 12.6° ($p = 0.002$). The arc of motion and AKS knee, AKS function and Lysholm scores before OWHTO were significantly increased than them after OWHTO ($p = 0.037$, $p < 0.001$, $p < 0.001$ and $p < 0.001$, respectively).

Table 3 shows the postoperative radiographic and CT data. The change in TPS was 0.9°. The coronal osteotomy plane angle was 16.6°, and the sagittal osteotomy plane angle was 6.2°. The osteotomy plane angle, which had an anterior-widening proximal tibial fragment in the sagittal view, had a positive value in 78% of knees (64/82). The coronal opening gap angle was 13.7°. The sagittal opening gap angle was − 0.7°. The opening gap angle, which showed the small posterior-opening in the sagittal view, had a negative value in 49% of knees (40/82).

There was no significant difference between the sagittal osteotomy plane angle and the change in TPS. The sagittal opening gap angle and the AP hinge position ratio were significantly correlated with the change in the TPS ($r = 0.477$ $p < 0.001$ and $r = -0.342$, $p = 0.002$, respectively) (Figs. 4 and 5).

The ICCs of the intra-observer agreement for the AP and lateral hinge position ratios were 0.902–0.888 and 0.907–0.838, respectively. The ICCs of the inter-observer agreement for the AP and lateral hinge position ratios were 0.875 and 0.833, respectively. The hinge position was located at a mean of 16.0% (10.0 mm) from the lateral tibial edge, and a mean of 48.6% (21.9 mm) from the posterior tibial edge on the upper osteotomy plane (Fig. 6).

Table 1 Patient characteristics. Presented as mean (confidence intervals) or number

Variable	Mean (95% CI)
Age (yrs)	65.2 (63.5 to 66.8)
Height (cm)	157.4 (155.5 to 159.3)
Weight (kg)	63.4 (61.0 to 65.9)
Body mass index	25.5 (24.8 to 26.2)
Sex (women / men)	58 / 24
Side (Left / Right)	38 / 44
Ahlbäck grade 0/1/2	1 / 61 / 20

Table 2. Preoperative and postoperative radiographic and clinical data. Presented as mean (confidence intervals)

p-value	Preoperation	2 years after surgery
aFTA (°) < 0.001[a]	181.6 (180.8 to 182.5)	168.5 (167.8 to 169.2)
WBL ratio (%) < 0.001[b]	14.7 (11.3 to 18.2)	69.8 (66.6 to 73.0)
TPS (°) 0.002[a]	11.9 (11.0 to 12.7)	12.6 (11.7 to 13.5)
aLDFA (°) 0.289[a]	81.3 (80.7 to 81.9)	81.1 (80.6 to 81.6)
JLCA (°) < 0.001[a]	4.6 (4.2 to 5.0)	3.6 (3.2 to 4.0)
aMPTA (°) < 0.001[b]	85.3 (84.3 to 86.2)	95.1 (94.0 to 96.3)
Arc of motion (°) 0.037[b]	125 (122 to 128)	128 (125 to 131)
AKS knee score (point) < 0.001[b]	51 (49 to 53)	86 (85 to 88)
AKS function score (point) < 0.001[b]	72 (69 to 75)	97 (96 to 99)
Lysholm score (point) < 0.001[b]	47 (44 to 50)	89 (87 to 91)

aFTA anatomical femorotibial angle, *WBL* weightbearing line, *TPS* tibial posterior slope, *aLDFA* anatomical lateral distal femoral agle, *JLCA* joint line convergence angle, *aMPTA* anatomical medial proximal tibial angle, *AKS* American Knee Society

[a]t-test

[b]Wilcoxon test

Discussion

The sagittal osteotomy plane angle with an anterior-widening proximal tibial fragment was not related with increased TPS. The sagittal opening gap angle and the AP hinge position ratio were significantly correlated with the change in the TPS. The hinge position was located a mean

Table 3 Postoperative radiographic and computed tomography data. Presented as mean (confidence intervals) or number (%)

Variable	Mean (95% confidence intervals)
Change in TPS (°)	0.9 (0.4 to 1.3)
Coronal osteotomy plane angle (°)	16.6 (15.5 to 17.7)
Sagittal osteotomy plane angle (°)	6.2 (4.4 to 8.1)
Positive / negative value (knees)	64 (78%) / 18 (22%)
Coronal opening gap angle (°)	13.7 (13.0 to 14.5)
Sagittal opening gap angle (°)	−0.7 (−1.4 to 0)
Positive / negative value (Knees)	40 (49%) / 42 (51%)

Sagittal osteotomy plane angle with an anterior-widening proximal tibial fragment is showed as a positive value

Sagittal opening gap angle with an anterior-opening gap is showed as a positive value

TPS tibial posterior slope

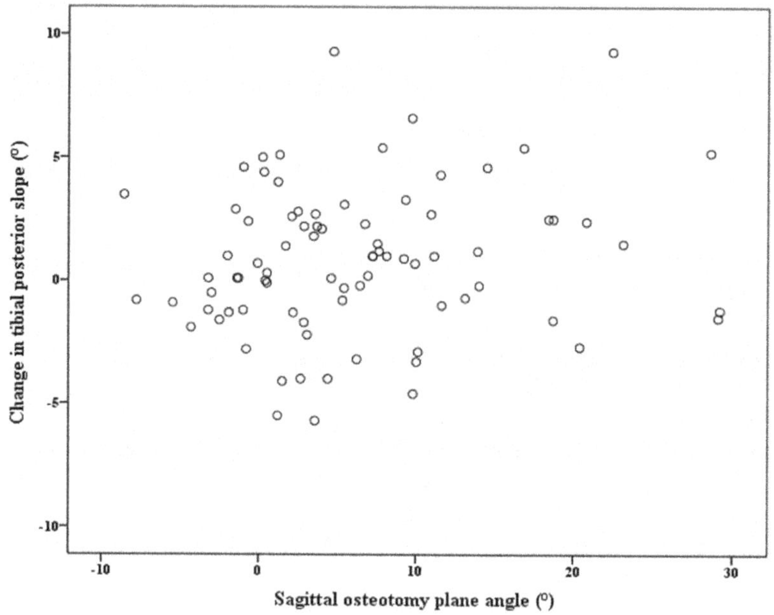

Fig. 4 Scatter graph showing the relationship between sagittal osteotomy plane angle and change in tibial posterior slope. The sagittal osteotomy plane was not related with the tibial posterior slope

of 16% from the lateral edge and a mean of approximately 50% from the posterior edge on the upper osteotomy plane of the proximal tibia.

In the current study, the mean sagittal osteotomy plane angle in 3DCT was 6.2° and 78.0% of knees had an anterior-widening proximal tibial fragment, a sagittal osteotomy plane angle with an anterior-widening fragment was not related to an increased change in TPS. Meanwhile, Lee et al. [4] reported that the mean sagittal osteotomy plane angle in lateral radiograph was 15.1°, and 87.1% of knees had an anterior-widening proximal tibial fragment. They also showed that the sagittal osteotomy

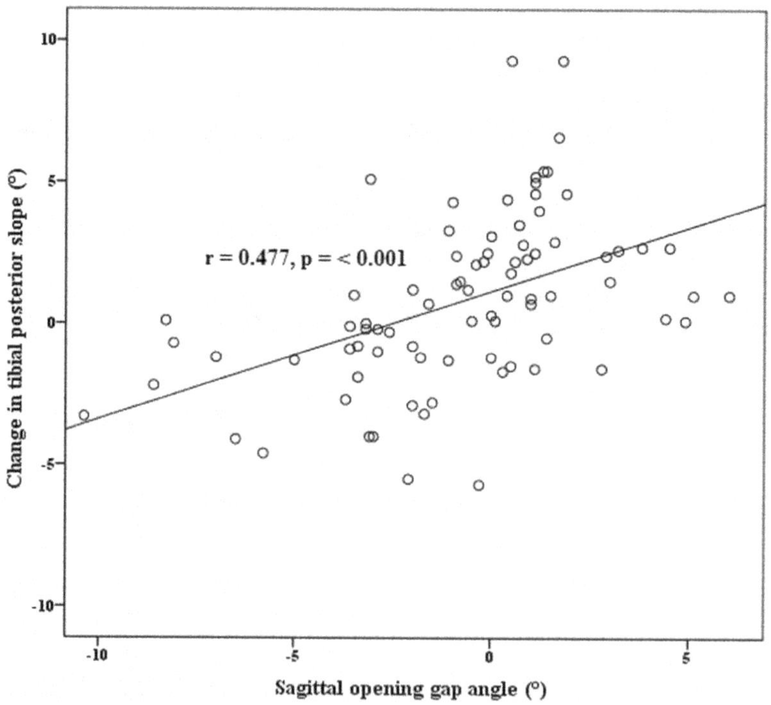

Fig. 5 Scatter graph showing the relationship between sagittal opening gap angle and change in tibial posterior slope

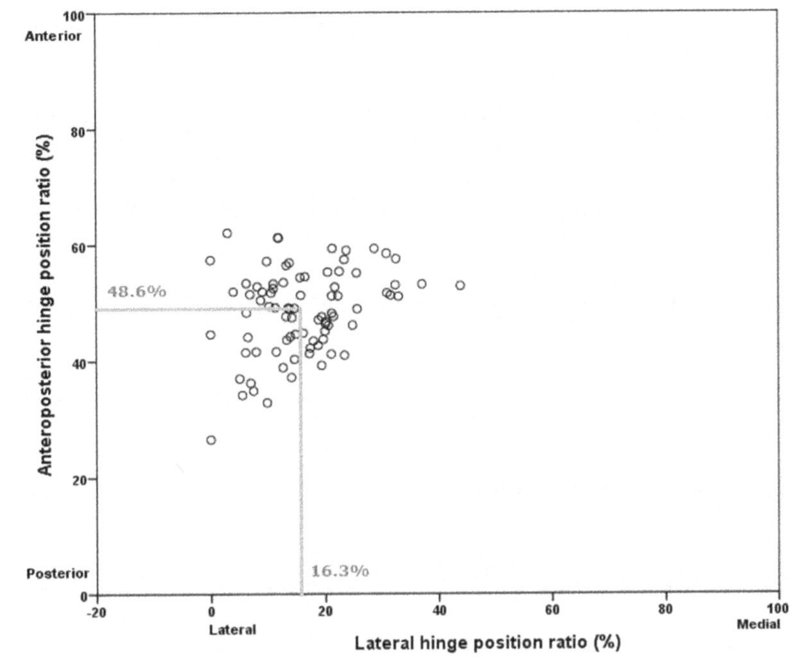

Fig. 6 Scatter graph showing the relationship between anteroposterior hinge position ratio and lateral hinge position ratio

plane angle was positively correlated with the change in TPS. The relationship between the sagittal osteotomy plane angle with an anterior-widening fragment and increased change in TPS was different between our and their studies [4]. Possible reasons for the difference between our and their studies might be related to the smaller mean value in the sagittal osteotomy plane angle, the difference in measurement method between radiograph and CT, or the difference in the treatment of the MCL and soft tissue. In addition, the operative technique that the anterior and posterior limits of the medial tibial plateau under fluoroscopy and inserted two K-wires in the osteotomy plane parallel to the medial TPS was superposed might be one of the reasons.

Regarding to the hinge position in the sagittal view, a previous study using 19 knees on 3D CT defined the direction of the hinge line compared with the AP axis on 3D CT axial view as the hinge axis, and reported that the hinge axis was located 4.9° posterolaterally compared with the AP axis [9]. They concluded that a posterolateral hinge position led to a significant increase in TPS. We showed the hinge position ratio using a coordinate system, which was calculated from the hinge line and the lateral tibial cortex on the upper osteotomy plane. This method is applicable to three-dimensional (2D) AP radiographs. Unlike their finding, we found that the hinge position ratio was located a mean of approximately 50% from the anterior edge on the upper osteotomy plane of the proximal tibia. We performed osteotomy from the medial proximal tibial surface after the release of the superficial MCL with an intact pes anserinus [17]. In addition, the release of the posteromedial soft tissue from the periosteum was adjusted according to the tightness of the posteromedial gap. Therefore, an adequate release of the MCL and posterior soft tissues might enable the hinge position to be located centrally in the sagittal view.

The hinge position ratio in the coronal view was located to the medial side of 16% from the lateral cortex on the upper osteotomy plane. A preoperative planning was measured on the AP standing whole leg radiograph of 2D, and the posteromedial corner was opened as a hinge of the lateral cortical edge. A previous study [9] and our results showed that the medial opening of the proximal tibia had been made at the axis of the hinge line where the upper and lower osteotomy planes intersected. Therefore, our findings showed that the postoperative WBL ratio moved more laterally than template during the preoperative planning. In addition, unintended decrease of the JLCA [18, 19] might result in a little more laterally postoperative WBL ratio. The medial movement of hinge position from most lateral had also affected a little more WBL ratio than 62% after OWHTO. Conversely, the hinge position near to the lateral cortical edge would more affect the risk of the lateral cortical fracture.

The opening gap angle and hinge position ratio in the sagittal view was correlated with an increased change in TPS. One study to 12 knees using cadavers [8] investigated whether the variable hinge position actually affected the change in TPS, and concluded that unintentional change in TPS could be avoided if a true lateral hinge position was achieved by performing a complete posterior osteotomy and inspecting the osteotomy using the gap ratio. They also stated that the osteotomy of the proximal tibia using the lateral location as a cortical hinge affected the change in TPS less than using the posterolateral location as a cortical hinge. In our study, the lateral hinge position ratio was located a mean of approximately 50% from the posterior edge. However, our findings were consistent with previous findings that the posterolateral hinge position led to an increase in TPS after OWHTO, and the posterior hinge position was related to anterior-opening gap. The control of AP hinge position must minimize the change in TPS. Conversely, the mean sagittal opening gap angle in our study was – 0.7° and the upper and lower osteotomy were almost opened parallel on the sagittal reference plane in the tibia. The aiming of the horizontal cut in the posterior 2/3 of the tibia and anterior gap of 2/3 of the posterior gap in the sagittal view enabled us to make an almost paralleled opening gap in the sagittal view [2].

We acknowledge the limitations of this study, which the various angles between the two planes were measured on 3D CT with the patients in the supine position, but the alignment was measured on AP whole leg radiographs with the patients in the standing position. In addition, the hinge position, osteotomy plane and opening gap angles were measured using the CT images taken 3 months after OWHTO, but radiographic and clinical evaluations were performed at 2 years after OWHTO.

Conclusions

Contrary to our expectation, the osteotomy plane did not need to be parallel to the tibial plateau plane in the sagittal view. However, the osteotomy gap should be rectangular in the sagittal view. The hinge position located nearly in the center of the sagittal view.

Abbreviations

3DCT: Three-dimensional computed tomography; aFTA: Anatomical femorotibial angle; AKS: American Knee Society; aLDFA: Anatomical lateral distal femoral angle; aMPTA: Anatomical medial proximal tibial angle; AP: Anteroposterior; CT: Computed tomography; ICCs: Interclass correlation coefficients; JLCA: Joint line convergence angle; MCL: Medial collateral ligament; OWHTO: Open wedge high tibial osteotomy; TPS: Tibial posterior slope; WBL: Weight bearing line; β-TCP: Beta-Tricalcium phosphate

Authors' contributions

YA: study design, data collection, interpreting the data and writing the paper. HK: data collection. MT, SN, KK, TS: interpretation. All authors read and approved the final manuscript.

Consent for publication

Not applicable.

Competing interests

The authors declare that they have no competing interests.

References

1. Staubli AE, De Simoni C, Babst R, Lobenhoffer P. TomoFix: a new LCP-concept for open wedge osteotomy of the medial proximal tibia--early results in 92 cases. Injury. 2003;34(Suppl 2):B55–62.
2. Song EK, Seon JK, Park SJ, Seo HY. Navigated open wedge high tibial osteotomy. Sports Med Arthrosc. 2008;16:84–90.
3. Miller BS, Downie B, McDonough EB, Wojtys EM. Complications after medial opening wedge high tibial osteotomy. Arthroscopy. 2009;25:639–46.
4. Lee SY, Lim HC, Bae JH, Kim JG, Yun SH, Yang JH, Yoon JR. Sagittal osteotomy inclination in medial open-wedge high tibial osteotomy. Knee Surg Sports Traumatol Arthrosc. 2017;25:823–31.
5. Noyes FR, Goebel SX, West J. Opening wedge tibial osteotomy: the 3-triangle method to correct axial alignment and tibial slope. Am J Sports Med. 2005;33:378–87.
6. Hinterwimmer S, Beitzel K, Paul J, Kirchhoff C, Sauerschnig M, von Eisenhart-Rothe R, Imhoff AB. Control of posterior tibial slope and patellar height in open-wedge valgus high tibial osteotomy. Am J Sports Med. 2011;39:851–6.
7. Jacobi M, Wahl P, Jakob RP. Avoiding intraoperative complications in open-wedge high tibial valgus osteotomy: technical advancement. Knee Surg Sports Traumatol Arthrosc. 2010;18:200–3.
8. Wang JH, Bae JH, Lim HC, Shon WY, Kim CW, Cho JW. Medial open wedge high tibial osteotomy: the effect of the cortical hinge on posterior tibial slope. Am J Sports Med. 2009;37:2411–8.
9. Moon SW, Park SH, Lee BH, Oh M, Chang M, Ahn JH, Wang JH. The effect of hinge position on posterior tibial slope in medial open-wedge high tibial osteotomy. Arthroscopy. 2015;31:1128–33.
10. Akamatsu Y, Sotozawa M, Kobayashi H, Kusayama Y, Kumagai K, Saito T. Usefulness of long tibial axis to measure medial tibial slope for opening wedge high tibial osteotomy. Knee Surg Sports Traumatol Arthrosc. 2016;24:3661–7.
11. Akamatsu Y, Kobayashi H, Kusayama Y, Kumagai K, Saito T. Comparative study of opening wedge high tibial osteotomy with and without combined CT-based and image-free navigation systems. Arthroscopy. 2016;32:2072–81.
12. Akagi M, Oh M, Nonaka T, Tsujimoto H, Asano T, Hamanishi C. An anteroposterior axis of the tibia for total knee arthroplasty. Clin Orthop Relat Res. 2004;420:213–21.
13. Insall JN, Dorr LD, Scott RD, Scott WN. Rationale of the knee society clinical rating system. Clin Orthop Relat Res. 1989;248:13–4.
14. Tegner Y, Lysholm J. Rating systems in the evaluation of knee ligament injuries. Clin Orthop Relat Res. 1985;198:43–9.
15. Takeuchi R, Ishikawa H, Aratake M, Bito H, Saito I, Kumagai K, Akamatsu Y, Saito T. Medial opening wedge high tibial osteotomy with early full weight bearing. Arthroscopy. 2009;25:46–53.
16. Lobenhoffer P, Agneskirchner JD. Improvements in surgical technique of valgus high tibial osteotomy. Knee Surg Sports Traumatol Arthrosc. 2003;11:132–8.
17. Seo SS, Kim CW, Seo JH, Kim DH, Lee CR. Does superficial medial collateral ligament release in open-wedge high tibial osteotomy for varus osteoarthritic knees increase valgus laxity? Am J Sports Med. 2016;44:908–15.
18. Heijens E, Kornherr P, Meister C. The coronal hypomochlion: a tipping point of clinical relevance when planning valgus producing high tibial osteotomies. Bone Joint J. 2016;98-B:628–33.
19. Lee DH, Park SC, Park HJ, Han SB. Effect of soft tissue laxity of the knee joint on limb alignment correction in open-wedge high tibial osteotomy. Knee Surg Sports Traumatol Arthrosc. 2016;24:3704–12.

21

Effect of high body mass index on knee muscle strength and function after anterior cruciate ligament reconstruction using hamstring tendon autografts

Wei-Hsiu Hsu[1,2,3*], Chun-Hao Fan[1], Pei-An Yu[1,2], Chi-Lung Chen[1,2,3], Liang-Tseng Kuo[1,2,3] and Robert Wen-Wei Hsu[1,2]

Abstract

Background: Increased body mass index (BMI) has been associated with poorer function in patients who have undergone anterior cruciate ligament (ACL) reconstruction. However, the effect of high BMI on muscle strength in these patients remained unclear. The current study aimed to compare knee muscle strength and Knee injury and Osteoarthritis Outcome Score (KOOS) in ACL-reconstructed patients with a variety of different BMIs.

Methods: From November 2013 to March 2016, we prospectively enrolled 30 patients who underwent ACL reconstruction (18–60 years of age). Anthropometric parameters, body compositions, isokinetic muscle strength and KOOS were assessed preoperatively, and at post-operative 16th week and 28th week. The patients were stratified into two groups by BMI, i.e. normal BMI (18.5–24.9 kg/m^2) and high BMI (≥25.0 kg/m^2).

Results: Twelve patients in the normal BMI group completed the follow-up, while sixteen patients did so in the high BMI group. In comparison of muscle strength between baseline and 28th week follow-up, the normal BMI group had significant increases in overall knee muscle strength, while the high BMI group only had increases in extensors of uninjured knee and flexors of the injured knee. However, there were significant increases in all KOOS subscales for the high BMI group. The high BMI patients reported increased KOOS, which may reflect the contribution of ligament stability in the presence of inadequate muscle strength.

Conclusions: The normal BMI patients had improvement in all knee muscle strength following ACL reconstruction, while high BMI patients only had increases in certain knee muscles. High BMI patients had a decreased quadriceps muscle symmetry index, as compared to their normal BMI counterparts. Increases in quadriceps muscle strength of the uninjured knee and ACL reconstruction were associated with improvements in KOOS in high BMI patients.

Keywords: Body composition, BMI, Leg symmetry index

Background

Anterior cruciate ligament (ACL) reconstruction surgery aims to re-establish the stability in the knee joint and allow patients to return to their previous activities after a period of muscle training [1]. Many factors have been suggested as contributing to self-reported function results for ACL reconstruction, including quadriceps index, pain intensity, and flexion motion deficit [2]. The effect of body mass index (BMI) on long-term outcome for ACL reconstruction patients remained unclear [3]. Increased BMI has been associated with poorer functional outcomes following ACL reconstruction [4, 5]. Meanwhile, ACL reconstruction has also been suggested as an effective treatment irrespective of preoperative BMI [6].

Whether the quadriceps recovers well is a major concern for function following ACL injury and reconstruction, as well as a determining factor in the development

* Correspondence: 7572@cgmh.org.tw
[1]Sports Medicine Center, Chang Gung Memorial Hospital at Chia Yi, Chia Yi, Taiwan
[2]Department of Orthopaedic Surgery, Chang Gung Memorial Hospital at Chia Yi, No 6 West section, Chia Pu Road, Puzih, Chia Yi Hsien 613, Taiwan
Full list of author information is available at the end of the article

of knee osteoarthritis [7–9]. The quadriceps of the injured knee weakens profoundly after anterior cruciate ligament injury and subsequent reconstruction [7, 9–11]. This weakness of the quadriceps muscle has been attributed to arthrogenic inhibition, incomplete voluntary activation of the muscle, and altered quadriceps corticomotor excitability [12–14]. It is generally accepted that the aim of postoperative care should be focused on the recovery of muscle strength after ACL reconstruction [15–17]. In fact, quadriceps strength did affect self-reported knee function [2, 18, 19].

Although it has been found that increased BMI is associated with slower muscle recovery as well as lower quadriceps muscle force in patients following total knee arthroplasty [20], whether this slow recovery occurs in ACL patients was previously unclear. Therefore, the purpose of this study was to compare body compositions, knee muscle strength, and Knee Injury and Osteoarthritis Outcome Score (KOOS) after ACL reconstruction in patients with different BMIs.

Methods

Between November 2013 and March 2016, we prospectively enrolled 30 patients who underwent anterior cruciate ligament reconstructions (aged 18–60 years) using hamstring tendon autografts. The individuals were excluded if they (1) had a history of surgery to either knee, (2) had a previous partial ACL tear, (3) had other ligamentous damage concurrent with ACL injury, (4) had any complications or additional surgery during follow-up. Since return to activity were usually advised 6 months after ACL reconstruction, end-point assessments were performed at 28 weeks after ACL reconstruction [21, 22]. To understand the temporal changes following ACL reconstruction, 16 weeks were further selected. The anthropometric parameters, body compositions, muscle strength and KOOS were assessed preoperatively, and then 16 weeks and 28 weeks post operatively. All participants were Taiwanese from the southern part of the country. The present study was approved by the institutional review board of Chang Gung Foundation (IRB102-0977B), and all study participants provided informed consent to be involved in the study.

Muscle strength

The muscle strength of the lower extremity including knee flexor/extensor was tested via the HUMAC NORM system (CSMi, U.S.A.), with the mode of concentric/concentric contraction at the angular velocity of 60 degrees/s [11, 15, 23]. The knee flexor/extensor was tested in a seated position. Isokinetic tests were performed 5 times for each examination, and each trial was separated by a rest period of 3 min. In the present study, muscle strength was then normalized for body weight [11]. Leg symmetry index was calculated via the equation ((Injured side maximum force/uninjured side maximum force) × 100%), and compared [12, 24].

Body composition

Body composition was assessed using an eight-polar tactile-electrode impedance meter (InBody 720; Biospace, Seoul, Korea), which simultaneously recorded body weight, total body fat mass, and lean body mass [25]. BMI (kg/m^2) was calculated as follows: BMI = weight/height^2. The participants were divided into two groups stratified by BMI. The classification of high BMI was based on BMI cut-points established by the World Health Organization. Two levels were determined: the normal BMI group (18.5–24.9 kg/m^2) and the high BMI goup (≥25.0 kg/m^2) [6, 26].

Questionnaire

The Knee Injury and Osteoarthritis Outcome Score is a 42-item self-administered knee-specific questionnaire assessing pain (9 items), symptoms (7 items), activities of daily living (ADL, 17 items), function, sports and recreational activities (Sports/Rec, 5 items) and knee-related quality of life (QOL, 4 items) in five separate subscales. All items are scored 0 to 4; for each subscale the scores are converted to a 0 to 100 scale (0 representing extreme knee problems and 100 representing no knee problems) [27].

The Marx activity rating scales is a patient-reported instrument which is determined by measuring some components of physical function that are common to the most sporting activities [28].

Exercise protocol

It was suggested the importance of improving lower limb muscle strength, starting at an date (2–6 weeks) early after surgery [29–31]. The participants were prescribed home based rehabilitation protocol that started at 4 weeks after surgery. Telephone to track the implementation of this rehabilitation protocol was performed weekly. The rehabilitation program was 1 h stretching and resistance training, with the use of a resistive band instead of weights, 3–5 times per week for 24 weeks. The stretching consisted of eight movements (lower back stretch, upper back stretch, hip stretch, quadriceps stretch, abdomen stretch, lower leg stretch, arm stretch and groin stretch), each held for 20–30 s. The resistance exercises were completed by side bending, biceps curl, leg extension, seated dip, shoulder press, hip abductor/adductor, chest press and leg press. To minimize fatigue, the exercises were alternated between the upper and lower body. Each movement was 4 sets of 15 repetitions. There was a rest interval between sets of 60 s, but no pauses between repetitions.

Table 1 Subject characteristics

	Normal BMI group (*N* = 12) Mean±SD	High BMI group (*N* = 16) Mean±SD	*p* value
Age (years)	41±13	35±13	0.270
Height (cm)	164±9	171±8	0.092
Time from injury to baseline test (mon)	17±28	5±5	0.319
Marx activity rating scales (score)	7±6	7±6	0.700
Male:Female ratio	7: 5	13: 3	0.085
Meniscal damage Yes:No ratio	7: 5	11: 5	0.143
Cause of injury Sport:Other ratio	8: 4	10: 6	0.558

Statistical analysis

All data analyses were performed using the Statistical Package for the Social Sciences for Windows (v 20.0; SPSS Inc., Chicago, IL, USA). All continuous data is presented as the mean ± standard deviation (SD). A two-way analysis of variance (ANOVA; group × time) with repeated measures was used to determine the effects of BMI group and time on the dependent measures. The level of significance was set at $p \leq 0.05$. A power of 95% and relevant effect size of 0.31 was calculated.

Results

Twenty-eight patients completed the follow-up test at 28 weeks, including twelve patients in the normal BMI group (BMI = 18.5–24.9 kg/m^2) and sixteen in the high BMI group (BMI ≥25.0 kg/m^2) (i.e., at least 75% of the training sessions). The reasons for loss of follow-up in the present study were personal factors, such as moving house. The demographic data showed no differences between both groups other than body weight (Table 1). However, it was found that high BMI patients underwent surgical interventions in a shorter interval after injury, and suffered an increased rate of concomitant meniscal injury. Causes of initial injury include: sports (basketball, volleyball and badminton), falling or car accident.

In body composition analysis, we observed a temporary increase in body fat in both the normal and high BMI groups at 16 weeks following ACL reconstruction, then returning to previous level at 28 weeks. Interestingly, an increase in lean body mass was shown in the high BMI group at 28 weeks after ACL reconstruction, which resulted in a corresponding increase in body weight. On the other hand, no difference was shown in the normal BMI group in either lean body weight or fat mass (Table 2).

In isokinetic muscle strength assessment, knee muscle strength increased for both knee flexor and extensor in the injured knee for the normal BMI group at the 28-

Table 2 Body composition

		Baseline Mean±SD	16 weeks Mean±SD	28 weeks Mean±SD	$^‡p$ value	$^§p$ value	^δp value
Weight (kg)	Normal BMI group	61±9 †	62±10‡†	62±10†	0.028	0.175	0.263
	High BMI group	85±12	86±12	86±12	0.134	0.214	0.938
	$^†p$ value	< 0.001	< 0.001	< 0.001			
BMI (kg/m^2)	Normal BMI group	23±2†	23±2†	23±2†	0.641	0.528	0.326
	High BMI group	29±3	29±4	29±3	0.277	0.414	0.775
	$^†p$ value	< 0.001	< 0.001	< 0.001			
LBM (kg)	Normal BMI group	45±8†	45±8†	45±8†	0.672	0.553	0.326
	High BMI group	60±9	60±10	61±10 ^{§δ}	0.682	0.017	0.049
	$^†p$ value	0.002	0.003	0.001			
Body fat (kg)	Normal BMI group	16±3†	17±3‡†	16±4†	0.012	0.735	0.141
	High BMI group	25±8	26±8 ‡	25±8 δ	0.034	0.865	0.036
	$^†p$ value	0.004	0.004	0.005			
LBM/ body fat ratio (%)	Normal BMI group	291±55	267±60‡	291±71δ	0.002	0.994	0.042
	High BMI group	260±84	252±86‡	263±86	0.042	0.678	0.073
	$^†p$ value	0.391	0.624	0.391			

LBM Lean body mass
$^†p \leq 0.05$ between normal and high BMI group
$^§p \leq .05$ between baseline and 28 weeks
$^‡p \leq .05$ between baseline and 16 weeks
$^δp \leq .05$ between 16 weeks and 28 weeks

Table 3 Modulus knee muscle strength (N-m)

			Baseline Mean±SD	16 weeks Mean±SD	28 weeks Mean±SD	‡p value	§p value	δp value
Injury side	Extensor	Normal BMI group	42±31	65±33‡	75±40§δ	0.028	0.011	0.042
		High BMI group	64±35	66±36	76±36	0.777	0.213	0.181
		†p value	0.152	0.937	0.938			
	Flexor	Normal BMI group	35±18†	51±12	66±25 §	0.066	0.011	0.072
		High BMI group	58±26	61±23	73±25	0.671	0.055	0.065
		†p value	.034	0.287	0.520			
Uninjured side	Extensor	Normal BMI group	76±40	99±30	96±36§	0.097	0.004	0.754
		High BMI group	101±39	120±46	131±42§	0.068	0.003	0.296
		†p value	0.152	0.271	0.058			
	Flexor	Normal BMI group	48±16†	66±14‡	67±20§	0.015	0.002	0.921
		High BMI group	75±26	85±29	89±32	0.088	0.094	0.648
		†p value	0.016	0.109	0.054			

†$p \le 0.05$ between normal and high BMI group
§$p \le .05$ between baseline and 28 weeks
‡$p \le .05$ between baseline and 16 weeks
δ$p \le .05$ between 16 weeks and 28 weeks

week follow-up. At the same time, an increase was shown only in the knee flexor muscle in the high BMI group. For the uninjured knee, the normal BMI group had simultaneously increased strength in both the knee extensor and flexor. On the contrary, an increase was demonstrated in extensor muscle strength for the uninjured knee in the high BMI group, as well as an increase in flexor muscle strength of the injured knee (Tables 3 and 4). When the symmetry index was calculated and compared, the normal BMI group had a significant increase in the symmetry index as compared to the high BMI group at the 28-week follow-up (Fig. 1).

In the functional assessment via KOOS, there were no differences in any category between the normal and high BMI groups, except in QOL score. The high BMI group had a decreased QOL score as compared to those in the normal BMI group at baseline ($p \le 0.05$). These differences in QOL became insignificant at 28 weeks after ACL reconstruction (Table 5). For the high BMI group, the KOOS increased from baseline to 28 weeks after ACL reconstruction in all categories. The symptom score increased from 62 ± 17 to 74 ± 15 ($p \le 0.05$). Similar increases were found in pain, ADL and QOL score (Table 5). Meanwhile, the sport/recreational activity

Table 4 Relative knee muscle strength (N-m/ kg)

			Baseline Mean±SD	16 weeks Mean±SD	28 weeks Mean±SD	‡p value	§p value	δp value
Injury side	Extensor	Normal BMI group	0.71±0.48	1.05±0.45‡	1.23±0.56§δ	0.025	0.017	0.050
		High BMI group	0.75±0.37	0.77±0.40	0.88±0.40	0.816	0.224	0.191
		†p value	0.903	0.105	0.105			
	Flexor	Normal BMI group	0.58±0.30	0.83±0.18‡	1.06±0.29 §δ	0.050	0.012	0.012
		High BMI group	0.68±0.27	0.70±0.24	0.84±0.25§	0.737	0.019	0.079
		†p value	0.358	0.209	0.092			
Uninjured side	Extensor	Normal BMI group	1.24±0.53	1.61±0.44	1.58±0.50§	0.093	0.017	0.889
		High BMI group	1.18±0.37	1.38±0.45	1.52±0.44§	0.098	0.004	0.301
		†p value	0.759	0.178	0.806			
	Flexor	Normal BMI group	0.80±0.21	1.08±0.24‡	1.09±0.25§	0.028	0.012	1.000
		High BMI group	0.87±0.25	0.98±0.27	1.02±0.31	0.098	0.070	0.756
		†p value	0.426	0.462	0.602			

†$p \le 0.05$ between normal and high BMI group
§$p \le .05$ between baseline and 28 weeks
‡$p \le .05$ between baseline and 16 weeks
δ$p \le .05$ between 16 weeks and 28 weeks

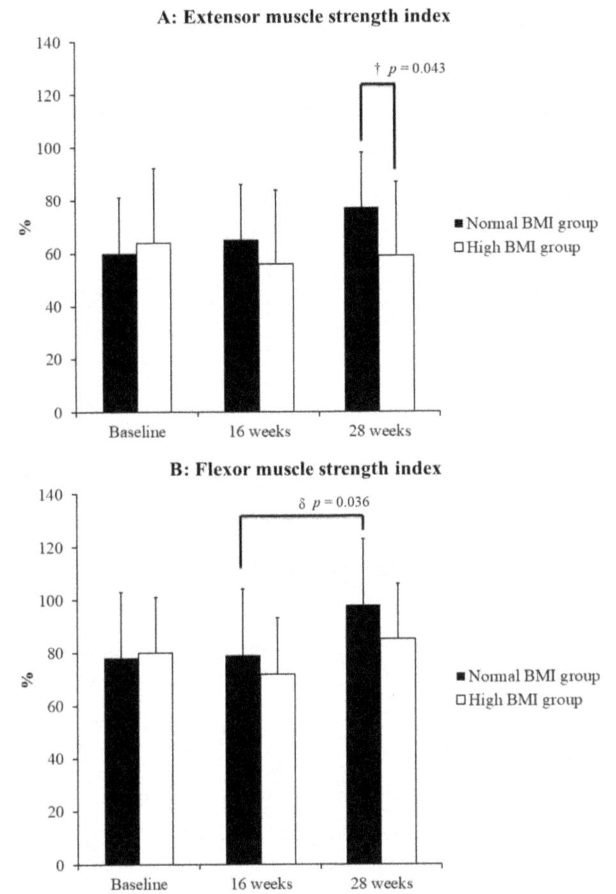

Fig. 1 Knee muscle strength index (Injured side/Uninjured side*100%); **a** extensor muscle strength index; **b** flexor muscle strength index. †$p < 0.05$ between normal and high BMI group; δ $p < .05$ between 16 weeks and 28 weeks

score increased from 36 ± 20 to 52 ± 22 at 16 weeks after surgery and further to 64 ± 17 at 28 weeks ($p \leq 0.05$). For the normal BMI group, an increase in the pain subcategory was demonstrated from 75 ± 15 at 16 weeks to 84 ± 13 at the 28-week follow-up (Table 5).

Discussion

The present study found that high BMI patients (BMI ≥ 25) had improving quadriceps muscle strength in the un-injured knee, while normal BMI patients had improvements in the both injured and uninjured knees. This study parallels the literature, in that normal BMI patients have an extensor symmetry index approaching 80% at 6-month follow-up [15, 32, 33]. However, such improvement was not shown in high BMI patients. Second, preoperative quality of life was shown inferior in the high BMI group as compared to the normal BMI group, and improved at 28 weeks after ACL reconstruction. Similarly, the score improved in symptoms, pain, sports, and ADL in the high BMI patients. Interestingly, the normal BMI group had only improvement in the pain subcategory, despite recovery of better muscle strength.

Utilizing strength/body weight ratio, we observed that both the normal and high BMI groups have similar flexor and extensor strength for the uninjured knee at 28 weeks follow-up. It seemed that the strength/ body weight would reach a plateau either in the high or normal BMI patients in the uninjured knee, while a persistent deficit was observed in the injured knee and to a greater extent in the high BMI group. The injured knee showed a pattern where the normal BMI group had progressive increases in both knee flexors and extensors, reaching symmetry indexes of 77% and 90%, respectively, while the high BMI group had no significant increases in extensor strength. Hence, the symmetry index for the extensor muscle was shown a significant difference between the high and normal BMI groups at the 28 week follow-up.

Literature suggests that the deficit in quadriceps strength for ACL deficient patients is greater than the deficit in hamstring strength [32, 34, 35]. This deficit in strength can be improved by an exercise program after ACL reconstruction, and recovery of strength in the flexor is faster than in the extensor [36, 37]. The present study exhibited similar patterns, and further showed that high BMI patients had a slower recovery of extensor muscle strength. The muscle strength deficit may result from arthrogenic muscle inhibition or quadriceps corticospinal excitability [13, 14]. It has been suggested that the cortical silent period (cSP) duration is longer in the injured limb of the ACL group, as compared to the uninjured limb [13]. The current study has shown that high BMI was associated with a greater duration of muscle strength deficit. Changed activation of quadriceps and with altered neuromuscular control was shown in obese patients [38]. The quadriceps symmetry index did not reach the desired high quadriceps index (> 90%) that which is suggested to be biomechanically advantageous after ACL reconstruction [8, 19, 21]. Neuromuscular training incorporating motor learning principles, such as eccentric training which was most effective in restoring quadriceps strength, should be added to strength training to optimize outcome measurements [39].

Increasing BMI was associated with a progressive reduction in physical functions [40, 41]. The deficit extended to those patients suffered from musculoskeletal disorders such as arthropathy and ACL ruptures. Surgical interventions, i.e. total knee arthroplasty (TKA) and ACL reconstructions, would result in comparable functional improvement irrespective of different BMIs [6, 42–44]. Interestingly, effect of BMI on pain for TKA and ACL reconstructed patients was shown a similar

Table 5 KOOS

		Baseline Mean±SD	16 weeks Mean±SD	28 weeks Mean±SD	‡p value	§p value	δp value
Symptoms	Normal BMI group	67±16	68±19	71±16	0.889	0.483	0.528
	High BMI group	62±17	65±18	74±15 §δ	0.594	0.023	0.023
	†p value	0.407	0.519	0.690			
Pain	Normal BMI group	78±17	75±15	84±13 δ	0.735	0.400	0.027
	High BMI group	74±19	80±14	87±10 §δ	0.605	0.001	0.008
	†p value	0.602	0.481	0.407			
ADL	Normal BMI group	83±19	87±12	91±11	0.401	0.128	0.108
	High BMI group	78±20	81±18	91±8§δ	0.326	0.012	0.004
	†p value	0.443	0.408	0.443			
Sports/Rec	Normal BMI group	50±30	55±17	71±19	0.623	0.089	0.090
	High BMI group	36±20	52±22+	64±19§	0.018	0.001	0.097
	† p value	0.207	0.517	0.422			
QOL	Normal BMI group	53±16†	58±18	65±12	0.344	0.131	0.235
	High BMI group	38±11	52±19‡	58±23§	0.008	0.002	0.274
	†p value	0.010	0.338	0.306			

ADL Activities of Daily Living, *Sports/Rec* function, sports and recreational activities, *QOL* knee-related Quality of Life
†$p \leq 0.05$ between normal and high BMI group
§$p \leq .05$ between baseline and 28 weeks
‡$p \leq .05$ between baseline and 16 weeks
δ$p \leq .05$ between 16 weeks and 28 weeks

pattern. In TKA patients, preoperative WOMAC (Western Ontario and McMaster Universities Osteoarthritis Index) pain score was worse as the BMI increased. TKA surgery resulted in a faster improvement in the higher BMI group at 6 month but reached a comparable level across all BMIs at 2 year [45]. In ACL reconstructed patients, faster improvement of pain score was also observed in high BMI patients [6]. In the present study, we demonstrated a significant improvement in KOOS pain subscales in 6 month follow up in the high BMI groups. In addition, we further showed that the high BMI group had improvement in all KOOS subscales, along with an increased muscle strength in the flexor of the injured knee. This could be attributed to, as least in part, the fact that the high BMI group had lower preoperative scores. In the high BMI group, ACL reconstruction providing for re-establishment of static stabilization, along with increased flexor muscle strength, may contribute to the improvement of KOOS. Increased knee muscle strength, mainly in the knee flexors, has been associated with lower activity limitations [46].

The current study was limited by the small number of patients and the relatively short follow-up. Longer-term follow-up is warranted to investigate muscle strength and functional recovery after ACL reconstruction for both normal and high BMI groups. However, this study demonstrated decreased quadriceps muscle strength recovery in the ACL reconstructed knee for higher BMI patients than for normal BMI patients at 6 months follow-up. It is suggested that further rehabilitation should include resistance training and neuromuscular facilitation in high BMI ACL reconstruction patients.

Conclusion

In the current study, the normal BMI patients had improvement in all knee muscle strength following ACL reconstruction, while high BMI patients only had increases in certain knee muscles. High BMI patients had a decreased quadriceps muscle symmetry index, as compared to their normal BMI counterparts. Increases in quadriceps muscle strength of the uninjured knee and ACL reconstruction were associated with improvements in KOOS in high BMI patients.

Abbreviations

ACL: Anterior cruciate ligament; ADL: Activities of daily living; BMI: Body mass index; cSP: Cortical silent period; KOOS: Knee injury and Osteoarthritis Outcome Score; QOL: Knee-related quality of life; Sports/Rec: Function, sports and recreational activities; TKA: Total knee arthroplasty; WOMAC: Western Ontario and McMaster Universities Osteoarthritis Index

Funding

Financial support from Chang Gung Memorial Hospital Grant CORPG6C0033 and CORPG6G0271 are appreciated. There was no external funding.

Authors' contributions
WHH and CHF designed the study and drafted the manuscript. WHH revised it critically. CHF and PAY performed the assessments and statistical analysis. CLC, LTK, and RWWH contributed substantially to the conception and design of the study. All authors have read and approved the final manuscript.

Consent for publication
Not applicable.

Competing interests
The authors declare that they have no competing interests.

Author details
[1]Sports Medicine Center, Chang Gung Memorial Hospital at Chia Yi, Chia Yi, Taiwan. [2]Department of Orthopaedic Surgery, Chang Gung Memorial Hospital at Chia Yi, No 6 West section, Chia Pu Road, Puzih, Chia Yi Hsien 613, Taiwan. [3]School of Medicine, Chang Gung University, Tao-Yuan, Taiwan.

References

1. Mohtadi N. Development and validation of the quality of life outcome measure (questionnaire) for chronic anterior cruciate ligament deficiency. Am J Sports Med. 1998;26(3):350–9.
2. Lentz TA, Tillman SM, Indelicato PA, Moser MW, George SZ, Chmielewski TL. Factors associated with function after anterior cruciate ligament reconstruction. Sports Health. 2009;1(1):47–53.
3. Magnussen RA, Spindler KP. The effect of patient and injury factors on long-term outcome after anterior cruciate ligament reconstruction. Curr Orthop Pract. 2011;22(1):90–103.
4. Kowalchuk DA, Harner CD, Fu FH, Irrgang JJ. Prediction of patient-reported outcome after single-bundle anterior cruciate ligament reconstruction. Arthroscopy. 2009;25(5):457–63.
5. Lebel B, Hulet C, Galaud B, Burdin G, Locker B, Vielpeau C. Arthroscopic reconstruction of the anterior cruciate ligament using bone-patellar tendon-bone autograft: a minimum 10-year follow-up. Am J Sports Med. 2008;36(7): 1275–82.
6. Ballal MS, Khan Y, Hastie G, Hatcher A, Coogan S, McNicholas MJ. Functional outcome of primary hamstring anterior cruciate ligament reconstruction in patients with different body mass index classes. Arthroscopy. 2013;29(8): 1314–21.
7. Lynch AD, Logerstedt DS, Axe MJ, Snyder-Mackler L. Quadriceps activation failure after anterior cruciate ligament rupture is not mediated by knee joint effusion. J Orthop Sports Phys Ther. 2012;42(6):502–10.
8. Lewek M, Rudolph K, Axe M, Snyder-Mackler L. The effect of insufficient quadriceps strength on gait after anterior cruciate ligament reconstruction. Clin Biomech. 2002;17(1):56–63.
9. Snyder-Mackler L, De Luca PF, Williams PR, Eastlack ME, Bartolozzi AR, 3rd. Reflex inhibition of the quadriceps femoris muscle after injury or reconstruction of the anterior cruciate ligament. J Bone Joint Surg Am. 1994;76(4):555–60.
10. Hiemstra LA, Webber S, MacDonald PB, Kriellaars DJ. Knee strength deficits after hamstring tendon and patellar tendon anterior cruciate ligament reconstruction. Med Sci Sports Exerc. 2000;32(8):1472–9.
11. Thomas AC, Villwock M, Wojtys EM, Palmieri-Smith RM. Lower extremity muscle strength after anterior cruciate ligament injury and reconstruction. J Athl Train. 2013;48(5):610–20.
12. Chmielewski TL, Stackhouse S, Axe MJ, Snyder-Mackler L. A prospective analysis of incidence and severity of quadriceps inhibition in a consecutive sample of 100 patients with complete acute anterior cruciate ligament rupture. J Orthop Res. 2004;22(5):925–30.
13. Ward SH, Pearce A, Bennell KL, Peitrosimone B, Bryant AL. Quadriceps cortical adaptations in individuals with an anterior cruciate ligament injury. Knee. 2016;23(4):582–7.
14. Kuenze C, Hertel J, Hart JM. Effects of exercise on lower extremity muscle function after anterior cruciate ligament reconstruction. J Sport Rehabil. 2013;22(1):33–40.
15. de Jong SN, van Caspel DR, van Haeff MJ, Saris DB. Functional assessment and muscle strength before and after reconstruction of chronic anterior cruciate ligament lesions. Arthroscopy. 2007;23(1):21–8 28 e21–23.
16. Eitzen I, Holm I, Risberg MA. Preoperative quadriceps strength is a significant predictor of knee function two years after anterior cruciate ligament reconstruction. Br J Sports Med. 2009;43(5):371–6.
17. Zwolski C, Schmitt LC, Quatman-Yates C, Thomas S, Hewett TE, Paterno MV. The influence of quadriceps strength asymmetry on patient-reported function at time of return to sport after anterior cruciate ligament reconstruction. Am J Sports Med. 2015;43(9):2242–9.
18. Logerstedt D, Lynch A, Axe MJ, Snyder-Mackler L. Pre-operative quadriceps strength predicts IKDC2000 scores 6 months after anterior cruciate ligament reconstruction. Knee. 2013;20(3):208–12.
19. Palmieri-Smith RM, Lepley LK. Quadriceps strength asymmetry after anterior cruciate ligament reconstruction alters knee joint biomechanics and functional performance at time of return to activity. Am J Sports Med. 2015;43(7):1662-69.
20. Pua YH, Seah FJ, Seet FJ, Tan JW, Liaw JS, Chong HC. Sex differences and impact of body mass index on the time course of knee range of motion, knee strength, and gait speed after Total knee arthroplasty. Arthritis Care Res (Hoboken). 2015;67(10):1397–405.
21. Di Stasi SL, Logerstedt D, Gardinier ES, Snyder-Mackler L. Gait patterns differ between ACL-reconstructed athletes who pass return-to-sport criteria and those who fail. Am J Sports Med. 2013;41(6):1310–8.
22. Laboute E, Savalli L, Puig P, Trouve P, Sabot G, Monnier G, Dubroca B. Analysis of return to competition and repeat rupture for 298 anterior cruciate ligament reconstructions with patellar or hamstring tendon autograft in sportspeople. Ann Phys Rehabil Med. 2010;53(10):598–614.
23. Konishi Y, Fukubayashi T. Relationship between muscle volume and muscle torque of the hamstrings after anterior cruciate ligament reconstruction. J Sci Med Sport. 2010;13(1):101–5.
24. Lepley LK, Wojtys EM, Palmieri-Smith RM. Combination of eccentric exercise and neuromuscular electrical stimulation to improve biomechanical limb symmetry after anterior cruciate ligament reconstruction. Clin Biomech (Bristol, Avon). 2015;30(7):738-47.
25. Hsu WH, Hsu RW, Lin ZR, Fan CH. Effects of circuit exercise and tai chi on body composition in middle-aged and older women. Geriatr Gerontol Int. 2015;15(3):282–8.
26. World HO. Obesity: preventing and managing the global epidemic. Report of a WHO consultation. In: WHO technical report series 894. Geneva: WHO; 2000.
27. Roos EM, Roos HP, Lohmander LS, Ekdahl C, Beynnon BD. Knee injury and osteoarthritis outcome score (KOOS)--development of a self-administered outcome measure. J Orthop Sports Phys Ther. 1998;28(2):88–96.
28. Marx RG, Stump TJ, Jones EC, Wickiewicz TL, Warren RF. Development and evaluation of an activity rating scale for disorders of the knee. Am J Sports Med. 2001;29(2):213–8.
29. Sekir U, Gur H, Akova B. Early versus late start of isokinetic hamstring-strengthening exercise after anterior cruciate ligament reconstruction with patellar tendon graft. Am J Sports Med. 2010;38(3):492–500.
30. Shaw T, Williams MT, Chipchase LS. Do early quadriceps exercises affect the outcome of ACL reconstruction? A randomised controlled trial. Aust J Physiother. 2005;51(1):9–17.
31. Hooper DM, Morrissey MC, Drechsler W, Morrissey D, King J. Open and closed kinetic chain exercises in the early period after anterior cruciate ligament reconstruction. Improvements in level walking, stair ascent, and stair descent. Am J Sports Med. 2001;29(2):167–74.
32. Lee DH, Lee JH, Jeong HJ, Lee SJ. Serial changes in knee muscle strength after anterior cruciate ligament reconstruction using hamstring tendon autografts. Arthroscopy. 2015;31(5):890–5.
33. Lepley LK. Deficits in quadriceps strength and patient-oriented outcomes at return to activity after ACL reconstruction: a review of the current literature. Sports Health. 2015;7(3):231–8.
34. Eriksson K, Hamberg P, Jansson E, Larsson H, Shalabi A, Wredmark T. Semitendinosus muscle in anterior cruciate ligament surgery: morphology and function. Arthroscopy. 2001;17(8):808–17.
35. Kim HJ, Lee JH, Ahn SE, Park MJ, Lee DH. Influence of anterior cruciate ligament tear on thigh muscle strength and hamstring-to-quadriceps ratio: a meta-analysis. PLoS One. 2016;11(1):e0146234.
36. Blanpied P, Carroll R, Douglas T, Lyons M, Macalisang R, Pires L. Effectiveness of lateral slide exercise in an anterior cruciate ligament reconstruction

rehabilitation home exercise program. J Orthop Sports Phys Ther. 2000; 30(10):602–8 discussion 609-611.
37. Sasaki S, Tsuda E, Hiraga Y, Yamamoto Y, Maeda S, Sasaki E, Ishibashi Y. Prospective randomized study of objective and subjective clinical results between double-bundle and single-bundle anterior cruciate ligament reconstruction. Am J Sports Med. 2016;44(4):855–64.
38. Amiri P, Hubley-Kozey CL, Landry SC, Stanish WD, Astephen Wilson JL. Obesity is associated with prolonged activity of the quadriceps and gastrocnemii during gait. J Electromyogr Kinesiol. 2015;25(6):951–8.
39. Gokeler A, Bisschop M, Benjaminse A, Myer GD, Eppinga P, Otten E. Quadriceps function following ACL reconstruction and rehabilitation: implications for optimisation of current practices. Knee Surg Sports Traumatol Arthrosc. 2014;22(5):1163–74.
40. Derraik JG, de Bock M, Hofman PL, Cutfield WS. Increasing BMI is associated with a progressive reduction in physical quality of life among overweight middle-aged men. Sci Rep. 2014;4:3677.
41. Giuli C, Papa R, Bevilacqua R, Felici E, Gagliardi C, Marcellini F, Boscaro M, De Robertis M, Mocchegiani E, Faloia E, et al. Correlates of perceived health related quality of life in obese, overweight and normal weight older adults: an observational study. BMC Public Health. 2014;14:35.
42. Stevens-Lapsley JE, Petterson SC, Mizner RL, Snyder-Mackler L. Impact of body mass index on functional performance after total knee arthroplasty. J Arthroplast. 2010;25(7):1104–9.
43. Singh JA, Gabriel SE, Lewallen DG. Higher body mass index is not associated with worse pain outcomes after primary or revision total knee arthroplasty. J Arthroplast. 2011;26(3):366–74 e361.
44. Jarvenpaa J, Kettunen J, Soininvaara T, Miettinen H, Kroger H. Obesity has a negative impact on clinical outcome after total knee arthroplasty. Scand J Surg. 2012;101(3):198–203.
45. Gillespie GN, Porteous AJ. Obesity and knee arthroplasty. Knee. 2007;14(2): 81–6.
46. Sanchez-Ramirez DC, van der Leeden M, van der Esch M, Roorda LD, Verschueren S, van Dieen J, Lems WF, Dekker J. Increased knee muscle strength is associated with decreased activity limitations in established knee osteoarthritis: two-year follow-up study in the Amsterdam osteoarthritis cohort. J Rehabil Med. 2015;47(7):647–54.

22

Arthroscopic debridement of anterior ankle impingement in patients with chronic lateral ankle instability

Qining Yang[1,2], Yongwei Zhou[2] and Youjia Xu[1,3*]

Abstract

Background: The aim of this study was to determine the functional and radiological outcomes of arthroscopic treatment of anterior ankle impingement (AAI) in patients with chronic lateral ankle instability (CAI).

Methods: All patients with CAI between June 2012 and May 2015 were invited to participate in this investigation. All of them accepted open modified Broström repair of lateral ankle ligaments and were divided into two groups: AAI group (with anterior ankle impingement) and pure CAI group (without anterior ankle impingement). All of them were followed up using American Orthopaedic Foot and Ankle Society Score (AOFAS), Karlsson Ankle Functional Score and Tegner activity score. Ankle dorsiflexion was also examined. X-ray examination was applied to investigate anterior tibiotalar osteophytes.

Results: Finally, a total of 60 patients were followed up at a mean of 37 ± 10 months, including 22 patients in the AAI group and 38 patients in the pure CAI group. Preoperatively, the AAI group had significant lower AOFAS score (62.9 ± 11.7 vs 72.9 ± 11.1; $p = 0.002$) and Tegner activity score (1.5 ± 0.8 vs 2.1 ± 1.0; $p = 0.04$) respectively when compared with the pure CAI group. The ankle dorsiflexion of the AAI group (13 ± 2.1) was also significantly lower than that of the pure CAI group (26.2 ± 2.1) ($p = 0.001$). However, there was no significant difference in the AOFAS score or the Karlsson score or the Tegner score or the Ankle dorsiflexion between the two groups postoperatively. The postoperative X-ray images demonstrated complete osteophyte resection in all patients, and no recurrence of osteophyte.

Conclusion: The functional outcome scores and dorsiflexion had significantly improved postoperatively. Combined treatment of chronic ankle instability and anterior ankle impingement produced satisfactory surgical outcomes in patients with CAI accompanied by anterior ankle impingement symptom.

Keywords: Ankle instability, Anterior ankle impingement, Osteophyte, Repair, Functional outcomes, ROM

Background

Lateral ankle sprains occur most commonly in both sports and daily activities, and usually result in the ruptures of anterior talofibular ligament (ATFL) and calcaneofibular ligament (CFL) [1]. Although with some conservative treatment, a few injured ankles will still be unstable and have repeated sprains [2]. In ankles with chronic ankle instability (CAI), it is common to observe ankle impingement with soft tissue or osteophyte [3–6]. Previously, Odak et al. [4] reported that 63% patients had soft tissue impingement and 12% patients had anterior bony (osteophyte) impingement in a cohort of 100 CAI patients. Similarly, Hua et al. [5] reported an incidence of 86% CAI patients with soft tissue impingement and 26% CAI patients with bony impingement. Thus, it can be seen that anterior ankle impingement (AAI) had a high correlation with CAI.

According to a previous report [7], ankle impingement in anterior tibiotalar joint is caused by either mechanical macrotrauma or recurrent microtrauma associated with CAI. In particular, CAI is associated with the formation

* Correspondence: youjiaxu12@sina.com
[1]Department of Orthopaedics, The Second Affiliated Hospital of Soochow University, Sanxiang Road No.1055, Suzhou 215004, Jiangsu, China
[3]Department of Orthopedics, 2nd Affiliated Hospital of Soochow University, Sanxiang Road No.1055, Suzhou, Jiangsu 215000, People's Republic of China
Full list of author information is available at the end of the article

in medial ankle osteophyte, which originates from distal tibia protruding to joint line [8, 9]. Anterior ankle joint capsule is just located at proximal end of the anterior talotibial osteophyte originate [10]. In the medial part of anterior talus, osteophyte development occurs in an intraarticular location [11].

In particular, anterior tibiotalar osteophyte is a headache problem that causes severe AAI syndrome, leading to anterior ankle pain or reduction of dorsiflexion [6, 7]. Pure conservative treatment cannot easily treat the persisting bony impingement syndrome [12]. However, anterior soft tissue and bony impingement can be effectively treated arthroscopically [7, 13, 14]. After surgical debridement, the ankle function can be improved thus to allow an early return to sports activity [15]. Previously, Walsh et al. [16] evaluated functional and radiological outcomes after arthroscopic treatment of anterior ankle impingement, and demonstrated a significant improvement in the functional outcome scores (Foot Functional Index) postoperatively despite a recurrence of radiographic osteophyte. To date, there has been a lack of clinical research investigating the clinical effect of AAI debridement in CAI patients.

Therefore, the aim of this study was to investigate the functional and radiological outcomes after arthroscopic treatment of anterior ankle impingement (AAI) in patients with mechanical chronic lateral ankle instability.

Methods

This retrospective study was approved by the Health Sciences Institutional Review Committee of Jinhua Hospital of Zhejiang University, and all participants signed a written consent form. All patients who underwent modified Broström-Gould to repair the lateral ankle ligament from June 2012 to May 2015 were required to participate in the study. Clinical diagnosis of CAI is according to a clinical history (pain or concession, repetitive varus sprain for more than 3 months), physical examination (anterior drawer test (ADT)) and MRI. Inclusion criteria were: (1) modified Broström-Gould to repair the lateral ankle ligament, and (2) follow-up for at least 2 years. Patients should be excluded if they had (1) significant cartilage lesions undergoing microfracture or autologous osteochondral transplantation, (2) prior surgery, (3) neuromuscular disease, and (4) lateral ligament reconstruction.

All patients underwent direct ATFL/CFL repair and debridement of bone and soft tissue under arthroscopy in the event of a anterior impingement. Patients underwent standard arthroscopy to evaluate the ankle joint before lateral ligament repair. Assessment and treatment of intra-articular lesions, debridement or microfracture of cartilage damage, removal of impacted soft tissue or synovial membrane, and removal of loose body. For anterior tibial impingement, the anterior lateral and anterior medial arthroscopy portals were used to remove the anterior osteophytes on the distal tibia and anterior lip of the talus. The ablation is completed until the ankle joint dorsiflexion recovered.

Then, the ATFL / CFL is repaired using the open modified Broström program according to the previous method [5]. After making a curved incision on the lateral side, the ATFL residue was identified and exposed. One or two suture anchors were inserted into the fibular (2.9-mm Loopine [DePuy Mitek, Raynham, MA]). The ankle was slightly everted. The ATFL is sutured, tensioned, and fixed onto the fibular. The proximal extensor support band is also used to strengthen the repair of the lateral ligament. All patients followed the same postoperative rehabilitation protocol. After the operation, the ankle was fixed in a slightly eversion position by using a casting. Rehabilitation training was started from the second day after surgery, including isometric contraction of muscle groups around the ankle joint, and weight bearing was allowed after 4 weeks. The casting was removed 4 weeks after the operation and changed to a sacral stent, and the range of passive motion was started.

At least 24 months after surgery, all patients were invited to this follow-up during outpatient service. Functional scores were assessed preoperatively and postoperatively, including American Orthopaedic Foot and Ankle Society (AOFAS), Karlsson Ankle Functional Score and Tegner activity score. Physical examinations, including ankle dorsiflexion and anterior drawer test (ADT), were also performed by an experienced orthopedic surgeon. The X-ray examination (lateral view) was performed to investigate the anterior tibiotalar osteophyte. Scranton and McDermott classification (SMC) grade was used to assess the osteophytes: Grade 1, tibial spur less than 3 mm; Grade 2, tibial spur more than 3 mm; Grade 3, significant tibial exostosis with secondaryspur on the neck of the talus, with eventual fragmentation of the osteophytes; Grade 4, osteophytes associated with arthritic joint destruction [16].

Statistical analysis was performed using Stata 10.0 software (Stata Corp, USA), and the data are reported as means and standard deviations. The categorical variables were compared using a χ^2 test, and the continuous variables were compared using a two-sample t test or two-sample Wilcoxon rank-sum test. A paired students t-test was performed to compare the results between pre-op and post-op within each group. The correlation between the functional scores and various factors (gender, age, BMI, injury time, follow-up time) was analyzed using Spearman's correlation coefficient. The significance level was set at 0.05.

Results

A total of 60 Broström-Gould repair patients participated in this study. Among them, 22 patients had anterior ankle impingement (AAI group) and the other 38 patients had no impingement (pure CAI group). In the AAI group, all the patients had synovitis and 18 patients had osteophytes in the anterior ankle compartment. Preoperative ankle X-ray images revealed a mean SMC grade of 2 (range 1–3). Actually, most patients had only ATFL tear. Three patients (14%) in the AAI group and 5 patients (13%) in the pure CAI group had both ATFL and CFL tears. Moreover, five patients in the AAI group and 8 patients in the pure CAI group had the associated cartilage lesions. These cartilage lesions were only with a rough surface or fibrillation (Grade I), and only debridement was performed. The Patients' demographic data was shown in Table 1. The average follow-up time was 37 months for both of the groups.

At final follow-up, no patient complained ankle instability, and ADT of all the ankles revealed negative. All these patients return to previous activity. After surgery, both groups had an increase of the functional scores. Preoperatively, the AAI group had a significant lower AOFAS score (62.9 ± 11.7 vs 72.9 ± 11.1; $p = 0.002$) and Tegner activity score (1.5 ± 0.8 vs 2.1 ± 1.0; $p = 0.04$) respectively when compared with the pure CAI group. The ankle dorsiflexion of the AAI group (13 ± 2.1°) was also significantly lower than that of the pure CAI group (26.2 ± 2.1°) ($p = 0.001$). After surgery, each functional score (AOFAS, Karlsson, Tegner activity) significantly increased ($p < 0.05$). The ankle dorsiflexion of the AAI group significantly increased from 13 ± 2.1° preoperatively to 25.9 ± 2.4° postoperatively ($p < 0.001$). There was no significant change of ankle dorsiflexion in the pure CAI group after surgery. At the final follow-up, there was no significant difference in postoperative AOFAS or Karlsson score or Tegner score or Ankle dorsiflexion between the two groups (Table 2). The postoperative X-ray images showed complete removal of the osteophytes in all patients (Fig. 1). No recurrence of osteophytes was found. There was also no statistically significant association between functional scores

Table 1 Participant demographic data between the anterior ankle impingement (AAI) group and pure CAI group

	AAI group ($n = 22$)	pure CAI group ($n = 38$)
Age, mean SD, y	31.2 ± 8.8	27.6 ± 8.5 n.s.
Body mass index (kg/m^2)	24.5 ± 3.0	23.2 ± 2.4 n.s.
Gender, n	Males, $n = 16$	Males, $n = 31$
	Females, $n = 6$	Females, $n = 7$
Side, n	Left, $n = 12$	Left, $n = 15$
	Right, $n = 10$	Right, $n = 23$
Injury time, months	37 ± 42	26 ± 36 n.s.
Follow-up time, months	37 ± 10 (24 ~ 56)	37 ± 10 (24 ~ 53) n.s.

AAI anterior ankle impingement. n.s. indicated there was no significant difference between groups

Table 2 Functional scores and Ankle dorsiflexion between the anterior ankle impingement (AAI) group and the pure CAI group pre-operatively and post-operatively

Variable		AAI group ($n = 22$)	pure CAI group ($n = 38$)	*P* value
AOFAS score	Pre-op	62.9 ± 11.7	72.9 ± 11.1	0.002
	Post-op	93.4 ± 7.4	92.3 ± 9.4	n.s.
Karlsson Score	Pre-op	57.3 ± 12.4	63.1 ± 16.5	n.s.
	Post-op	90.0 ± 9.1	89.6 ± 12.5	n.s.
Tegner score	Pre-op	1.5 ± 0.8	2.1 ± 1.0	0.04
	Post-op	4.4 ± 1.3	5.2 ± 1.8	n.s.
Ankle dorsiflexion (°)	Pre-op	13 ± 2.1	26.2 ± 2.1	< 0.001
	Post-op	25.9 ± 2.4	26 ± 2.1	n.s.

AAI anterior ankle impingement, *AOFAS* American Orthopaedic Foot and Ankle Society; *Pre-op* pre-operatively, *Post-op* post-operatively "*p* value" indicated the comparison between the AAI group and the pure CAI group

(AOFAS, Karlsson score, or Tegner score) and gender, age, BMI, injury time, and follow-up time ($p > 0.05$).

Regarding the complications, one patient in the AAI group and two patients in the pure CAI group presented numbness. They recovered within one year after surgery. At two weeks after surgery, superficial wound infection was observed in 1 patients in the AAI group and 2 patients in the pure CAI group. With anti-infective treatment, these three cases recovered at one months after surgery.

Discussion

In this study, it was found that the AAI group had a comparable results with the pure CAI group at a mean follow-up of three years. Furthermore, the postoperative X-ray images demonstrated complete osteophyte removal in all patients, and no recurrence of osteophyte was observed.

Combined lateral ligament repair and anterior ankle impingement treatment are safe and allow most patients to resume exercise [17]. Murawski et al. [18] investigated 41 patients who underwent arthroscopic treatment of AAI, and found that 38 patients (93%) were satisfied with the resection procedure. The AOFAS score increased from 62.83 points preoperatively to 91.17 points postoperatively. In the present study, most patients had osteophytes in anterior ankle compartment. It is indicated that the osteophytes were the main cause of decreased dorsiflexion. After surgical removal of the impinged osteophytes and soft tissue, patients obtained an increase of functional scores.

In the present study, the ankle dorsiflexion of the AAI group significantly increased from 13 ± 2.1° preoperatively to 25.9 ± 2.4° postoperatively. Previously, Cannon and Hackney [19] investigated 13 CAI patients with AAI and found that mean improvement of dorsiflexion was 12.4°. Previously, Ahn et al. [20] investigated 20 CAI

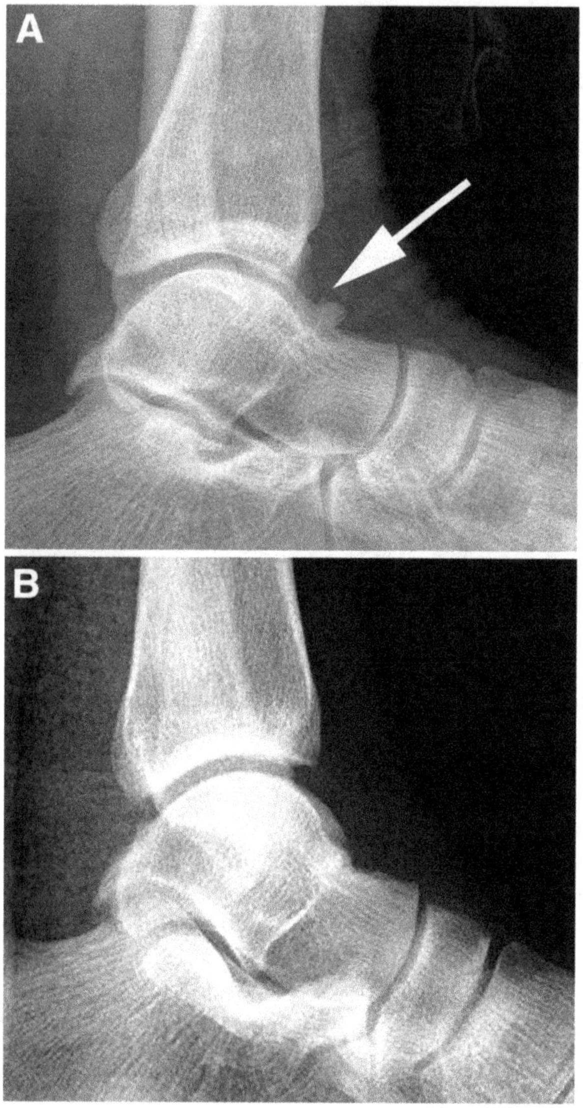

Fig. 1 X-ray images of an ankle with bony anterior ankle impingement preoperatively (**a**) and postoperatively (**b**). White arrow indicates osteophytes

patients with AAI, and the mean dorsiflexion improvement was 7.9 degrees in the impingement group at a mean follow-up of 1.4 years. In the present study, the mean improvement of dorsiflexion was almost 12 degrees. It was presumed that different dorsiflexion improvement might be due to different severity of osteophytes.

In this study, all the patients in the AAI group underwent open modified Broström procedure to repair ATFL and CFL. At the final follow-up, the ankle stability of all the patients recovered. It is well known that removal of the anterior osteophytes may reduce tibial coverage of talus [21]. The patient developed an impingement again after debridement alone if without ankle instability. Therefore, it is very important to ensure that the ankle joint is stable to avoid micro-trauma of the tibialtalar joint. ATFL and CFL repair using suture anchors is an effective method for the treatment of CAI [22]. In addition, it has recently been reported that arthroscopic repair of the lateral ankle ligament may produce similar beneficial results compared with open ankle repair [23]. Arthroscopic ATFL repair as a minimally invasive technique may provide more favorable results.

Previously, Walsh et al. [16] assessed functional and radiological outcomes after arthroscopic treatment of AAI, and reported a recurrence of radiological osteophyte in 84% of patients. In the present study with a mean follow-up of 3 years, no recurrence of osteophyte was found and the postoperative X-ray images showed complete osteophyte resection in all patients. The difference might be due to all the patients had ankle stability after repair surgery in the present study, while the patients only accepted debridement of ankle impingement in that study by Walsh et al. [16].

There are three limitations that need to be addressed. The first limitation is the small sample size of the AAI group and the pure CAI group. Other studies with larger sample sizes may be needed to determine differences in clinical outcomes between groups. The study documented short-term results and more research was needed to determine long-term outcomes for this patient population. In addition, there was a lack of comparison in the AAI group without surgery or placebo.

Conclusions

Functional outcome scores and dorsiflexion were significantly improved after 3 years of ligament repair and impingement treatment. Comprehensive treatment of CAI and AAI produces satisfactory clinical results in patients with CAI associated with anterior impingement symptoms.

Level of evidence

level III. Cohort study.

Abbreviations

AAI: Anterior ankle instability; ADT: Anterior drawer test; AOFAS: American Orthopaedic Foot and Ankle Society; ATFL: Anterior talofibular ligament; CAI: Chronic ankle instability; CFL: Calcaneofibular ligament

Authors' contributions

QY and YZ performed the follow-up experiments. YX gave the experiment guidance during this study and revised this paper critically for important intellectual content. QY analyzed and interpreted the data and was a major contributor in writing the manuscript. All authors read and approved the final manuscript.

Consent for publication
not applicable.

Competing interests
The authors declare that they have no competing interests.

Author details
[1]Department of Orthopaedics, The Second Affiliated Hospital of Soochow University, Sanxiang Road No.1055, Suzhou 215004, Jiangsu, China. [2]Department of joint orthopaedic surgery, Jinhua hospital of Zhejiang University (Jinhua municipal central hospital), Jinhua, Zhejiang 321000, People's Republic of China. [3]Department of Orthopedics, 2nd Affiliated Hospital of Soochow University, Sanxiang Road No.1055, Suzhou, Jiangsu 215000, People's Republic of China.

References
1. Ferran NA, Oliva F, Maffulli N. Ankle instability. Sports Med Arthrosc. 2009; 17(2):139–45.
2. Takao M, Miyamoto W, Matsui K, Sasahara J, Matsushita T. Functional treatment after surgical repair for acute lateral ligament disruption of the ankle in athletes. Am J Sports Med. 2012;40(2):447–51.
3. Cha SD, Kim HS, Chung ST, Yoo JH, Park JH, Kim JH, Hyung JW. Intra-articular lesions in chronic lateral ankle instability: comparison of arthroscopy with magnetic resonance imaging findings. Clin Orthop Surg. 2012;4(4):293–9.
4. Odak S, Ahluwalia R, Shivarathre DG, Mahmood A, Blucher N, Hennessy M, Platt S. Arthroscopic evaluation of impingement and osteochondral lesions in chronic lateral ankle instability. Foot & ankle international. 2015;36:1045–9.
5. Hua Y, Chen S, Li Y, Chen J, Li H. Combination of modified Brostrom procedure with ankle arthroscopy for chronic ankle instability accompanied by intra-articular symptoms. Arthroscopy. 2010;26:524–8.
6. Lavery KP, McHale KJ, Rossy WH, Theodore G. Ankle impingement. J Orthop Surg Res. 2016;11:97.
7. Baums MH, Kahl E, Schultz W, Klinger HM. Clinical outcome of the arthroscopic management of sports-related "anterior ankle pain": a prospective study. Knee Surg Sports Traumatol Arthrosc. 2006;14:482–6.
8. Ross KA, Murawski CD, Smyth NA, Zwiers R, Wiegerinck JI, van Bergen CJ, Dijk CN, Kennedy JG. Current concepts review: arthroscopic treatment of anterior ankle impingement. Foot Ankle Surg. 2017;23:1–8.
9. Tol JL, Slim E, van Soest AJ, van Dijk CN. The relationship of the kicking action in soccer and anterior ankle impingement syndrome. A biomechanical analysis Am J Sports Med. 2002;30:45–50.
10. Tol JL, van Dijk CN. Etiology of the anterior ankle impingement syndrome: a descriptive anatomical study. Foot Ankle Int. 2004;25:382–6.
11. Hayeri MR, Trudell DJ, Resnick D. Anterior ankle impingement and talar bony outgrowths: osteophyte or enthesophyte? Paleopathologic and cadaveric study with imagingcorrelation. AJR Am J Roentgenol. 2009;193: W334–8.
12. Arnold H. Posttraumatic impingement syndrome of the ankle--indication and results of arthroscopic therapy. Foot Ankle Surg. 2011;17:85–8.
13. Miyamoto W, Takao M, Matsui K, Matsushita T. Simultaneous ankle arthroscopy and hindfoot endoscopy for combined anterior and posterior ankle impingement syndrome in professional athletes. J Orthop Sci. 2015;20:642–8.
14. van Dijk CN, Tol JL, Verheyen CC. A prospective study of prognostic factors concerning the outcome of arthroscopic surgery for anterior ankle impingement. Am J Sports Med. 1997;25:737–45.
15. Edmonds EW, Chambers R, Kaufman E, Chambers HG. Anterolateral ankle impingement in adolescents: outcomes of nonoperative and operative treatment. J Pediatr Orthop. 2010;30:186–91.
16. Walsh SJ, Twaddle BC, Rosenfeldt MP, Boyle MJ. Arthroscopic treatment of anterior ankle impingement: a prospective study of 46 patients with 5-year follow-up. Am J Sports Med. 2014;42:2722–6.
17. Maffulli N, Del Buono A, Maffulli GD, Oliva F, Testa V, Capasso G, Denaro V. Isolated anterior talofibular ligament Broström repair for chronic lateral ankle instability: 9-year follow-up. Am J Sports Med. 2013;41:858–64.
18. Murawski CD, Kennedy JG. Anteromedial impingement in the ankle joint: outcomes following arthroscopy. Am J Sports Med. 2010;38:2017–24.
19. Cannon LB, Hackney RG. Anterior tibiotalar impingement associated with chronic ankle instability. J Foot Ankle Surg. 2000;39:383–6.
20. Ahn JY, Choi HJ, Lee WC. Talofibular bony impingement in the ankle. Foot & ankle international. 2015;36:1150–5.
21. Frigg A, Frigg R, Hintermann B, Barg A, Valderrabano V. The biomechanical influence of tibio-talar containment on stability of the ankle joint. Knee Surg Sports Traumatol Arthrosc. 2007;15:1355–62.
22. Petrera M, Dwyer T, Theodoropoulos JS, Ogilvie-Harris DJ. Short- to medium-term outcomes after a modified Brostrom repair for lateral ankle instability with immediate postoperative Weightbearing. Am J Sports Med. 2014;42: 1542–8.
23. Li H, Hua Y, Li H, Ma K, Li S, Chen S. Activity level and function 2 years after anterior Talofibular ligament repair: a comparison between arthroscopic repair and open repair procedures. Am J Sports Med. 2017;45:2044–51.

Pilot randomized controlled trials in the orthopaedic surgery literature

Bijal Desai[1], Veeral Desai[1], Shivani Shah[2], Archita Srinath[3], Amr Saleh[1], Nicole Simunovic[4,5*], Andrew Duong[5], Sheila Sprague[4,5] and Mohit Bhandari[4,5]

Abstract

Background: The primary objective of this systematic review is to examine the characteristics of pilot randomized controlled trials (RCTs) in the orthopaedic surgery literature, including the proportion framed as feasibility trials and those that lead to definitive RCTs. This review aim to answer the question of whether pilot RCTs lead to definitive RCTs, whilst investigating the quality, feasibility and overall publication trends of orthopaedic pilot trials.

Methods: Pilot RCTs in the orthopaedic literature were identified from three electronic databases (EMBASE, MEDLINE, and Pubmed) searched from database inception to January 2018. Search criteria included the evaluation of at least one orthopaedic surgical intervention, research on humans, and publication in English. Two reviewers independently screened the pool of pilot trials, and conducted a search for corresponding definitive trials. Screened pilot RCTs were assessed for feasibility outcomes related to efficiency, cost, and/or timeliness of a large-scale clinical trial involving a surgical intervention. The quality of the pilot and definitive trials were assessed using the Checklist to Evaluate a Report of a Non-Pharmacological Trial (CLEAR NPT).

Results: The initial search for pilot RCTs yielded 3857 titles, of which 49 articles were relevant for this review. 73.5% (36/49) of the orthopaedic pilot RCTs were framed as feasibility trials. Of these, 5 corresponding definitive trials (10.2%) were found, of which four were published and one ongoing. Based on author responses, the lack of a definitive RCT following the pilot trial was attributed to a lack of funding, inadequacies in recruitment, and belief that the pilot RCT sufficiently answered the research question.

Conclusions: Based on this systematic review, most pilot RCTs were characterized as feasibility trials. However, the majority of published pilot RCTs did not lead to definitive trials. This discrepancy was mainly attributed to poor feasibility (e.g. poor recruitment) and lack of funding for an orthopaedic surgical definitive trial. In recent years this discrepancy may be due to researchers saving on time and cost by rolling their pilot patients into the definitive RCT rather than publish a separate pilot trial.

Keywords: Orthopaedic, Surgery, RCT, Feasibility, Pilot study, Definitive trial

* Correspondence: simunon@mcmaster.ca
[4]Department of Health Research Methods, Evidence, and Impact (HEI), Division of Orthopaedic Surgery, McMaster University, Hamilton, ON, Canada
[5]Department of Surgery, Division of Orthopaedic Surgery, McMaster University, Hamilton, ON, Canada
Full list of author information is available at the end of the article

Background

Definitive randomized controlled trials (RCTs) exist to demonstrate unmistakable evidence of a certain inventions benefit on a patient [1]. Although they are very impactful for clinical practice are typically expensive and time-consuming [2]. Given the resources and time, investigators often conduct pilot trials designed with an aim to demonstrate the feasibility of the larger-scale definitive trial [3]. Pilot trials can identify possible challenges, predict costs, and fine-tune study design. In addition, by demonstrating feasibility, a successful pilot trial can be used to leverage momentum and definitive trial funding [2].

Effective pilot trials have a well-defined set of objectives to assess feasibility.[3] Feasibility is assessed in terms of whether the intervention of interest, trial design, and protocol can be successfully implemented and completed by the researchers [3]. Feasibility can be determined at the program level, study level, and site or investigator level. Program level feasibilities include determining the prevalence of particular diseases in a particular region and include clinical and epidemiological trials [4]. Study level feasibilities are centered on assessing whether a specific clinical trial can be conducted in a country or region [3]. Site or investigator level feasibility trials focus on identifying challenges and probable solutions with respect to the investigator and clinical aspects of the trial (drug dosages, actual study population, recruitment and follow-up, usage of assessment tools, etc.) [4].

Despite the benefits of pilot trials, previous literature has demonstrated that they do not always lead to a definitive trial. In 2004, Lancaster et al reviewed four general medicine journals and three specialist journals and identified 90 pilot studies published from 2000 to 2001; of which 45 reported the intention to carry out further work [1]. However, in 2010, Arain et al. found that only eight out of the 45 were followed by a larger, definitive study [5]. The impact of pilot data and subsequent research remains to be evaluated in the orthopaedic surgical literature.

This systematic review assessed the quality of pilot RCTs and frequency of ensuing definitive RCTs in the orthopaedic surgical literature. The primary objectives of this review were to: 1) assess feasibility outcomes across pilot trials in the orthopaedic surgery literature; 2) identify the proportion of pilot trials that lead to and how they inform definitive RCTs, and 3) evaluate the quality and frequency of pilot trials over time.

Methods

Identification of RCTs

EMBASE, MEDLINE and Pubmed were searched for relevant articles published from database inception until January 25, 2018 (Additional file 1). All search results were imported into the Mendeley Reference Manager software (Elsevier Publishing, 2013) to remove all duplicate trials.

Once the final pool of included pilot RCTs was determined, an additional search was conducted in the same electronic databases in an attempt to find corresponding definitive trials. If a literature search of titles was unsuccessful, other trials conducted by at least one of the authors after the pilot were considered. The secondary search was conducted using key terms used in the pilot RCT. Additionally, clinicaltrials.gov, an online database of ongoing clinical trials, was reviewed to determine if the previously identified pilot RCTs had a definitive trial in progress. Finally, if no definitive trial was found using these methods, the pilot RCT authors were contacted by email and asked whether a definitive trials was ongoing, published, or submitted for publication.

Eligibility criteria

Trails had to be defined explicitly and reported as pilot trials within the paper itself to be included in this review. Trials reported as pilot RCTs were deemed eligible for this review if they: 1) included an orthopaedic surgical intervention, 2) included a drug that was used intra-operatively at the site of surgery/fracture, or 3) evaluated the difference between two surgical interventions or surgical vs. non-surgical orthopaedic interventions. Only clinical trials in humans published in English were included. RCTs were excluded if they were: 1) non-pilot RCT designs (including small trials not reported as pilot trials) 2) trial interventions were exclusively non-surgical including physiotherapy, exercise regimens, post-operative rehabilitation, anesthesia, post-operative pain management interventions, or 3) trial interventions were surgical procedures not related to orthopaedics (e.g. oral, urology, and ocular surgeries), and 4) drugs and supplements administered orally (intravenously administered during surgery were included).

Screening

Articles were independently screened in duplicate at the title, abstract, and full-text stage by decisions were independently recorded in a spreadsheet (Microsoft Excel, 2015). In order to ensure comprehensive screening, an article was progressed to the next screening stage if at least one reviewer had noted that the article should be included, and illustrated as a flow diagram and checklist in Fig. 1 below. All disagreements were resolved by consensus during the full-text screening phase in consultation with a third senior reviewer (AD).

Data abstraction

Pilot and definitive trial data, such as the country, number of patients in the RCT, orthopaedic condition being treated, orthopaedic intervention(s), controls, primary and secondary outcomes, percentage of patients that were lost to follow-up, follow-up schedule, and feasibility objectives were abstracted. In addition, for the definitive trials, any

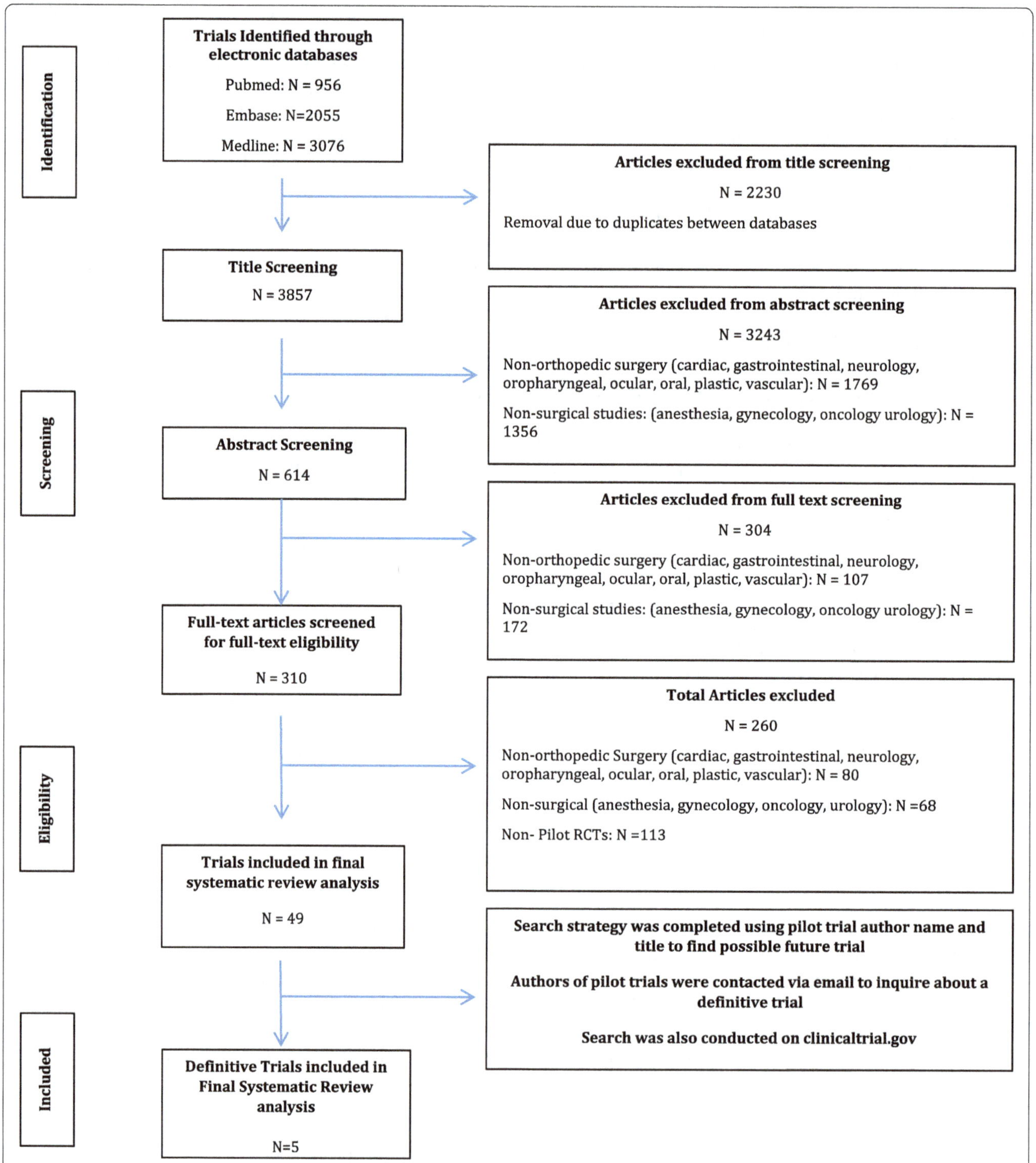

Fig. 1 Flow diagram of the search and screening strategies to define the final pool of trails

changes in interventions, controls, primary and secondary outcomes, or patient sample from the pilot trial were noted. For definitive RCTs, the time elapsed between the date of publication of the pilot and definitive trial and whether or not the sample size was calculated based on event rates from the pilot trial were determined.

Assessment of feasibility

Feasibility trials were defined as trials with a primary purpose of piloting the protocol to inform a definitive trial. In order to distinguish between pilot trials created solely for investigating the efficacy of interventions compared to feasibility trials, specific reference to feasibility objectives were evaluated. Feasibility objectives include determining the preliminary efficacy of a surgical intervention as well as the safety of the intervention, accurate event rates for a definitive sample size, the cost of a large scale clinical trial, patient recruitment rates, trial design, randomization procedure, and ability to maintain blinding.

Assessment of methodological quality

The reviewers (BD, VD, ALS, and SS) independently assessed the quality of each included pilot and definitive trial in duplicate using the Checklist to Evaluate A Report of Non-Pharmacological Trial (CLEAR NPT). The CLEARN NPT is designed for the critical appraisal of RCTs in nonpharmacological and surgical trials [6]. The original checklist was modified, where the question regarding patient adherence was omitted as all our trials evaluated a single, one-time surgical intervention. As the original checklist did not provide a scoring method, the criteria employed by Somford et al. was adopted to provide a modified CLEAR NPT (Additional file 2) [6]. The maximum CLEAR NPT score was 18, whereby a score of 0–6 indicated a low quality trial, 7–12 indicated a medium quality trial, and 13–18 indicated a high quality trial.

Statistical analysis

A kappa (κ) statistic was used to determine agreement at all stages of article screening with 95% confidence intervals (CI) [7]. An intraclass correlation coefficient (ICC) was calculated for the purpose of evaluating inter-rater reliability for the CLEAR NPT quality assessment. Agreement for both the κ and ICC was categorized as follows: > 0.90 indicated an almost perfect level of agreement, 0.80 < 0.90 strong agreement, 0.60 < 0.79 moderate agreement, 0.40 < 0.59 weak agreement, 0.21 < 0.39 minimal agreement, and 0.0 < 0.20 no agreement [8].

A t-test was performed using an online statistical calculator (Vassal Stats) to compare trial quality between pilot and definitive trials and a Pearson's r correlation was calculated to determine if there was a relationship between number of studies and quality of pilot RCTs over time. A *p*-value less than 0.05 was considered significant. Descriptive statistics including means, proportions, standard deviations, and CIs are reported. A meta-analysis was not performed given the broad heterogeneity of the trial designs, interventions, and outcome measures.

Results

Screening

The initial screening of online databases yielded 3857 articles after the removal of 2230 duplicates. After title, abstract, and full text screening, 49 pilot RCTs were included (Fig. 1 and Additional file 3). Of these, we identified five definitive trials (one of which is still ongoing) that corresponded to the original published pilot trial. Inter-reviewer agreement was high at all stages of screening (title, κ = 0.886 (95% CI 0.878 to 0.893); abstract, κ = 0.740 (95% CI 0.693 to 0.780); and full text, κ = 0.792 (95% CI 0.737 to 0.835)).

Pilot trial characteristics

Pilot trials were commonly published from the UK and Canada (22 and 16%, respectively) (Tables 1 and 2). A total of 2117 patients were recruited across all pilot RCTs, and 5.84 ± 10.9% of patients, on average, were lost to follow up. The greatest proportion of pilot trials (59.2%, 29/49) focused on surgical fracture repair, including long bone, knee, spinal, foot and hip fractures (Fig. 2). As classified by the World Bank, 40 of the pilot trails were conducted in high-income countries, 6 were classified as middle income and 3 were classified as low income [9].

Primary and secondary outcomes of the pilot trials were divided into physician-reported and patient-reported outcomes. 65.3% (32/49) of all pilot RCTs used radiographic analysis, such as x-rays, MRIs, ultrasounds and CT scans. Patient-reported outcomes were recorded through self-reporting or interview style questionnaires. Questionnaires addressed outcomes such as quality of life, pain, function/independence, and emotional health. Of the pilot trials, 67.3% (33/49) made use of patient-reported questionnaires as tools for monitoring trial outcomes.

Overall, 73.5% (36/49) of the pilot RCTs found in the orthopaedic surgery literature were framed as feasibility trials (Table 1). The two most commonly explored feasibility objectives were safety and efficacy of an orthopaedic surgical intervention (Fig. 3). 26.5% (13/49) of pilot RCTs explored more than one feasibility objective. The pilot trials CLEAR NPT rating varied from 10 to 18. Only 3 of the 5 definitive RCTs included in this review determined their sample size based on their corresponding pilot trial. None of the definitive RCTs enrolled the pilot patients into the definitive trial. Additionally, 22.4% (11/49) of the pilot trials listed the efficacy/effectiveness of the surgical intervention as a primary outcome. Of these, only one led to a definitive trial.

Definitive trial characteristics

Of the 49 identified pilot RCTs, five (10.2%) corresponding definitive RCTs were found (Table 2). On average, definitive trials were published at a mean of 4.25 years (3–7 years) after the pilot trial. The sample size of the pilot trial was 7.2% of the definitive trials. The total number of patients recruited to definitive RCTs was 4016, with one trial still recruiting participants (Table 2). Only one of these definitive trials was ongoing according to clinicaltrials.gov (31). Authors from 17 pilot trials (34.7%) responded to our email confirming that a definitive trial had not been published. Of these, 8 authors cited the following reasons for not conducting a

Table 1 Characteristics of the Included Pilot RCTs

Title	Country	# of patients	Condition	Type of Surgery	Control	Patient-Reported Outcomes	Clinician Reported Outcomes
Hamdy, R. C et al., (2009) [15]	Canada	52	Lower extremity limb lengthening and deformity correction.	Ilizarov technique	Sterile saline solution	Faces Pain Scale-revised, Adolescent Pediatric Pain Tool, Pediatric Quality of Life Inventory, Gillette Functional Assessment Questionnaire	n/a
Vaccaro, A. R et al., (2005) [16]	USA	12	Iliac crest autograft in posterolateral lumbar fusions	Op-1 putty (rhbmp-7) as an adjunct	No control group	Oswestry scale and SF-36	Radiographic
Ekrol, I et al., (2008) [17]	UK	30	Distal radial fractures.	RhBMP-7 as an alternative to bone graft healing	No control group	n/a	Radiographic, clinical and functional outcomes
Lerner, T et al., (2009) [18]	Germany	40	Adolescent idiopathic scoliosis.	Graft extenders in scoliosis surgery	No Control Group	VAS pain score	Biopsies
Marks, P et al., (2008) [19]	Canada	40	ACL reconstruction	Comparing the Mitek bone–tendon– bone cross pin and bioabsorbable screw	No control - comparative trial	International Knee Documentation Committee (IKDC) Knee Ligament Standard Evaluation, Mohtadi's ACL Deficiency Quality of Life	Lateral x-Ray
Shamji, M. F et al., (2014) [20]	Canada	23	Thoracolumbar burst	Applying a brace to treat thoracolumbar bursts	No brace	VAS pain score	Radiographic, clinical & functional outcome
Carson, J. L et al., (1998) [21]	UK	84	Hip fracture	Blood transfusion during hip fracture	No Control-comparative trial	Phone interviews of family or patient	Various methods to evaluate adverse effects (CT scan, ultrasound, autopsy)
Vaccaro, A. R et al., (2003) [22]	USA	12	Iliac crest autograft in posterolateral lumbar fusions	Op-1 putty (rhbmp-7) as an adjunct	No control group	n/a	Radiographic & clinical
Vaccaro, A. R et al., (2004) [23]	USA	36	Symptomatic degenerative spondylolisthesis	Spinal stenosis	Autograft	n/a	Radiographic & clinically
Glazebrook, M et al., (2013) [24]	Canada	24	Ankle and Hindfoot Arthrodesis	B2A-Coated Ceramic Granules (Amplex) Compared to Autograft	Autograft	Computerized tomography & Ankle Osteoarthritis Scale scores	n/a
Mauffrey, C et al., (2012) [25]	UK	24	Tibial fracture	Arthrodesis surgery	No control - comparative trial	Functional outcome questionnaire (DRI)	n/a
Darmanis, S et al., (2007) [26]	UK	40	Knee arthroplasty	Knee arthroplasty	No laser	Fisher's Exact test and the Mann-Whitney U test	n/a
Buse, G. L et al., (2014) [27]	Canada	60	Hip fracture	Accelerated surgery	No	Functional Independence Measure & SF-36	Troponin measurement & confusion Assessment Method.
Adolfsson, L et al., (2001) [28]	Sweden	53	Waist	Percutaneous Acutrak screw fixation.	Immobilization in a below elbow plaster cast for 10 weeks	n/a	Radiographic

Table 1 Characteristics of the Included Pilot RCTs *(Continued)*

Title	Country	# of patients	Condition	Type of Surgery	Control	Patient-Reported Outcomes	Clinician Reported Outcomes
Kang, P et al., (2012) [29]	China	77	Femoral	Multiple drilling core decompression combined with systemic alendronate as a femoral head-preserving procedure	Multiple drilling core decompression	THA & Harris score	Radiographic
Moseley, J. B et al., (1996) [30]	USA	10	knee	Arthroscapic surgery of the knee	Placebo (sterile saline)	Arthritis Impact Measurement Scale 34 and the SF-36	n/a
Chhabra, H. S et al., (2009) [31]	India	5	Spinal cord	Olfactory mucosal transplantation into the spinal cord	No	American Spinal Injury Association (ASIA) Impairment Scale (AIS), Spinal Cord Independence Measure, Beck Depression Inventory scores and life impact scores on International Spinal Cord Injury Scale	MRI
Wang, Y et al., (2015) [32]	China	21	Foot	Total-contact casting (TCC)	No	Quantitive sensory Testing (temperature, pain, light touch, perception)	Radiographic
Zou, J et al., (2013) [33]	China	94	Tibial	Minimally invasivepercutaneous plate osteosynthesis	Comparative trial, control group was treated with ORIF	n/a	Radiographic
Zehir, S et al., (2015) [34]	Turkey	45	Clavicular	Minimally invasive plating fixation	Mini invasive plating	(DASH) Quick Disability of the Arm, Shoulder and Hand	Radiographic
Pang, H. N et al., (2011) [35]			Singapore	140	Knee	Knee arthroplasty	Resection technique
No	18						
Wondrasch, B et al., (2009) [36]	Austria	21	Femoral	Matrix associated autologous chondrocyte implantation	Delayed weightbearing	Knee Documentation Committee (IKDC), the Tegner activity scale, and the Knee Injury and Osteoarthritis Outcome Score (KOOS)	Radiological outcome was evaluated by the MOCART score and the size and amount of bone marrow edema and effusion
De Sèze, M. P et al., (2011) [11]	France	28	ankle	ankle foot orthosis	Standard ankle-foot orthosis	Pain evaluation on an analogical visual scale	n/a
Kraus, V. B et al., (2012) [37]	USA	11	Knee	ACL	Placebo (sterile saline)	Standardized Knee Injury and Osteoarthritis Outcome Score (KOOS) questionnaire	n/a
Flow Investigators (2011) [38]	Canada	111	General open fractures	Fracture healing	Saline	SF-12 and EQ-5D, respectively (12-item questionnaire that measures health-related quality of life in 8 domains)	n/a
Lindsey, R. W et al., (2006) [39]	USA	10	General long bone fractures	Grafting long bone fractures	No	n/a	Radiographic
Costa, M. L et al., (2003) [40]	UK	28	Achilles tendon	Achilles tendon ruptures	Serial plaster casting	n/a	Ultrasound

Table 1 Characteristics of the Included Pilot RCTs *(Continued)*

Title	Country	# of patients	Condition	Type of Surgery	Control	Patient-Reported Outcomes	Clinician Reported Outcomes
Mahowald, M. L et al., (2009) [41]	USA	11	Advanced rheumatoid arthritis and osteoarthritis	IA-BONT/A	Saline Placebo	Patient global assessment of change was measured with a validated 7-point verbal descriptor scale & WOMAC	n/a
Paterson, K et al., (2013) [42]	Australia	37	Knee	PA-PRP	Hyaluronic acid	VAS pain score	n/a
Zehir, S et al., (2014) [43]	Turkey	64	Distal radius fractures	Sonoma Wrx	Standard volar locking plate fixation	n/a	Radiographic
Hey, H et al., (2013) [44]			Singapore	7	Spinal	Hybrid surgery	Anterior cervical discectomy and fusion + artificial disc replacement
No	10.5						
Kuo, L. C et al., (2013) [45]	Taiwan	22	Radial	Early digit mobilization	Home programmes	Manual Ability Measure-36 (MAM-36) to assess their self-awareness of manual abilities	Radiographic
Abbott, A et al., (2013) [46]	Sweden	17	Cervical	With post-operative cervical collar usage	Without post-operative cervical collar usage	Falls Efficacy Scale (patients measuring completing tasks without falling)	Radiographic
McMorland, G et al., (2010) [47]	Canada	120	SCIATICA	Surgical microdiskectomy	Standardized chiropractic spinal manipulation	McGill Pain Questionnaire, Aberdeen Back Pain Scale, and Roland-Morris Disability Index)	n/a
Ringel, F et al., (2012) [48]	Germany	60	Spinal	Robot-assisted (RO) implantation	Freehand (FH) conventional technique	n/a	CT scan
Boonen, S et al., (2002) [49]	Belgium	33	Proximal Femoral Fracture	Administration of rhIGF-I/IGFBP-3	Placebo	Kerr-Atkins score for pain and function	Radiographic
Griffin, D et al., (2014) [50]	UK	151	Calcaneal fractures	Surgery by open reduction and internal fixation	Non-operative treatment	Kerr-Atkins calcaneal fracture score	Radiographic
Guo, Q et al., (2013) [51]	China	90	Intertrochanteric fractures	Percutaneous compression plate	Proximal femoral nail anti-rotation	n/a	Radiographic
Storey, P et al., (2013) [52]	UK	49	Carpal Tunnel	C-Trac splints	Conventional resting splint	n/a	Radiographic
Zhang, Y. Z et al., (2011) [53]	China	22	Abnormalities with hip joint	Navigation template implantation	Conventional THA	n/a	CT scan
Nejrup, K et al., (2008) [54]	Denmark	43	Knee osteoarthritis	Gold implantation	Sham implantation	WOMAC, Knee Society Clinical Rating System	Radiographic
Eskander, M. B. F et al., (1997) [55]	UK	44	Femoral neck fractures	Enoxaparin	Application of intermittent calf compression garments	n/a	CT scan

Table 1 Characteristics of the Included Pilot RCTs *(Continued)*

Title	Country	# of patients	Condition	Type of Surgery	Control	Patient-Reported Outcomes	Clinician Reported Outcomes
Jordan, R et al., (2014) [56]	UK	24	Tibial plateau fractures	Balloon osteoplasty	Traditional methods	Oxford Knee score and SF12 questionnaire at 3, 6 and 12 month	CT scan
Kearney, R. S et al., (2011) [57]	UK	52	Achilles tendon rupture	Surgical repair	Non-surgical repair	Disability rating index EQ-5D, Achilles Total Rupture Score	n/a
Sabeti, M et al., (2014) [58]	Austria	20	Calcific rotator cuff tendinitis	Intraoperative ultrasound	Needling and palpating techniques	n/a	Radiographic
Dutton, T et al., (2012) [59]	UK	48	Knee fractures	Retransfusion drain	No drain	n/a	Measure of transfusion rate
Sardar, Z et al., (2015) [60]	Canada	24	Spinal fracture	B2A peptide–enhanced ceramic granules (Prefix)	Autogenous iliac crest bone graft (ICBG)	n/a	Radiographic
Capa-Grasa, A et al., (2014) [61]	Spain	40	Carpal Tunnel	Ultra-MIS	Mini-open Carpal Tunnel Release	Quick-DASH questionnaire	n/a
Okcu, G et al., (2013) [62]	Turkey	40	Reverse obliquity fractures of the proximal femur	Long nail implant	Standard nail implant	n/a	Radiographic

Table 1 Characteristics of the Included Pilot RCTs *(Continued)*

Title	Primary Outcome	Secondary Outcome	Loss to follow-up (%)	Length of follow-up	Feasibility Category	Framed as feasibility?	Definitive Trial Published?	CLEAR-NPT Score
Hamdy, R. C et al., (2009) [15]	Pain, quality of life, functional mobility	Adverse effects	3%	3 mo	Study design	Yes	Yes	17
Vaccaro, A. R et al., (2005) [16]	Fusion success rate	Cost effectiveness and pain	0%	24 mo	Safety & efficacy	Yes	No	11
Ekrol, I et al., (2008) [17]	Functional outcome	Complications	0%	12 mo	Efficacy	Yes	No	18
Lerner, T et al., (2009) [18]	Fusion success rate	Pain	0%	48 mo	Efficacy	Yes	No	15.5
Marks, P et al., (2008) [19]	Clinical outcomes	Length of surgery	20%	24 mo	Efficacy	Yes	No	16.5
Shamji, M. F et al., (2014) [20]	Average length of hospital stay & cost	Pain & adverse effects	0%	6 mo	Efficacy	Yes	No	14.5
Carson, J. L et al., (1998) [21]	Mortality & ability to walk 10 ft across a room	Functional status, residence status, in-hospital myocardial infarction, thromboembolism, stroke and pneumonia.	3%	60 days	Patient recruitment	Yes	No	16.5
Vaccaro, A. R et al., (2003) [22]	Fusion success rate	Adverse effects	0%	24 mo	Safety & efficacy	Yes	No	13.5
Vaccaro, A. R et al., (2004) [23]	Fusion success rate	Well-being/Quality of life	5%	1 yr	Safety	Yes	No	18
Glazebrook, M et al., (2013) [24]	Bone healing at site of fusion	n/a	0%	12 mo	Safety & efficacy	Yes	No	17
Mauffrey, C et al., (2012) [25]	DRI	Olerud and Molander Ankle Score (OMAS)10 and the EuroQol EQ-5D generalized health outcome questionnaire	0%	12 mo	Efficacy	Yes	No	18
Darmanis, S et al., (2007) [26]	Fisher's Exact test and the Mann-Whitney U test	n/a	0%	n/a	Efficacy	Yes	No	15.5
Buse, G. L et al., (2014) [27]	Proportion of eligible patients randomly assigned, completeness of follow-up & timelines of accelerated surgery	Major perioperative complication	0%	18 mo	Sample size	Yes	No- Ongoing Definitive Trial	15
Adolfsson, L et al., (2001) [28]	Assessment of union	Failure	1%	10 wks	Efficacy	Yes	No	16.5
Kang, P et al., (2012) [29]	Efficacy of combined treatment	Reduction in disease progression	10%	48 mo	Safety & efficacy	Yes	No	17
Moseley, J. B et al., (1996) [30]	Evaluate the placebo effect as part of a pilot trial preceding a randomized, controlled trial of arthroscopic treatment of osteoarthritis	Ability to find and recruit eligible subjects; developing and testing measurement instruments; ability to retain patients for at least 6 months; determine feasibility of completing trial	0%	12 mo	Ability of patients to complete the trial; ability to maintain blindness	Yes	No	18

Table 1 Characteristics of the Included Pilot RCTs *(Continued)*

Title	Primary Outcome	Secondary Outcome	Loss to follow-up (%)	Length of follow-up	Feasibility Category	Framed as feasibility?	Definitive Trial Published?	CLEAR-NPT Score
Chhabra, H. S et al., (2009) [31]	Autologous olfactory mucosal transplantation therapy	n/a	0%	18 mo	Safety & efficacy	Yes	No	16
Wang, Y et al., (2015) [32]	Comparing the effectiveness of arthrodesis plus TCC with TCC alone for the prevention, treatment and recurrence of midfoot ulcerations	Sample size	0%	12 mo	n/a	No	No	18
Zou, J et al., (2013) [33]	Functional status	Sample size	0%	12 mo	n/a	No	No	16.5
Zehir, S et al., (2015) [34]	Efficacy	Sample size	0%	12 mo	Efficacy	Yes	No	16.5
Pang, H. N et al., (2011) [35]	Efficacy	Unclear	0%	24 mo	Efficacy	Yes	No	18
Wondrasch, B et al., (2009) [36]	Efficacy	n/a	0%	24 mo	Efficacy	Yes	No	14
De Sèze, M. P et al., (2011) [11]	Gain ratio at day 30		0%		Efficacy	Yes	No	16
Kraus, V. B et al., (2012) [37]	Efficacy	Sample size	0%	1 mo	Efficacy	Yes	No	16
Flow Investigators (2011) [38]	Reoperation rates	Infection & wound healing problems	11%	12 mo	Efficacy & large scale trial	Yes	Yes	18
Lindsey, R. W et al., (2006) [39]	Effectiveness of a composite graft consisting of demineralized bone matrix (DBM) putty enriched with aspirated bone marrow	Sample size	0%	24 mo	Efficacy	Yes	No	16
Costa, M. L et al., (2003) [40]	Safety	Sample size	29%	12 mo	Safety	Yes	Yes	18
Mahowald, M. L et al., (2009) [41]	Efficacy and safety of IA-BoNT/	Decreases in pain and functional improvement	13%	1 mo	Safety & efficacy	Yes	No	12
Paterson, K et al., (2013) [42]	Recruitment and safety data	Symptomatic and functional changes following treatment	17%	4 and 12 wks	Efficacy	Yes	No	18
Zehir, S et al., (2014) [43]	Reliability and efficacy	Complication prevention	0%	12–13 mo	Efficacy	Yes	No	13.5
Hey, H et al., (2013) [44]	Clinical differences between three groups	n/a	0%	2 wks	Safety & efficacy	Yes	No	10.5
Kuo, L. C et al., (2013) [45]	Differences in functional outcome	n/a	0%	12 wks	Efficacy & cost	Yes	No	18
Abbott, A et al., (2013) [46]	Sample size feasibility	Physical, functional, and quality of life-related outcomes	45%	6 wks	Cost & sample size	Yes	No	12

Table 1 Characteristics of the Included Pilot RCTs *(Continued)*

Title	Primary Outcome	Secondary Outcome	Loss to follow-up (%)	Length of follow-up	Feasibility Category	Framed as feasibility?	Definitive Trial Published?	CLEAR-NPT Score
McMorland, G et al., (2010) [47]	Recruitment and randomization process, choice of outcome measures, and effect size for definitive trial	Compare the clinical efficacy	0%	1 yr	Sample size patient recruitment randomization	Yes	No	18
Ringel, F et al., (2012) [48]	Evaluate accuracy of techniques	n/a	0%	No follow up	Efficacy	Yes	No	16
Boonen, S et al., (2002) [49]	Pain and function	Musculoskeletal effects	0%	6 mo	Safety	Yes	No	17
Griffin, D et al., (2014) [50]	Pain and function	Complications	5%	24 mo		No	No	18
Guo, Q et al., (2013) [51]	Clinical effectiveness	Complications	0%	2 yrs		No	No	16.5
Storey, P et al., (2013) [52]	Levine questionnaire scores	Grip, pinch and sensation scores	0%	1 yr		No	No	14
Zhang, Y. Z et al., (2011) [53]	Unclear	Unclear	0%	12 to 18 mo		No	No	13
Nejrup, K et al., (2008) [54]	Knee pain, stiffness and function	Time from implant until effect and migration potential of implanted gold beads.	7%	0, 6 and 12 mo		No	No	18
Eskander, M. B. F et al., (1997) [55]	Unclear	Unclear	0%	6 wks		No	No	16.5
Jordan, R et al., (2014) [56]	Quality of reduction based on the post-operative CT scan	Surgical complication & patient satisfaction	Not stated	3, 6 and 12 mo		No	No	18
Kearney, R. S et al., (2011) [57]	Estimate of effect size for the functional outcome	Assess the use of a comprehensive cohort research design	10%	2 wks, 6 wks, 3 mo, 6 mo & 9 mo	Study design	Yes	No	10
Sabeti, M et al., (2014) [58]	Notable potential clinical differences between the two groups	Clinical improvement using ultrasound	10%	2 and 6 wks and the 9 mo		No	No	13
Dutton, T et al., (2012) [59]	Which patients benefit most from drains	n/a	0%	No follow up		No	No	12.5
Sardar, Z et al., (2015) [60]	Safety and efficacy	Fusion rate	0%	6 wks, 3, 6, and 12 mo after surgery.		No	No	14.5
Capa-Grasa, A et al., (2014) [61]	Safety and efficacy	Recruitment rates, compliance, completion, treatment blinding, personnel resources and sample size calculation	0%	3 mo	Safety, sample size & cost	Yes	Yes	17
Okcu, G et al., (2013) [62]	Reoperation (fixation failure), 1 year mortality rate, function and mobility & union rate	Implant success	18%	12 to 20 mo		No	No	16

Table 2 Characteristics of Included Definitive trials

Pilot RCT Author	Definitive RCT Author	Country of Publication	Number. Of Patients	Change in Condition/ Intervention	Primary Outcomes	Secondary Outcomes	Loss to Follow up (%)	Were Pilot Patients rolled into the definitive sample size?	Was the sample size calculation based on data from the pilot?	Number of months between publication of pilot trial and definitive trial	CLEAR NPT score:
Buse G. et al. (2014) [27]	Manach, Y. L. et al.,(ongoing) [63]	Canada	1200 (still recruiting)	No change	Major perioperative complication	Mortality, myocardial infarction, cardiac revascularization procedure	0.00	Unclear	Yes	68 (projeted end date July 2018)	18
Hamdy, R. C. et al. (2009) [15]	Hamdy, R. C. et al. (2016) [64]	Canada	125	No change	Quality of life (questionaires, filled out by parents and children) 4 PedsQL scales.	n/a	4.00	Unclear	No	78	18
Flow Investigators (2011) [38]	Bhandari M. et al. (2015) [65]	Canada	2551	No change	Reoperation, to treat an infection at the operative site or contiguous to it, manage a wound-healing problem or promote bone healing.	n/a	0.00	No	No	51	18
Costa, M. et al. (2003) [40]	Costa, M. et al. (2006) [66]	UK	48	No change	Time taken to return to normal activities, as reported by the patient	Complication rate in the treatment group	10.40	No	Yes	26	18
Capa-Grasa. et al. (2014) [61]	Rojo-Manaute, J. et al. (2016) [67]	Spain	92	No change	To compare the clinical outcomes of two surgical outcomes with primary carpal tunnel syndrome.	n/a	0.00	No	Yes	4	18

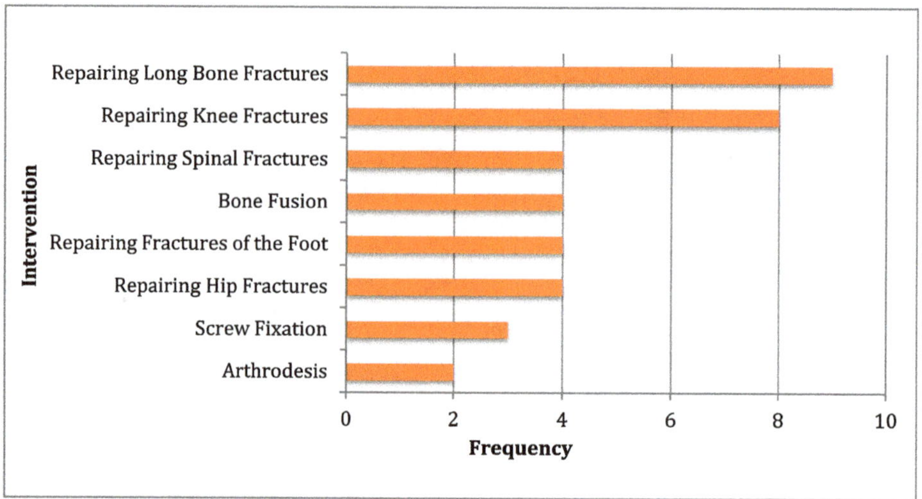

**Only one of the 49 pilot trials respectively, examined general fracture, deformity correction, carpal tunnel, orthosis, electronically assisted surgery and intraoperative interventions and were therefore not included in this figure.*

Fig. 2 Frequency of various types of pilot RCT interventions in each intervention category

definitive RCT: a lack of funding (12.5%), inability to meet recruitment targets (12.5%), preliminary efficacy of the intervention was not demonstrated (25.0%), the pilot study was thought to yield reliable results therefore eliminating the need for further investigation (50.0%).

Trial quality

There was no correlation ($r = -0.1508$, $p = 0.5655$) between number of studies and quality of pilot RCTs over time (Table 3). The overall quality of the pilot RCTs was relatively high (mean CLEAR NPT score 15.9 ± 1.53). Based on the CLEAR NPT scale, the highest quality pilot RCTs involved the treatment of arthrodesis and repair of knee fractures. All of the definitive RCTs were given a score of 18 and were therefore 2.6 points higher on the CLEAR NPT scale than their corresponding pilot trials ($p < 0.01$). The agreement among reviewers for the quality assessment was very high (ICC = 0.969 (95% CI 0.948 to 0.982)).

Discussion

Results from this systematic review demonstrate that the majority of orthopaedic surgical pilot RCTs were framed as feasibility trials, and that the pilot trials mostly

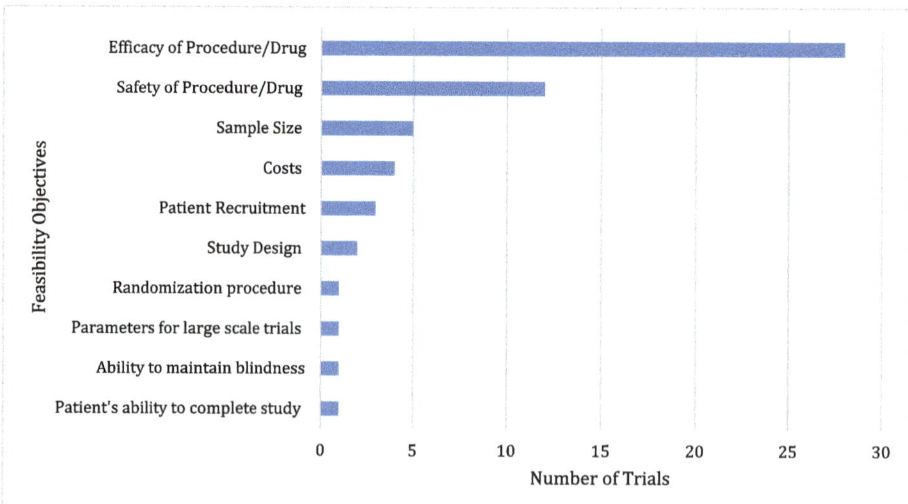

**One trial may define more than one feasibility objective and can therefore belong to more than one category.*

Fig. 3 Number of RCTs that define each of these feasibility objectives in their pilot RCT

Table 3 Number and average quality of pilot RCTs over time of publication

Year	Number of Trials	Mean Clear NPT Score
1996	1	18.0
1997	1	16.5
1998	1	16.5
2001	1	16.5
2002	1	17.0
2003	3	16.5
2005	1	11.0
2006	1	16.0
2007	1	15.5
2008	3	17.5
2009	5	14.9
2010	2	17.0
2011	5	15.0
2012	4	15.9
2013	10	15.3
2014	6	15.7
2015	3	16.3
2016	0	n/a
2017	0	n/a
2018	0	n/a

evaluated site or investigator level feasibility. As expected, the quality of the corresponding definitive RCTs was higher than their respective pilot trial. Despite the majority (87%) of pilot RCTs being conducted in the high-income countries, the majority of the included pilot trials however, did not lead to a definitive RCT. In these cases, reasons cited included: a lack of funding, inadequate sample sizes, and that research questions were sufficiently answered in the pilot phase.

Similar to other fields of medicine, the majority of orthopaedic surgical pilot trials were not followed by a definitive trial. Arain et al. reviewed seven medical journals, including four general medicine journals (British Medical Journal, Lancet, the New England Journal of Medicine and the Journal of American Medical Association) and three specialist journals (British Journal of Surgery, British Journal of Cancer, British Journal of Obstetrics and Gynecology) to identify 54 pilot studies [5]. The authors reported a very low number of follow up studies, wherein only 14.8% (8/54) pilot studies yielded published definitive studies. Additionally, a systematic review published in 2017 by Kaur et al., looked at the quality of pilot studies within the Clinical Rehabilitation journal over the past 30 years, and they concluded that only 12% of their pilot studies led to a definitive trial [10].

The limited number of published pilot trials and corresponding definitive trials may be attributed to numerous factors. Firstly, the pilot may have demonstrated that a definitive trial was not feasible based on criteria established a priori (e.g. ability to recruit patients). However, we would expect that in some of these cases, researchers would amend their trial design, interventions, and outcomes to ensure feasibility in the definitive trial. Secondly, if found to be feasible, investigators may refrain from publishing their pilot trial and instead, roll the pilot patients into the definitive RCT to help save on time and costs. Trial methods papers and online registries are often used to first describe these trials. Thirdly, based on author responses in this review, definitive trials may not be feasible due to a lack of funding. In one case, the authors noted that their research question was answered by the pilot trial [11]. However, the published pilot did not provide a sample size calculation, and therefore, we cannot determine if the statistical power threshold was met for the primary outcome [12].

The majority of the orthopaedic surgical pilot trials found in this review posited feasibility objectives and were of relatively high quality. The first published pilot surgical trial was found in 1996, and since then, there has been an increase in the number of pilot RCTs published over time, with a relatively constant quality of trials up until 2013, with a decline in publications up until 2016. From 2016 to the end of our search in 2018, there were no orthopaedic surgical pilot RCTs published. This may be due to a more recent trend of trialists to roll their pilot patients into a definitive trial to save on costs and maximize recruitment. There may also be a lag in pilot publications in the past 3 years.

Strengths and limitations

Strengths of this review include a broad systematic search and high agreement at all stages of screening and quality assessment. The main limitation is the minimal data available regarding the reasons why pilot trials have not led to definitive RCTs. There was a lack of response from authors, limiting further insight into barriers to definitive trials. Within the past 5 years, 13 of the 49 pilot RCTs and 4 of the 5 definitive trials were published. Thus, the inclusion of more recent pilot RCTs may be a limitation, as their current definitive trials may be underway, and/or not yet published. This potential source of bias was mitigated by searching the clinical trial registry, clinicaltrials.gov, for any records of ongoing definitive RCTs.

This review includes the use of the CLEAR NPT checklist to evaluate each pilot trial. Specifically within orthopedic literature, the quality of reporting RCTs using the CLEAR NPT is suboptimal, and that there is a need for improved surgical reporting [13]. However, in comparison to the CONSORT statement, the CLEAR

NPT scale proves to be more useful in its analysis in interventions that require technical skill, with unique considerations in both conducting and reporting trials [14]. In this review, to account for methodological considerations, a modified CLEAR NPT scale was used instead to increase reliability and remove the necessity of including the Cochrane Risk of Bias Tool. The CLEAR NPT scale was modified, tested and optimized for orthopaedic trials, which was the focus of this paper.

Conclusion

While the majority of pilot RCTs found in the surgical orthopaedic literature are framed as feasibility trials, most did not lead to definitive trials. The reported reasons include: minimal funding, the inability to recruit an adequate sample size and that the research questions were sufficiently answered in the pilot phase. Although, most pilot RCTs did not result in a definitive trial, this does not diminish the value of the pilot trial in determining feasibility.

Abbreviations

CI: Confidence intervals; CLEAR NPT: Checklist to Evaluate A Report of Non-Pharmacological Trial; ICC: Intraclass correlation coefficient; n/a: Not applicable; RCT: Randomized controlled trial

Acknowledgements

The authors would like to thank Ajaykumar Shanmugaraj for his assistance with the article's submission.

Funding

Not applicable.

Authors' contributions

BD, VD, SS, AS and AS all contributed to paper screening, data abstraction, data validation, and writing of the paper. NS, AD, SS, and MB contributed to study design, manuscript revision, study supervision, and have critically reviewed all content during the preparation of the final paper. All authors have made substantial contributions to the paper, including study conduct, manuscript drafting, have given final approval for this version to be published, and have agreed to be accountable for all aspects of the work.

Consent for publication

Not applicable.

Competing interests

The authors declare that they have no competing interests.

Author details

[1]Faculty of Health Sciences, McMaster University, Hamilton, ON, Canada. [2]Schulich School of Medicine and Dentistry, Western University, London, ON, Canada. [3]Faculty of Medicine, University of Toronto, Toronto, ON, Canada. [4]Department of Health Research Methods, Evidence, and Impact (HEI), Division of Orthopaedic Surgery, McMaster University, Hamilton, ON, Canada. [5]Department of Surgery, Division of Orthopaedic Surgery, McMaster University, Hamilton, ON, Canada.

References

1. Hujoel P. Definitive vs. exploratory periodontal trials: a survey of published studies. J Dent Res. 1995;74(8):1453–8.
2. Lancaster GA, Dodd S, Williamson PR. Design and analysis of pilot studies: recommendations for good practice. J Eval Clin Pract. 2004;10(2):307–12.
3. Feeley N, Cossette S, Côté J, Héon M, Stremler R, Martorella G, et al. The importance of piloting an RCT intervention. Can J Nurs Res. 2009;41(2):84–99.
4. Rajadhyaksha V. Conducting feasibilities in clinical trials: an investment to ensure a good study. Perspect Clin Res. 2010;1(3):106–9.
5. Arain M, Campbell MJ, Cooper CL, Lancaster GA. What is a pilot or feasibility study? A review of current practice and editorial policy. BMC Med Res Methodol. 2010;10(1):67.
6. Somford MP, Van Deurzen DF, Ostendorf M, Eygendaal D, Van den Bekerom MP. Quality of research and quality of reporting in elbow surgery trials. J Shoulder Elb Surg. 2015;24(10):1619–26.
7. McGinn T, Wyer P, Newman T, Keitz S, Leipzig R. Tips for learners of evidence-based medicine: 3. Measures of observer variability (kappa statistic). CMAJ. 2004;171(11):1369–73.
8. Sackett DL, Haynes RB, Guyatt GH, Tugwell P. Clinical Epidemiology. 2nd ed. Boston: Little, Brown and Company; 1991.
9. How does the World Bank classify countries. The World Bank. 2018.
10. Kaur N, Figueiredo S, Bouchard V, Moriello C, Mayo N. Where have all the pilot studies gone? A follow-up on 30 years of pilot studies in clinical rehabilitation. Clin Rehabil. 2017;31(9):1238–48.
11. De Sèze MP, Bonhomme C, Daviet JC, Burguete E, Machat H, Rousseaux M, et al. Effect of early compensation of distal motor deficiency by the chignon ankle-foot orthosis on gait in hemiplegic patients: a randomized pilot study. Clin Rehabil. 2011;25(11):989–98.
12. Nayak B. Understanding the relevance of sample size calculation. Indian J Ophthalmol. 2010;58(6):469.
13. Mundi R, Chaudhry H, Singh I, Bhandari M. Checklists to improve the quality of orthopaedic literature. IJO. 2008;42(2):150.
14. Chan S, Bhandari M. The quality of reporting of orthopaedic randomized trials with use of a checklist for nonpharmacological therapies. JBJS. 2007; 89(9):1970–8.
15. Hamdy R, Montpetit K, Raney E, Aiona M, Fillman R, MacKenzie W, et al. Botulinum toxin type a injection in alleviating postoperative pain and improving quality of life in lower extremity limb lengthening and deformity correction: a pilot study. J Pediatr Orthop. 2009;29(5):427–34.
16. Vaccaro AR, Patel T, Fischgrund J, Anderson DG, Truumees E, Herkowitz H, et al. A 2-year follow-up pilot study evaluating the safety and efficacy of op-1 putty (rhbmp-7) as an adjunct to iliac crest autograft in posterolateral lumbar fusions. Eur Spine J. 2005;14(7):623–9.
17. Ekrol I, Hajducka C, Court-Brown C, McQueen MM. A comparison of RhBMP-7 (OP-1) and autogenous graft for metaphyseal defects after osteotomy of the distal radius. Injury. 2008;39:S73–82.
18. Lerner T, Bullmann V, Schulte TL, Schneider M, Liljenqvist U. A level-1 pilot study to evaluate of ultraporous β-tricalcium phosphate as a graft extender in the posterior correction of adolescent idiopathic scoliosis. Eur Spine J. 2009;18(2):170–9.
19. Marks P, O'Donnell S, Yee G. A pilot clinical evaluation comparing the Mitek bone–tendon–bone cross pin and bioabsorbable screw in anterior cruciate ligament reconstruction fixation, a randomized double blind controlled trial. Knee. 2008;15(3):168–73.
20. Shamji MF, Roffey DM, Young DK, Reindl R, Wai EK. A pilot evaluation of the role of bracing in stable thoracolumbar burst fractures without neurological deficit. J Spinal Disord Tech. 2014;27(7):370–5.
21. Carson JL, Terrin ML, Barton FB, Aaron R. Greenburg, AG, heck DA, et al. a pilot randomized trial comparing symptomatic vs. hemoglobin-level-driven red blood cell transfusions following hip fracture. Transfusion. 1998;38(6): 522–9.
22. Vaccaro AR, Patel T, Fischgrund J, Anderson DG, Truumees E, Herkowitz H, et al. A pilot safety and efficacy study of OP-1 putty (rhBMP-7) as an adjunct

to iliac crest autograft in posterolateral lumbar fusions. Eur Spine J. 2003; 12(5):495–500.
23. Vaccaro AR, Patel T, Fischgrund J, Anderson DG, Truumees E, Herkowitz HN, et al. A pilot study evaluating the safety and efficacy of OP-1 putty (rhBMP-7) as a replacement for iliac crest autograft in posterolateral lumbar arthrodesis for degenerative spondylolisthesis. Spine. 2004;29(17):1885–92.
24. Glazebrook M, Younger A. Lalonde, KAA prospective pilot study of B2A-coated ceramic granules (Amplex) compared to autograft for ankle and hindfoot arthrodesis. Foot Ankle Int. 2013;34(8):1055–63.
25. Mauffrey C, McGuinness K, Parsons N, Achten J, Costa ML. A randomised pilot trial of "locking plate" fixation versus intramedullary nailing for extra-articular fractures of the distal tibia. J Bone Joint Surg Br. 2012;94(5):704–8.
26. Darmanis S, Toms A, Durman R, Moore D, Eyres K. A technical innovation for improving identification of the trackers by the LED cameras in navigation-assisted total knee arthroplasty. Comput Aided Surg. 2007; 12(4):247–51.
27. Buse GL, Bhandari M, Sancheti P, Rocha S, Winemaker M, Adili A, et al. Accelerated care versus standard care among patients with HIP fracture: the HIP ATTACK pilot trial. CMAJ. 2013;186(1):E52–60.
28. Adolfsson L, Lindau T, Arner M. Acutrak screw fixation versus cast immobilisation for undisplaced scaphoid waist fractures. J Hand Surg. 2001; 26(3):192–5.
29. Kang P, Pei F, Shen B, Zhou Z, Yang J. Are the results of multiple drilling and alendronate for osteonecrosis of the femoral head better than those of multiple drilling? A pilot study. Joint Bone Spine. 2012;79(1):67–72.
30. Moseley JB, Wray NP, Kuykendall D, Willis K, Landon G. Arthroscopic treatment of osteoarthritis of the knee: a prospective, randomized, placebo-controlled trial results of a pilot study. Am J Sports Med. 1996;24(1):28–34.
31. Chhabra HS, Lima C, Sachdeva S, Mittal A, Nigam V, Chaturvedi D, et al. Autologous mucosal transplant in chronic spinal cord injury: an Indian pilot study. Spinal Cord. 2009;47(12):887.
32. Wang Y, Zhou J, Yan F, Li G, Duan X, Pan H, et al. Comparison of arthrodesis with total contact casting for midfoot ulcerations associated with charcot neuroarthropathy. Med Sci Monit. 2015;21:2141–8.
33. Zou J, Zhang W, Zhang CQ. Comparison of minimally invasive percutaneous plate osteosynthesis with open reduction and internal fixation for treatment of extra-articular distal tibia fractures. Injury. 2013;44(8):1102–6.
34. Zehir S, Zehir R, Şahin E, Çalbıyık M. Comparison of novel intramedullary nailing with mini-invasive plating in surgical fixation of displaced midshaft clavicle fractures. Arch Orthop Trauma Surg. 2015;135(3):339–44.
35. Pang HN, Yeo SJ, Chong HC, Chin PL, Ong J, Lo NN. Computer-assisted gap balancing technique improves outcome in total knee arthroplasty, compared with conventional measured resection technique. Knee Surg Sports Traumatol Arthrosc. 2011;19(9):1496–503.
36. Wondrasch B, Zak L, Welsch GH, Marlovits S. Effect of accelerated weightbearing after matrix-associated autologous chondrocyte implantation on the femoral condyle on radiographic and clinical outcome after 2 years a prospective, randomized controlled pilot study. Am J Sports Med. 2009; 37(1-suppl):88–96.
37. Kraus VB, Birmingham J, Stabler TV, Feng S, Taylor DC, Moorman CT, et al. Effects of intraarticular IL1-Ra for acute anterior cruciate ligament knee injury: a randomized controlled pilot trial. Osteoarthr Cartil. 2012;20(4):271–8.
38. Investigators F. Fluid lavage of open wounds (FLOW): a multicenter, blinded, factorial pilot trial comparing alternative irrigating solutions and pressures in patients with open fractures. J Trauma Acute Care Surg. 2011;71(3):596–606.
39. Lindsey RW, Wood GW, Sadasivian KK, Stubbs HA, Block JE. Grafting long bone fractures with demineralized bone matrix putty enriched with bone marrow: pilot findings. Orthopedics. 2006;29(10):939–41.
40. Costa ML, Shepstone L, Darrah C, Marshall T, Donell ST. Immediate full-weight-bearing mobilisation for repaired Achilles tendon ruptures: a pilot study. Injury. 2003;34(11):874–6.
41. Mahowald ML, Krug HE, Singh JA, Dykstra D. Intra-articular botulinum toxin type a: a new approach to treat arthritis joint pain. Toxicon. 2009;54(5):658–67.
42. Paterson K, Nicholls M, Bates D. Intra-articular injection of platelet-rich plasma in patients with knee osteoarthritis: a randomised controlled pilot study. J Sci Med Sport. 2013;16:e90.
43. Zehir S, Calbiyik M, Zehir R, Ipek D. Intramedullary repair device against volar plating in the reconstruction of extra-articular and simple articular distal radius fractures; a randomized pilot study. Int J Orthop. 2014;38(8): 1655–60.
44. Hey HWD, Hong CC, Long AS, Hee HT. Is hybrid surgery of the cervical spine a good balance between fusion and arthroplasty? Pilot results from a single surgeon series. Eur Spine J. 2013;22(1):116–22.
45. Kuo LC, Yang TH, Hsu YY, Wu PT, Lin CL, Hsu HY, et al. Is progressive early digit mobilization intervention beneficial for patients with external fixation of distal radius fracture? A pilot randomized controlled trial. Clin Rehabil. 2013;27(11):983–93.
46. Abbott A, Halvorsen M, Dedering Å. Is there a need for cervical collar usage post anterior cervical decompression and fusion using interbody cages? A randomized controlled pilot trial. Physiother Theory Pract. 2013;29(4):290–300.
47. McMorland G, Suter E, Casha S, du Plessis SJ, Hurlbert RJ. Manipulation or microdiskectomy for sciatica? A prospective randomized clinical study. JMPT. 2010;33(8):576–84.
48. Ringel F, Stüer C, Reinke A, Preuss A, Behr M, Meyer B, et al. Accuracy of robot-assisted placement of lumbar and sacral pedicle screws: a prospective randomized comparison to conventional freehand screw implantation. Spine. 2012;37(8):E496–501.
49. Boonen S, Rosen C, Bouillon R, Sommer A, McKay M, Rosen D, et al. Musculoskeletal effects of the recombinant human IGF-I/IGF binding protein-3 complex in osteoporotic patients with proximal femoral fracture: a double-blind, placebo-controlled pilot study. J Clin Endocrinol Metab. 2002; 87(4):1593–9.
50. Griffin D, Parsons N, Shaw E, Kulikov Y, Hutchinson C, Thorogood M, et al. Operative versus non-operative treatment for closed, displaced, intra-articular fractures of the calcaneus: randomised controlled trial. BMJ. 2014;349:g4483.
51. Guo Q, Shen Y, Zong Z, Zhao Y, Liu H, Hua X, et al. Percutaneous compression plate versus proximal femoral nail anti-rotation in treating elderly patients with intertrochanteric fractures: a prospective randomized study. J Orthop Sci. 2013;18(6):977–86.
52. Storey P, Armstrong D, Dear H, Bradley M, Burke F. Pilot randomised controlled trial comparing C-Trac splints with beta wrist braces for the management of carpal tunnel syndrome. Hand Ther. 2013;18(2):35–41.
53. Zhang YZ, Chen B, Lu S, Yang Y, Zhao JM, Liu R, et al. Preliminary application of computer-assisted patient-specific acetabular navigational template for total hip arthroplasty in adult single development dysplasia of the hip. Int J Med Robot. 2011;7(4):469–74.
54. Nejrup K, de Fine ON, Jacobsen JL, Siersma V. Randomised controlled trial of extraarticular gold bead implantation for treatment of knee osteoarthritis: a pilot study. Clin Rheumatol. 2008;27(11):1363–9.
55. Eskander MBF, Limb D, Stone MH, Furlong AJ, Shardlow D, Stead D, et al. Sequential mechanical and pharmacological thromboprophylaxis in the surgery of hip fractures. Int Orthop. 1997;21(4):259–61.
56. Jordan R, Hao J, Fader R, Gibula D, Mauffrey C. Study protocol: trial of inflation osteoplasty in the management of tibial plateau fractures. EJOST. 2014;24(5):647–53.
57. Kearney RS, Achten J, Parsons NR, Costa ML. The comprehensive cohort model in a pilot trial in orthopaedic trauma. BMC Med Res Methodol (2011);11(1):1.
58. Sabeti M, Schmidt M, Ziai P, Graf A, Nemecek E, Schueller-Weidekamm C. The intraoperative use of ultrasound facilitates significantly the arthroscopic debridement of calcific rotator cuff tendinitis. Arch Orthop and Trauma Surg. 2014;134(5):651–6.
59. Dutton T, De-Souza R, Parsons N, Costa ML. The timing of tourniquet release and 'retransfusion'drains in total knee arthroplasty: a stratified randomised pilot investigation. Knee. 2012;19(3):190–2.
60. Sardar Z, Alexander D, Oxner W, Plessis SD, Yee A, Wai EK, et al. Twelve-month results of a multicenter, blinded, pilot study of a novel peptide (B2A) in promoting lumbar spine fusion. J Neurosurg Spine. 2015;22(4):358–66.
61. Capa-Grasa A, Rojo-Manaute JM, Rodríguez FC, Martín JV. Ultra minimally invasive sonographically guided carpal tunnel release: an external pilot study. OTSR. 2014;100(3):287–92.
62. Okcu G, Ozkayin N, Okta C, Topcu I, Aktuglu K. Which implant is better for treating reverse obliquity fractures of the proximal femur: a standard or long nail? Clin Orthop Relat Res. 2013;471(9):2768–75.
63. Manach YL, Collins G, Bhandari M, Bessissow A, Boddaert J, Khiami F, et al. Outcomes after hip fracture surgery compared with elective total hip replacement. JAMA. 2015;314(11):1159.

64. Hamdy RC, Montpetit K, Aiona MD, MacKenzie WG, van Bosse HJ, Narayanan U, et al. Safety and efficacy of botulinum toxin a in children undergoing lower limb lengthening and deformity correction: results of a double-blind, multicenter, randomized controlled trial. J Pediatr Orthop. 2016;36(1):48–55.
65. Bhandari M, Jeray KJ, Petrisor BA, Devereaux PJ, Heels-Ansdell D, Schemitsch EH, et al. A trial of wound irrigation in the initial management of open fracture wounds. N Engl J Med. 2015;373(27):2629.
66. Costa ML, MacMillan K, Halliday D, Chester R, Shepstone L, Robinson AH, et al. Randomised controlled trials of immediate weight-bearing mobilisation for rupture of the tendo Achillis. J Bone J Surg Br. 2006;88(1):69–77.
67. Rojo-Manaute J, Capa-Grasa A, Chana-Rodríguez F, Perez-Mañanes R, Rodriguez-Maruri G, Sanz-Ruiz P, et al. Ultra-minimally invasive ultrasound-guided carpal tunnel release. J Ultrasound Med. 2016;35(6):1149–57.

Long-term follow-up after anterior cruciate ligament reconstruction using a press-fit quadriceps tendon-patellar bone autograft

Alexander Barié[1*], Michael Köpf[1], Ayham Jaber[1], Babak Moradi[1], Holger Schmitt[3], Jürgen Huber[2] and Nikolaus Alexander Streich[2]

Abstract

Background: The use of a quadriceps tendon-patellar bone (QTPB) autograft provides an alternative procedure in primary reconstruction of the anterior cruciate ligament (ACL). Using the press-fit technique for femoral fixation and knotting over a bone bridge as well as additional spongiosa filling for tibial fixation can completely eliminate the need for fixation implants. The objective of this study was to evaluate the long-term clinical, functional and radiological results of this operating method.

Methods: Sixty-nine patients (27 female-42 male) were included in this study. Fifty-seven patients (83%) received a comprehensive follow-up review after an average period of 7.5 years (range: 7–8.7). All other patients were surveyed by telephone. Six patients (9%) suffered a re-rupture of the ACL graft caused by a new related trauma and were therefore excluded from the statistical analysis.

Results: Of all patients, 98% were satisfied with the operation. Normal or almost normal results were recorded in the subjective IKDC scores form by 88% of the patients. The Lysholm score demonstrated very good and good results in 83% of the patients. Only 1 patient reported minor complaints in the donor area. Seven (12%) patients developed Cyclops syndrome with limited knee extension. This complication was treated arthroscopically within the first year postoperatively. Their results on follow-up were not worse than the results of the patients without Cyclops syndrome. Regarding the 57 patients who received a comprehensive evaluation, the stability test with the KT-1000 Arthrometer yielded a difference of less than 3 mm in the contralateral comparison for 89% of the operated knees. The pivot-shift test was normal in 79% and almost normal in 21%. In the Single-leg Triple Hop Test, patients achieved an average of 98% of the hopping distance attained with the contralateral leg. The radiological examination revealed a slight deterioration in the Kellgren-Lawrence Score in 2 patients.

Conclusion: The ACL reconstruction using the QTPB autograft performed with the press-fit technique leads to good results in comparison with published results of established procedures for primary ACL surgery using other autografts. Further investigations should involve comparative studies with the objective of providing evidence-based, individually adapted therapy for ACL rupture.

Keywords: Knee, Anterior cruciate ligament, Reconstruction, Quadriceps tendon, Press-fit technique

* Correspondence: alexander.barie@med.uni-heidelberg.de
[1]Clinic for Orthopedics and Trauma Surgery, Center for Orthopedics, Trauma Surgery and Spinal Cord Injury, Heidelberg University Hospital, Schlierbacher Landstrasse 200a, 69118 Heidelberg, Germany
Full list of author information is available at the end of the article

Background

Anterior cruciate ligament (ACL) reconstruction is considered to be the gold standard in ACL insufficient knees. The aim of the surgery is to reduce the onset of secondary degenerative changes as well as to restore the ability to perform sport activities on a level comparable to that prior to incurring the injury. Due to the high incidence of ACL ruptures in the young and active patient population [1], there exists a growing interest in the advancement of the surgical technique. The goals of improvement include reducing donor site morbidity, providing an adequate knee function, as well as maintaining knee stability with a low complication rate on long-term follow-up.

The femoral press-fit fixation in ACL reconstruction was originally developed and described by Hertel in 1987. A following tibial press-fit fixation technique was then presented in 1989 [2]. Boszotta and colleagues described the procedure using an arthroscopic approach in 1997 [3]. Afterwards, several authors reported their experience with this surgical technique [4–8]. Advantages of the press-fit fixation include direct bone-to-bone healing, accelerated rehabilitation, absence of hardware related complications or allergic reactions, less costs and the ease of revision procedures since there is no metal removal or tunnel enlargement [9, 10].

The use of a quadriceps tendon-patellar bone (QTPB) autograft for anterior cruciate ligament (ACL) reconstruction was first described by Blauth in 1984 [11]. As a result, the suitability of the quadriceps tendon graft for ACL reconstruction was compared with the patellar tendon graft. Anatomical studies showed that a 10 mm wide tendon strip from the middle third of the quadriceps tendon has a significantly higher cross-sectional area than a 10 mm wide patellar tendon strip and that the attachment surface at the patella was significantly bigger in the quadriceps tendon graft with bone block [12]. Experimental attempts showed an equivalent or higher tear resistance for the quadriceps tendon graft [13]. In spite of these good experimental results, either hamstring tendon autografts or patellar tendon autografts remained to be the gold standard for ACL reconstruction [14]. In two recent reviews, a total of 24 clinical studies with a mid-to long-term follow-up using the QTPB autograft were identified and evaluated, leading to the conclusion that this graft is a safe alternative with good results and low donor site morbidity [15, 16]. The published results of ACL reconstruction using QTPB anchored using a press-fit technique with 1-year follow-up show promising results [17, 18]. The long-term outcome of this technique needs further evaluation. The objective of this study was therefore to examine the clinical results with a long term follow-up after ACL reconstruction with the QTPB autograft.

Methods

Study population and follow-up

The survey retrospectively included all patients operated on with a minimum of 7 years and a maximum of 9 years before the start of the study. Sixty-nine patients had received an arthroscopic reconstruction of the ACL using a QTPB autograft with hardware-free fixation and met the strict inclusion and exclusion criteria (Table 1). All patients were operated on by one senior surgeon (JH). Twenty-seven (39%) of the patients were female and 42 (61%) were male. The average age on operation day was 27 years (range: 14 to 43 years).

Six patients (9%) suffered a re-rupture of the ACL graft during the follow-up period as a result of a new trauma; these patients received a revision ACL reconstruction using a different surgical technique and were therefore excluded from the statistical analysis.

After the retrospective inclusion of the patients, we prospectively performed the collection of the data. A total of 6 patients (9%) did not attend for physical examination but all of them were reached and have completed the subjective surveys on the telephone.

The period between injury and operation was on average 4.3 months (range: 8 days to 15 months). The investigation was carried out after a mean follow-up interval of 7.5 years (range: 7.0 to 8.7) by two experienced orthopedic specialists (AB, NAS) who were not involved in the primary operation.

Mechanism and level of injury

Sixty-four (93%) patients incurred ACL injuries during sports: football (*n* = 23, 36%), skiing (*n* = 15, 24%), handball (*n* = 12, 18%), basketball (*n* = 5, 8%), tennis (*n* = 3, 5%), volleyball (n = 2, 3%), rugby (n = 2, 3%), fistball (n = 1, 1.5%), gymnastics (n = 1, 1.5%). Five patients (7%) were injured during the course of everyday physical activities. Additional lesions were identified with meniscus damage in 24 (35%) patients, cartilage damage in 8 (12%) patients and meniscus damage and cartilage damage in 16 (23%) patients. Two patients (3%) had a combination of ACL rupture, rupture of the medial collateral ligament, tear of the outer meniscus and cartilage damage. Only 19 (27%) patients had an isolated ACL rupture. Since meniscus repair was an exclusion criterion, only patients with partial meniscus resection (*n* = 34, 50%) or stable meniscus lesions which were not addressed (*n* = 8, 12%), were included. Interventions on the cartilage were not carried out in the case of articular cartilage damage °I (n = 8, 12%) and °II (*n* = 15, 22%). Higher grade cartilage damage led to exclusion from the study [19].

Surgical procedure

ACL reconstruction was performed using a technique in which fixation of the graft and the bony filling for the

Table 1 Criteria of patient selection for this study

Inclusion criteria	Exclusion criteria
Primary ACL rupture	Previous operations on both knee joints
Maximum 18 months between injury and operation	Injuries of the lateral collateral ligament and the posterior cruciate ligament
Maximum age at operation 45 years	Chondromalacia greater that grade II according to Outerbridge
Age of at least 18 years on investigation	Meniscal repair
Activity level before the injury ≥4 in the Tegner Score	Instability of the contralateral knee joint

tunnels can be done without the use of hardware. This is made possible by using oscillating hollow burrs (Additional file 1: Figure SA) and a special asymmetrically shaped spongiosa compactor. When harvesting the graft (Fig. 1 / Additional file 2: Figure SB), the diameter of the cylindrical patellar bone block can thereby be precisely defined to 9.4 mm (Fig. 2). The femoral press-fit anchoring is then done by using the bone block to plug the 8 mm femoral tunnel that has been drilled and slightly dilated (Fig. 3). A hollow burr is also used to create the tibial tunnel so that a spongiosa cylinder can be harvested. The tibial fixation is carried out as a hybrid technique. Blocking the tendon in the tibial tunnel with the harvested bone cylinder (Fig. 4) leads to rapid healing of the bone and the knotting of the threads reinforces the quadriceps tendon over a bone bridge (Additional file 3: Figure SC), ensuring primary stability. A detailed description of the individual steps to the surgical procedure and the standardized rehabilitation were described in 2013 [20].

Questionnaires / subjective activity level

A general questionnaire surveyed the patients' data for details of the trauma mechanism and the subjective satisfaction of the patient. Patients specified their satisfaction with the result of the operation on a Visual Analog Scale (VAS) of 0 to 10 [21].

The sporting activity level of the patients was surveyed before the injury and at the time of the follow-up investigation using the Tegner Score of 0 to 10. Level 0 corresponds to an inability to work, level 5 corresponds to the ability to do more intensive physical activities such as cross-country skiing, cycling and jogging two times a week, whereas level 10 corresponds to the ability to play football on a national or international level [22]. The Lysholm Score served to evaluate the subjectively perceived impairment of knee-joint function. It is scored using a point system that evaluates the knee joint in eight everyday stress situations. By adding the points a maximum of 100 points can be achieved. A score of 91–100 points refers to a very good knee function, 84–90 points is good, 65–83 points is moderate and 0–64 points refers to a bad knee function [23]. The Form of the IKDC Score 2000 (International Knee Documentation Committee) for subjective assessment of the knee in everyday and sporting activity was also assessed. It includes seven questions about the symptoms and two questions on activities and function of the knee joint. The result is a point value in which category A (90–100 points) represents a normal knee function, category B (80–89 points) is nearly normal, category C (70–79 points) is abnormal and category D (0–69 points) represents a strongly abnormal knee function [24].

Clinical investigation

The clinical investigation was carried out using the Form for investigation of the knee for the IKDC Score 2000 [24]. The instrumental measurement of the anterior-posterior stability was carried out using the KT-1000™ Knee Ligament Arthrometer® manufactured by MEDmetric® Corporation (http://www.medicalproductguide.com/companies/1364/medmetric_corp, MEDmetric® Corporation, 7542 Trade Street, San Diego, CA 92121; Patent

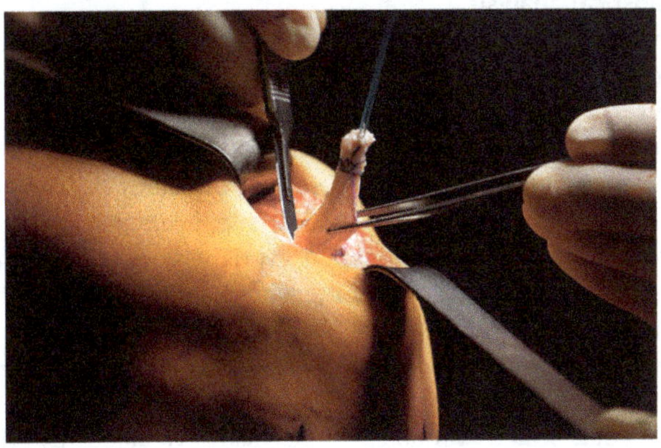

Fig. 1 A 5 cm long, 1 cm wide and 6 to 8 mm-thick strip of the quadriceps tendon is dissected out and reinforced with Mersilene threads

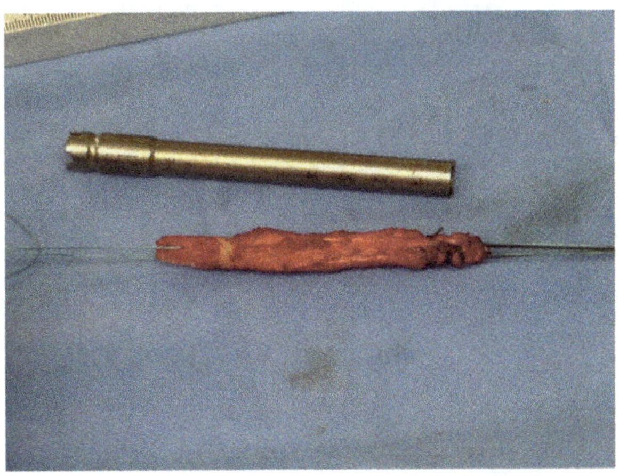

Fig. 2 The armed transplant before implantation

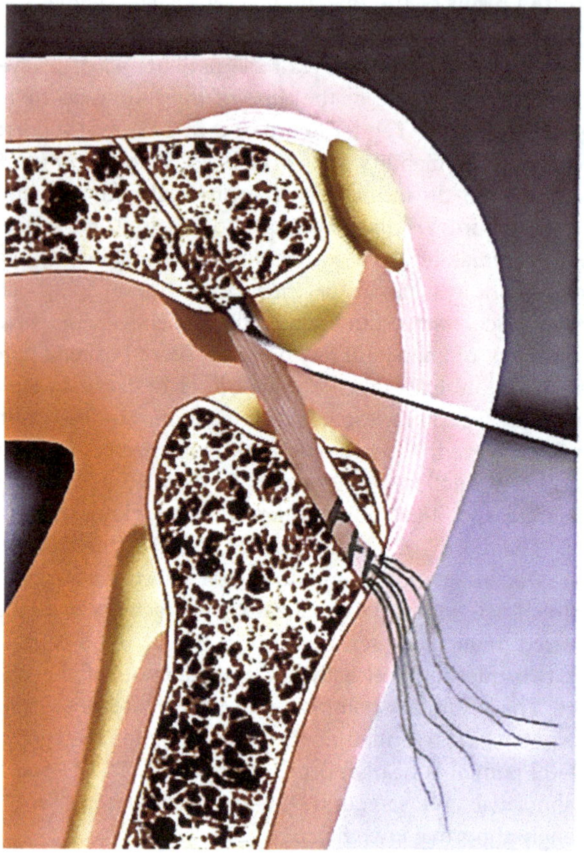

Fig. 3 Diagram showing the press-fit fixation of the patellar bone cylinder in the femoral tunnel

no. 4,583,555) and a tension force of 134 N. The clinical investigation was supplemented by thigh circumference measurements and the Single-Leg Triple-Hop Test [25]. Two measurements of the thigh circumference were done, 10 cm and 20 cm proximal to the joint line. Järvelä and colleagues showed a highly significant correlation ($p < 0.001$) between thigh measurement and the isokinetic strength test for knee extension [26].

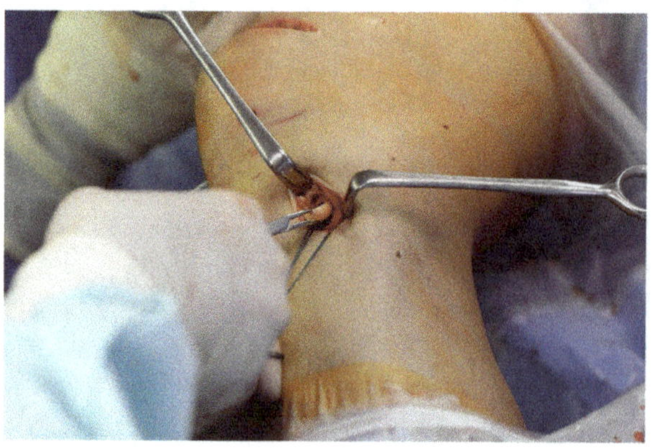

Fig. 4 Spongiosa transplantation filling up the tibial tunnel

Radiological investigation

Osteoarthritis stage was evaluated according to Kellgren -Lawrence classification [27]. Assessment of the tunnels involved X-rays of the knee taken immediately postoperatively in three planes (exercise X-ray according to Rosenberg in the posterior-anterior beam path at 25° knee bend, lateral view at 30° flexion standing and 1 patella-tangential view). The same views of X-rays were taken on follow-up and were compared with the postoperative X-rays.

Subgroup analysis

We further performed a subgroup analysis in order to investigate whether different clinical variables had an impact on the postoperative results. For this purpose, the patient collective was divided into two groups and analyzed statistically. The divisions were made according to sex (Male / Female), by age (< 30 years old on operation day / ≥ 30 years old on operation day), by Body Mass Index (< 25 / ≥ 25), period between injury and surgery (< 3 months ≥3 months), Tegner score before injury (< Level 8 / ≥ Level 8), accompanying injuries in the form of meniscal injuries (presence of meniscal injury / no meniscal injury), cartilage damage (presence of cartilage damage / no cartilage damage), difference in KT-1000 measurement (≤ 2 / > 2), result of the pivot shift test (no pivoting / pivoting), measurement of the thigh circumference (thigh circumference of operated leg ≥ thigh circumference of contralateral side) / thigh circumference of operated side < thigh circumference of contralateral side), and postoperative complications (patients without cyclops or other complications / patients with cyclops or other complications).

Statistical analysis

The entire data input and evaluation was carried out using the program IBM® SPSS® version 24. The normal distribution test was performed by the Kolmogorov-smirnoff, respectively by the Shapiro-Wilk test and the variance homogeneity by the Levine test. For the comparative statistics of the subgroups, statistical significance was calculated for the metric scaled variables according to distribution and variance homogeneity by the t-test or the Mann-Whitney U-test. For the ordinal scaled variables, the evaluation was done using the Mann-Whitney U-test or by correlation with the spearman rank coefficient. Nominal scaled variables were also evaluated by the Mann-Whitney U-test or by cross-tabulation using the Chi-square test or fisher's exact test. The comparison of two measurement points recorded at two different times was done by the Wilcoxon test. For all the tests used, a p-value of less than 0.05 was considered as significant.

Results

Complications and revision interventions

There were no intraoperative complications. One patient (1.5%) had a wound infection postoperatively which was treated conservatively with antibiotics. One patient (1.5%) had a deep vein thrombosis which was treated with anticoagulant therapy. Seven patients (12%) experienced limited knee extension postoperatively. A consequent magnetic resonance imaging (MRI) scan identified the development of a Cyclops in all 7 cases. An arthroscopic operation with resection of the Cyclops and a notchplasty was carried out in all cases after approximately 6 months. Thereafter all patients achieved full extension of the knee joint. The 7-year results of the patients with complications differed neither in the subjective nor the objective parameters from the patients without complications.

Subjective questionnaires

On Follow up, 42 patients (74%) were very satisfied (VAS 9–10), 11 patients (19%) were satisfied (VAS 6–8), 3 patients (5%) were moderately satisfied (VAS 3–5) and 1 patient (2%) was dissatisfied (VAS 0–2).

The median level of physical activity measured by using the 11-stage Tegner Score (0–10) fell significantly from 7 (range: 4–9) before the injury to 6 (range: 1–9) at the time of the follow-up investigation ($p = 0.001$). On follow-up, 36 (63%) patients achieved at least the same activity level as before the injury and 21(37%) patients remained one to five stages below that.

The average value for the Lysholm Score at the follow-up examination was 92 ± 10.6 points (range: 60–100). Forty-two patients (74%) rated their knee function as very good (91–100 points), 5 (9%) had good knee function (84–90 points), 7 (12%) had moderate knee function (65–83 points) and 3 (5%) had poor knee function (≤ 64 points).

The average value of the scores for subjective assessment of knee-joint function for everyday activities and in sport (IKDC 2000 Form) was 90 ± 9.9 points (range: 47–100). Thirty-seven patients (65%) of the patients had normal knee function (90–100 points). Thirteen (23%) patients had almost normal knee function (80–89 points), 5 (9%) patients had abnormal knee function (70–79 points) and 2 (3%) patients had significantly abnormal knee function (≤69 points). The evaluation of question 9 of the subjective IKDC 2000 Form revealed no difficulties in kneeling or squatting in any of the patients.

Clinical investigation

Table 2 shows the results of clinical investigations using palpation and instruments based on the IKDC 2000 Form for clinical investigation of the knee. The posterior-anterior translation was measured using the KT-1000 Arthrometer and yielded an average value of 6.7 ± 1.7 mm (range: 2 to 11 mm) for the unoperated knee and an average value for the operated knee of 7.5 ± 1.7 mm (range: 3 to 12 mm). This increased sagittal translation of the operated knee from an average of 0.9 ± 1.3 mm (range: -2 mm to 4 mm) was statistically significant ($p = 0.004$). The circumference measured for the thigh 10 cm proximal to the base of the patella gave an average value for the operated knee of 46 ± 4.2 cm (range: 39-58 cm) and 47 ± 4.7 cm (range: 39-65 cm) for the unoperated knee. Twenty cm proximal to the patella yielded an average of 55 ± 4.7 cm (range: 45-69 cm) for measurement of the operated knee and 56 ± 4.7 cm (range: 47-75 cm) for the unoperated knee. However, the lower circumference for the operated thigh was not significant for both values ($p = 0.408$). In the Single-leg Triple-Hop Test, the hopping distance achieved in three consecutive single-leg hops was measured and the side-to-side difference was determined. Two patients did not want to take part in this test. The average hop distance for the operated leg was 416 ± 91 cm (range: 225-635 cm) and for the unoperated leg was 427 ± 93 cm (range: 200-635 cm). The difference was not statistically significant ($p = 0.570$). Furthermore, only one patient (1%) reported hypaesthesia (sensitivity to touch) at the donor site, none reported anterior knee pain. Meniscus tests were abnormal in 1 patient. This patient also had the worst functional results.

Radiological investigation

On follow-up, three patients were pregnant. As a result, the radiological examination could only be carried out in 54 (78%) patients. The X-rays were taken directly postoperatively and on follow-up for these patients. Assessment of osteoarthritis according to Kellgren-Lawrence showed deterioration by one stage in two patients (Table 2). The assessment of the drill tunnel diameter provided radiological evidence in all patients for complete bony filling of the femoral tunnel and almost complete bony filling of the tibial tunnel. No tunnel-widening occurred in any patients. None of the patients experienced a dislocation of the femoral bone block or dislocation of the tibial spongiosa cylinder.

Subgroup analysis

The following differences were revealed in the subgroup analysis:

Older patients had a greater loss of activity level in the Tegner Score than younger people ($p = 0.013$). Patients with a longer waiting time between injury and surgery achieved a poorer score in the Pivot-Shift Test than patients with a shorter waiting time ($p = 0.017$).

Table 2 Results of the clinical, instrumental and radiological investigations based on the IKDC 2000 Form for knee evaluation

N = 57	Number of patients (percent of patients)			
Investigation	Normal	Almost Normal	Abnormal	Significantly abnormal
1. Effusion	56 (98%)	1 (2%)	–	–
2. Movement deficit				
Extension deficit	57 (100%)	–	–	–
Flexion deficit	55 (96%)	2 (4%)	–	–
3. Ligament examination				
KT 1000 Arthrometer	51 (89%)	6 (11%)	–	–
Lachmann Test (manual)	50 (88%)	7 (12%)	–	–
Posterior Drawer Test	57 (100%)	–	–	–
Valgus stress	57 (100%)	–	–	–
Varus stress	57 (100%)	–	–	–
Pivot-shift Test	45 (79%)	12 (21%)	–	–
4. Crepitation	44 (77%)	8 (14%)	5 (9%)	–
5. Donor site morbidity	56 (98%)	1 (2%)	–	–
6. Joint space narrowing on X-ray				
Directly postoperative ($n = 54$)	54 (100%)	–	–	–
On follow-up ($n = 54$)	52 (96%)	2 (4%)	–	–
7. Single-leg Triple-Hop Test ($n = 55$)	49 (89%)	6 (11%)	–	–

Patients who had meniscus injuries achieved a poorer score in the KT-1000 stabilization measurement than patients without a meniscus injury ($p = 0.033$) and their difference in the thigh circumference was greater ($p = 0.028$). Patients who had cartilage damage had a knee flexion deficit more frequently than patients without cartilage damage ($p = 0.009$). No significant differences in outcome could be identified in regards to the following parameters: sex ($p = 0.74$), Body mass index ($p = 0.073$), Tegner level of sporting activity before the injury ($p = 0.334$), and complications ($p = 0.366$).

Discussion

The objective of this study was to evaluate the long-term outcome of the surgical technique for ACL reconstruction with a QTPB autograft fixated without the use of hardware. To date, only short-term results with a follow-up after 12 months are available with good clinical outcomes [17, 18]. Clinical studies with a long-term follow-up after ACL reconstruction using bone-patellar tendon-bone autograft using a press-fit fixation reported good results. As far as the authors are aware, only results with a maximum average follow-up of 5.6 years [28] are available for other techniques using hardware for fixation of the QTPB autograft.

Critics have expressed doubts about the stability of the fixation technique without the use of hardware fixation. In the biomechanical studies, the femoral press-fit fixation used here possessed adequate primary stability with ultimate load to failure at least equal to results for interference screws [29, 30]. The tibial hybrid fixation with bone bridge and spongiosa filling also demonstrated the same tear strengths under experimental conditions as interference-screw fixation [31]. This clinical study identified no complication in any patient which could be assessed as a consequence of the fixation technique. No tunnel expansion occurred comparable to that reported with other fixation materials [32]. This is comparable to other studies that report a decreased rate of tunnel expansion on follow-up after ACL-Reconstruction using this procedure [10]. Also in the 6 patients with re-rupture, the drill tunnels were filled with bony material so that a revision operation on one side without the need for spongioplasty was possible.

The clinical stability measurements yielded normal values for 88% of the patients in the Lachmann Test, for 89% in the KT-1000 Arthrometer measurement and for 79% in the Pivot-Shift Test. These values were within the range of values obtained for other techniques. It is described that normal values were obtained for the patellar-tendon graft with the Lachmann Test in 76–100% and with the Pivot-Shift Test in 81–100% of the patients. For the hamstring tendon graft, 64–100% of the patients obtained normal values with the Lachmann Test and 72–100% with the Pivot-Shift Test [33].

The average value of 92 points in the Lysholm Score was also within the range of the specified values for the patellar tendon graft (91–93) and for the hamstring tendon graft (80–94). Eighty-eight percent of the patients achieved a normal or almost normal value in the subjective IKDC 2000 Form. Comparable studies published 48–97% for the patellar tendon graft and 50–97% for the hamstring tendon graft [33].

All the parameters for knee-joint laxity and function that have been assessed were within the range of values similar to that achieved in the patellar tendon and hamstring tendon grafts that are most frequently used and are often designated as the Gold Standard [34, 35]. The primary targets of the ACL operation could therefore be achieved using this surgical procedure with good dependability even after 7.5 years.

Fractures of the patella and tears of the quadriceps tendon are specific complications giving rise to concerns when using the QTPB autograft [36]. However, these specific complications did not occur in the previous reports with short-term follow-up [17, 18] and also not in this study. It is therefore questionable as to whether these potential complications are of clinical relevance.

A complication brought to light in this study is the development of Cyclops syndrome in 12% of the patients. High rates of Cyclops syndrome were also specified for the patellar tendon graft at 11% [37] and 7% [3]. The rates for the hamstring tendon graft are generally lower at up to 3% [38]. Ultimately, the reason for this development is not clear. One possible and reasonable explanation is that the quadriceps tendon graft and the patellar tendon graft have a rougher texture than the hamstring tendon and fibers sloughing off during the process of ligamentization may lead to growths in the area of the tibial ACL insertion. MRI diagnostics is important in patients with persistent knee extension deficit followed by surgical revision using arthroscopic debridement of the hypertrophied tissue and if necessary supplementary notch graft. Full knee extension was achieved for all the patients participating in this study and there were no negative effects on the knee function at final follow-up. This confirms the previous clinical experience that there is generally no recurrence after the mechanical obstruction has been removed [39].

Most grafts do not seem to be significantly different on long-term follow-up. This is presumably a result of the intraarticular ligamentization process that all grafts undergo after reconstruction. This remodeling eventually leads to a ligamentous "ACL-like" structure which histologically resembles a normal ACL. Only ultrastructural differences regarding collagen fibril distribution persist [40]. The ligamentization process has been mainly described in the patellar tendon graft and the hamstring tendon graft. Studies that examine the ligamentization process of the QTPB autograft are lacking.

Measurements of thigh circumference were carried out to investigate muscular weakness. These revealed no significant differences between the operated and unoperated leg. The Single-Leg Triple Hop Test also demonstrated no significant statistical differences. Eighty-nine percent of the patients achieved at least 90% of the hop distance achieved with the unoperated leg. Essentially similar results of 80–93% were published in the literature for hamstring tendon graft and patellar tendon graft [38].

The donor site morbidity of the QTBP autograft is frequently the focus of discussion. The donor site morbidity in this study was very low (2%). This rate is significantly lower compared to the bone-patellar tendon-bone autograft using the same fixation technique [7, 8, 41]. The previous results for the quadriceps tendon graft using hardware fixation also revealed a low rate of anterior knee pain [15, 16].

The subgroup analysis confirmed the known negative influencing factors of the associated meniscus tear and the associated cartilage injury. An interesting finding was the fact that patients with a short interval between injury and operation performed significantly better in tests for rotational stability than patients with an interval of more than 2 months. One possible explanation for this could be that the anatomical footprints of the ACL may be easier to identify when the operation is done at an early stage. This makes it easier to carry out the anatomical reconstruction.

A limitation of this study is the lack of a control group. It is important to note for purposes of radiological evaluation that the X-ray images were not available in digital form and the assessment of the width of the joint space and tunnels therefore represent subjective assessments by the two follow-up investigators. However, the assessments by the two follow-up investigators were separate and blinded, and they were identical. The methods used to assess muscular weakness are hardly valid. An attempt to establish isokinetic power measurement in this study failed. A second investigation date would have been required at a different site and most patients rejected this.

Conclusions

The results of our evaluation suggest that this surgical method using a QTPB autograft with hardware-free graft fixation provides a reliable alternative for reconstruction of the anterior cruciate ligament. Advantages of press-fit fixation include avoidance of complications related to hardware fixation, direct bone-to-bone healing, cost effectiveness compared to other fixation techniques, and ease of revision surgery if needed. Furthermore, the use of the quadriceps tendon autograft showed lower donor site morbidity compared to other grafts. However, a complication in the form of Cyclops syndrome must always be considered.

Further investigation should involve short-term studies that describe the influence of QTPB autograft on short-term disability, second injury rates and quadriceps strength deficits. Comparative studies with different surgical techniques could focus on assessing muscular regeneration in the context of rehabilitation.

Additional files

Additional file 1: Figure SA. Two oscillating hollow burrs are used to harvest the patellar bone block and to create the tibial tunnel. A curved plunger is used to press the patellar bone block in the femoral tunnel.

Additional file 2: Figure SB. The oscillating hollow burr is pushed over the free tendon to saw out a cylinder, 22 mm in length, of the ventral upper pole of the patella.

Additional file 3: Figure SC. Knotting the Mersilene threads over the tibial bone bridge.

Acknowledgments
None.

Funding
This clinical study was internally funded. No external or 3rd party financial support was needed.

Authors' contributions
AB, NS and HS were responsible for the idea and conception of the study. AB, MK and HS planned the Study protocol. JH performed all operations and re-operations mentioned in the study. MK was responsible for the organization of all clinical trials as well as data acquisition. AB and NS performed the clinical examination for all study participants. AB, BM did the statistical analysis and interpreted the results. AB and AJ wrote the Manuscript. All authors read and approved the final manuscript.

Consent for publication
Not Applicable.

Competing interests
The authors declare that they have no competing interests.

Author details
[1]Clinic for Orthopedics and Trauma Surgery, Center for Orthopedics, Trauma Surgery and Spinal Cord Injury, Heidelberg University Hospital, Schlierbacher Landstrasse 200a, 69118 Heidelberg, Germany. Center for Joint Surgery and Sport Injuries, Sportopaedie Heidelberg, Clinic St. Elisabeth Heidelberg, Max Reger Strasse 5-7, 69121 Heidelberg, Germany. [3]Center for Orthopedics and Sports Trauma Surgery, Atos Clinic Heidelberg, Bismarckstraße 9-15, 69115 Heidelberg, Germany.

References
1. Sanders TL, et al. Incidence of anterior cruciate ligament tears and reconstruction: a 21-year population-based study. Am J Sports Med. 2016; 44(6):1502–7.
2. Hertel P (1990) Anatomic reconstruction of the ACL: a new technique for ACL replacement. Presented at the 4th ESSKA congress, S.
3. Boszotta H. Arthroscopic anterior cruciate ligament reconstruction using a patellar tendon graft in press-fit technique: surgical technique and follow-up. Arthroscopy. 1997;13(3):332–9.
4. Gobbi A, et al. Patellar tendon anterior cruciate ligament reconstruction with conical press-fit femoral fixation: 5-year results in athletes population. Knee Surg Sports Traumatol Arthrosc. 2002;10(2):73–9.
5. Al-Husseiny M, Batterjee K. Press-fit fixation in reconstruction of anterior cruciate ligament, using bone-patellar tendon-bone graft. Knee Surg Sports Traumatol Arthrosc. 2004;12(2):104–9.
6. Pavlik A, et al. Biomechanical evaluation of press-fit femoral fixation technique in ACL reconstruction. Knee Surg Sports Traumatol Arthrosc. 2004;12(6):528–33.
7. Widuchowski W, et al. Femoral press-fit fixation in ACL reconstruction using bone-patellar tendon-bone autograft: results at 15 years follow-up. BMC Musculoskelet Disord. 2012;13:115.
8. Hertel P, et al. ACL reconstruction using bone-patellar tendon-bone press-fit fixation: 10-year clinical results. Knee Surg Sports Traumatol Arthrosc. 2005; 13(4):248–55.
9. Felmet G. Implant-free press-fit fixation for bone-patellar tendon-bone ACL reconstruction: 10-year results. Arch Orthop Trauma Surg. 2010; 130(8):985–92.
10. Akoto R, et al. Press-fit fixation using autologous bone in the tibial canal causes less enlargement of bone tunnel diameter in ACL reconstruction--a CT scan analysis three months postoperatively. BMC Musculoskelet Disord. 2015;16:200.
11. Blauth W. 2-strip substitution-plasty of the anterior cruciate ligament with the quadriceps tendon. Unfallheilkunde. 1984;87(2):45–51.
12. U Stäubli H, et al. Quadriceps tendon and patellar ligament: Cryosectional anatomy and structural properties in young adults. Vol. 4; 1996. p. 100–10.
13. Harris NL, et al. Central quadriceps tendon for anterior cruciate ligament reconstruction. Part I: morphometric and biomechanical evaluation. Am J Sports Med. 1997;25(1):23–8.
14. Carmichael JR, Cross MJ. Why bone–patella tendon–bone grafts should still be considered the gold standard for anterior cruciate ligament reconstruction. Br J Sports Med. 2009;43(5):323.
15. Mulford JS, Hutchinson SE, Hang JR. Outcomes for primary anterior cruciate reconstruction with the quadriceps autograft: a systematic review. Knee Surg Sports Traumatol Arthrosc. 2013;21(8):1882–8.
16. Slone HS, et al. Quadriceps tendon autograft for anterior cruciate ligament reconstruction: a comprehensive review of current literature and systematic review of clinical results. Arthroscopy. 2015;31(3):541–54.
17. Barie A, et al. Anterior cruciate ligament reconstruction using quadriceps tendon autograft and press-fit fixation. Unfallchirurg. 2010;113(8):629–34.
18. Akoto R, Hoeher J. Anterior cruciate ligament (ACL) reconstruction with quadriceps tendon autograft and press-fit fixation using an anteromedial portal technique. BMC Musculoskelet Disord. 2012;13:161.
19. Outerbridge RE. The etiology of chondromalacia patellae. 1961. Clin Orthop Relat Res. 2001;389:5–8.
20. Barié A, Streich N, Jürgen H. Arthroscopic anterior cruciate ligament reconstruction using a quadriceps tendon-patellar bone autograft in press-fit fixation. Tech Orthop. 2013;28(2):145–8.
21. Voutilainen A, et al. How to ask about patient satisfaction? The visual analogue scale is less vulnerable to confounding factors and ceiling effect than a symmetric Likert scale. J Adv Nurs. 2016;72(4):946–57.
22. Tegner Y, Lysholm J. Rating systems in the evaluation of knee ligament injuries. Clin Orthop Relat Res. 1985;198:43–9.
23. Lysholm J, Gillquist J. Evaluation of knee ligament surgery results with special emphasis on use of a scoring scale. Am J Sports Med. 1982; 10(3):150–4.
24. Hefti F, et al. Evaluation of knee ligament injuries with the IKDC form. Knee Surg Sports Traumatol Arthrosc. 1993;1(3–4):226–34.
25. Sueyoshi T, et al. Single-leg hop test performance and isokinetic knee strength after anterior cruciate ligament reconstruction in athletes. Orthop J Sports Med. 2017;5(11):2325967117739811. https://doi.org/10.1177/2325967117739811. eCollection 2017 Nov.
26. Jarvela T, et al. Simple measurements in assessing muscle performance after an ACL reconstruction. Int J Sports Med. 2002;23(3):196–201.
27. Kellgren JH, Lawrence JS. Radiological assessment of osteo-arthrosis. Ann Rheum Dis. 1957;16(4):494–502.

28. Deangelis J, Fulkerson J. Quadriceps Tendon-A Reliable Alternative for Reconstruction of the Anterior Cruciate Ligament, vol. 26; 2007. p. 587–96.
29. Dargel J, et al. The effect of bone tunnel dilation versus extraction drilling on the initial fixation strength of press-fit anterior cruciate ligament reconstruction, vol. 127; 2007. p. 801–7.
30. Arnold MP, et al. The biomechanical strength of a hardware-free femoral press-fit method for ACL bone-tendon-bone graft fixation. Knee Surg Sports Traumatol Arthrosc. 2017;25(4):1234–40.
31. Jagodzinski M, et al. Biomechanical analysis of press-fit fixation of anterior cruciate ligament transplants. Unfallchirurg. 2010;113(7):532–9.
32. Fahey M, Indelicato PA. Bone tunnel enlargement after anterior cruciate ligament replacement. Am J Sports Med. 1994;22(3):410–4.
33. Magnussen RA, Carey JL, Spindler KP. Does autograft choice determine intermediate-term outcome of ACL reconstruction? Knee Surg Sports Traumatol Arthrosc. 2011;19(3):462–72.
34. West RV, Harner CD. Graft selection in anterior cruciate ligament reconstruction. J Am Acad Orthop Surg. 2005;13(3):197–207.
35. Pinczewski L, Roe J, Salmon L. Why autologous hamstring tendon reconstruction should now be considered the gold standard for anterior cruciate ligament reconstruction in athletes. Br J Sports Med. 2009;43(5):325–7.
36. Lee S, et al. Outcome of anterior cruciate ligament reconstruction using quadriceps tendon autograft. Arthroscopy. 2004;20(8):795–802.
37. Matsumoto A, et al. A comparison of bone-patellar tendon-bone and bone-hamstring tendon-bone autografts for anterior cruciate ligament reconstruction. Am J Sports Med. 2006;34(2):213–9.
38. Leo AP, et al. A 10-year comparison of anterior cruciate ligament reconstructions with hamstring tendon and patellar tendon autograft: a controlled, prospective trial. Am J Sports Med. 2007;35(4):564–74.
39. Bosch U, et al. Ätiologie der Arthrofibrose. Arthroskopie. 1999;12(5):215–21.
40. Claes S, et al. The "ligamentization" process in anterior cruciate ligament reconstruction: what happens to the human graft? A systematic review of the literature. Am J Sports Med. 2011;39(11):2476–83.
41. Riaz O, et al. Quadriceps Tendon-Bone or Patellar Tendon-Bone Autografts When Reconstructing the Anterior Cruciate Ligament: A Meta-analysis. Clin J Sport Med. 2018;28(3):316–24.

25

Comparison of 2 femoral tunnel drilling techniques in anterior cruciate ligament reconstruction

Yunhang Geng[1,2] and Pengzhou Gai[2*]

Abstract

Background: To evaluate the length and position of femoral tunnel,and exam whether knee stability and clinical functional outcomes are superior in AMP method.

Methods: From August 2014 to February 2015, we prospectively recruited 104 patients undergoing anterior cruciate ligament reconstruction. They were randomized to anteromedial portal or transtibial method. All patients underwent Lysholm score, International Knee Documentation Committee score,Tegner score at pre-operative and last follow-up point as subjective assessment of clinical function. The Lachman test, the Pivot-shift test and KT-1000 were performed at the last follow-up as a evaluation of knee joint stability. We measured the length of femoral tunnel intraoperatively and at 1 week post-operatively, CT-based three-dimensional reconstruction was used to assess femoral tunnel location.

Results: The average follow-up time of anteromedial portal group was 25.7 ± 6.8 months (range:12–36.5 months), and the average follow-up time of the transtibial group was 24.9 ± 6.0 months (range:12–37 months). There was no significant difference between the groups pre-operative Lysholm score, IKDC score and Tegner scores. Both groups showed significantly improvement in these clinical function scores at follow up for their ACL reconstruction. However, there was no significant difference in the function scores between the two groups at last follow up. However, the mean femoral tunnel length in the anteromedial portal group was significantly shorter than that in the transtibial group. And tunnel location was significantly lower and deeper with the anteromedial portal technique than with the transtibial technique.

Conclusion: The use of anteromedial portal method resulted in a significantly lower and deeper placement of the femoral tunnel, and a shorter tunnel length compared to the transtibial method. However, there was no statistical difference in terms of clinical function and knee joint stability between the anteromedial portal method and the transtibial method.

Keywords: Anterior cruciate ligament, Anteromedial portal, Transtibial, Femoral tunnel

* Correspondence: gpz1731@163.com
[2]Department of Orthopaedic Surgery, Qindao University Medical College Affiliated Yantai Yuhuangding Hospital, Yantai, Shandong, People's Republic of China
Full list of author information is available at the end of the article

Background

The anterior cruciate ligament (ACL) is an important static stabilizer of the knee joint and plays an important role in both anteroposterior and rotational stability [1]. Injury seriously affects this stability, requiring surgical reconstruction as the main method for restoring knee stability and function. The transtibial (TT) method is widely used for placing the femoral tunnel integral to ACL reconstruction. However, this approach can limit the accuracy of femoral tunnel placement, and failure of the reconstruction may be influenced most by inaccurate tunnel placement [2, 3]. The anteromedial portal (AMP) approach is becoming more popular as femoral tunnel placement is not limited by the tibial tunnel, resulting in easier and potentially more accurate location of the femoral tunnel in the ACL anatomical footprint [4–7]. Differences have been shown in femoral tunnel location between AMP and TT methods in previous retrospective studies [5, 8–10]. And Gadikota HR et al. [11] used a corpse-controlled study, and findings of this study indicated that a larger posterolateral bundle coverage was achieved by the AM portal than by the TT technique and center of the tunnel created by the AM portal was closer to the native ACL footprint center than the center of the TT technique tunnel. In addition to, meta-analysis of Riboh JC et al. [12] also demonstrated that more anatomic graft placement with AMP method.

Although graft placement with AMP method is more anatomic,the length of the femoral tunnel is statistically significantly shorter with the AMP approach compared to TT method [5, 8, 9, 13]. A shorter femoral tunnel (less than 25 mm) makes the femoral tendon - bone effective healing length shorter, and leading to the smaller the healing strength [14].

Nowadays, there is still controversy about the stability of the knee joint between two methods. Musahl V et al. [15] used a corpse-controlled study, and findings of this study indicated that knee kinematics was closer to the intact knee with the AMP technique. The prospective randomized comparative study of Hussein M et al. [16] demonstrated that anteroposterior and rotational stability of the knee was better with the AMP technique. The meta-analysis of Chen H et al. [17] and Riboh JC et al. [12] both demonstrated that with the AMP technique was better than that with the TT technique in terms of postoperative stability. However,retrospective study of Rezazadeh S et al. [1] demonstrated that anteroposterior and rotational stability did not differ statistically between two methods. And, the prospective randomized comparative study of Bohn MB et al. [18] demonstrated that no significant difference in rotational stability walking, running, and pivoting was seen between two techniques at 1-year follow-up.

Similarly, there is still controversy about the function of the knee between two methods. Previous retrospective studies [1, 6, 7, 19, 20] have not definitively demonstrated a resultant clinical superiority in knee function with AMP technique. And, the prospective randomized comparative study of Hussein M et al. [16] and meta-analysis of Riboh JC et al. [12] both demonstrated that there was no statistical difference between the two groups on knee function. However,the retrospective cohort study of Kilinc BE et al. [21] demonstrated that ACL reconstruction with AMP method was better than with the TT technique in term of clinical function. The meta-analysis of Chen H et al. [17] also demonstrated that with the AMP technique is better than that with the TT technique in terms of functional recovery of the knee.

Our research is to evaluate the length and position of femoral tunnel,and exam whether knee stability and clinical functional outcomes are superior in AMP method.

Methods

Patients

From August 2014 to February 2015, we prospectively recruited patients undergoing autologous hamstring tendon ACL reconstruction. ACL damage was diagnosed by clinical manifestations and MRI (GE3T) findings. Inclusion criteria were at least 1 year post-operative follow up, normal contralateral knee joint, no accompanying fracture. Exclusion criteria were combined anterior and posterior cruciate ligament injury, accompanying collateral ligament injury, osteoarthritis and revision surgery. Prior to the study, according to the literature and our own experience, it was calculated that there must be 48 patients in each group when we accepted the difference in tunnel location between groups being 2% (assuming a standard deviation of 3.5%, at 80% power and α error of 0.05). According to our own experience, considering almost 20% rate of lost of follow up, a total of 120 patients were required for the study. Randomisation was performed according to a random number table, with even numbers in the AMP group and odd numbers in the TT group. Initially there were 63 patients in AMP group and 57 patients in TT group. Because of lost of follow-up, 7 patients in AMP group were excluded and 9 patients in TT group were excluded. Finally, 56 were included in AMP group and 48 were included in TT group. The population assessed is predominantly male. This study was approved by the Qindao University Medical College Affiliated Yantai Yuhuangding Hospital Ethics Committee (Numbered:YHY2014065), and all patients signed informed consent. This study has been registered in Chinese Clinical Trial Registry (Numbered: ChiCTR1800014874. URL: http://www.chictr.org.cn/showproj.aspx?proj=25277. UTN: U1111-1210-8275 Registrant: Pengzhou Gai).

Surgical procedure

All operations were performed under general anesthesia or epidural anesthesia by the same orthopaedic surgeon. Arthroscopy was used to further confirm the diagnosis by conventional anteromedial and anterolateral portals. The ruptured ACL was cleaned using a planer. Contours of the intercondylar notch were observed with knee extension at 30 °. If the intercondylar notch was narrow, it was expanded with 5.5 mm drill to an inverted "U" shape, although this was not commonly required in our cohort. A medial longitudinal incision over the tibial tubercle was performed to harvest Semitendinosus and Gracilis tendon, which were dissected, woven, preprocessed and reserved. The tibial tunnel locator was placed with the outer end located at least 3 cm below the joint line and 1.5 cm medial to the tibial tubercle (inside the tendon incision), and the inner end located at the center of insertion of the anterior cruciate ligament. The guide pin was inserted, and the cannulated reamer was selected according to the graft diameter. Then the tunnel was drilled along the guide pin.

For TT method the femoral tunnel locator was placed via tibial tunnel under arthroscopy and for AMP method via anteromedial portal under arthroscopy. The posterior wall of the femoral tunnel is at least 2 mm from the posterior cortex of the femoral condyle. A guide pin is then placed and cannulated reamer selected according to the graft diameter. Tunnel depth of drilling is approximately 2.1 cm, then beyond this a 0.45 cm cannulated reamer is used. A depth gauge (Smith & Nephew) was used to hook the outer cortex of the femoral tunnel and total length of the tunnel recorded (Fig. 1). Grafts were transferred to the tunnel through wire and suture. Suitable Endobutton (Smith & Nephew) was used based on the length of the femoral tunnel. Intrafix (Depuy) was used according to the diameter of the tibial tunnel. Finally the ligament isometry and the intercondylar notch impingement was checked.

Evaluation methods

All evaluations were performed by one doctor who was blind to the treatment group. All patients underwent Lysholm score, International Knee Documentation Committee (IKDC) score and Tegner score at pre-operative and final follow-up points as subjective assessment of clinical function. The Lachman test, the Pivot-shift test and KT-1000 (MEDmetric Corporation, San Diego, California) were performed at the last follow-up as a evaluation of knee joint stability. We measured the length of femoral tunnel intraoperatively. And after 1 week post-operatively, all patients were performed CT-based three-dimensional reconstruction (GE64 CT AW4.3 workstation, MIMICS) to assess the location of the femoral tunnel. Measurement of femoral tunnel location used the quadrant method described by Bernard M et al. [22] (Fig. 2).

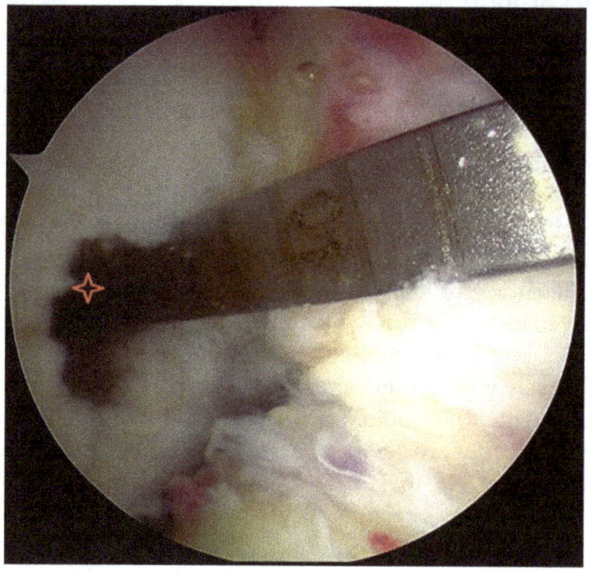

Fig. 1 A depth gauge was used to hook the outer cortex of the femoral tunnel and intraoperative measurement of femoral tunnel depth is seen(*)

Statistical analysis

SPSS 20.0 (SPSS Inc., Chicago, IL) software and G*Power (3.1.9.2) software was used for statistical analysis. To compare age, follow-up time, time from injury to surgery, body mass index (BMI), Lysholm score, IKDC score, Tegner

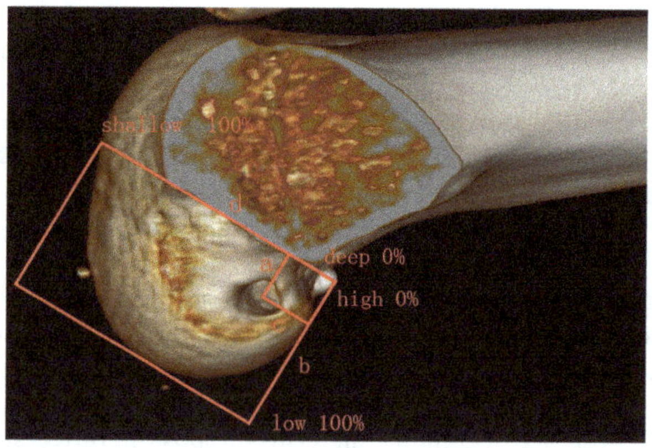

Fig. 2 Blumensaat's line is represented by 'd',with 'b' representing the line perpendicular to it. 'a' is the distance between the femoral tunnel center to Blumensaat's line, and 'c' is the distance between the femoral tunnel center to b. Thus, a/b represents the height ratio, i.e., the ratio of the distance between the femoral tunnel center and the top of intercondylar notch to the total height of intercondylar notch; and c/d represents the depth ratio, i.e., the ratio of the distance between the femoral tunnel center and posterior articular surface of femoral lateral condyle to the total depth of intercondylar notch

Table 1 General Information

Variate	AMP group	TT group	*P* value
Patient(n)	56	48	
Gender (male:female,n)	46:10	40:8	.873
Age (Mean ± SD, range, year)	29.6 ± 11.7 (18–65)	31.8 ± 11.0 (19–69)	.346
Follow-up time(Mean ± SD,range, months)	25.7 ± 6.8 (12–36.5)	24.9 ± 6.0 (12–37)	.529
Time from injury to surgery(Mean ± SD,range, weeks)	9.8 ± 6.3 (0.5–24)	10.6 ± 6.8 (0.5–28)	.557
Injured knee (left:right,n)	26:30	22:26	.952
BMI(Mean ± SD,range, kg/m^2)	24.1 ± 3.2 (20–32)	23.8 ± 3.1 (18–31)	.636

AMP:Anteromedial portal, *TT*:Transtibial, *BMI*:Body mass index

score, KT-1000, tunnel length and tunnel location, unpaired T test was used. For gender and injury side of the knee, chi-square test was selected, and Mann-Whitney rank test for the Lachman and Pivot-shift test comparisons. Statistical significance was at $P < 0.05$.

Results

The average follow-up time of anteromedial portal group was 25.7 ± 6.8 months (range:12–36.5 months), and the average follow-up time of the transtibial group was 24.9 ± 6.0 months (range:12–37 months). 24 underwent notchplasty in AMP group and 17 underwent notchplasty in TT group.

General demographic data were not significantly different between the two groups (Table 1).

There was no significant difference between the groups pre-operative Lysholm score, IKDC score and Tegner scores. Both groups showed significantly improvement in these clinical function scores at follow up for their ACL reconstruction. However, there was no significant difference in the function scores between the two groups at last follow up. (Table 2 and Table 3).

In terms of Lachman test, Pivot-shift test and KT-1000 for assessment of knee joint stability, there was no statistical difference at the last follow-up between the two groups (Table 4).

The mean femoral tunnel length in the AMP group was significantly shorter than that in the TT group. And tunnel location was significantly lower and deeper with the AMP technique than with the TT method (Table 5).

Discussion

Previous studies demonstrated that [5, 8–12] center of the tunnel created by the AM portal was closer to the native ACL footprint center than the center of the TT technique tunnel. And although graft placement with AMP method is more anatomic,the length of the femoral tunnel is statistically significantly shorter with the AMP approach compared to TT method [5, 8, 9, 13]. In addition to, controversy continues as to whether the AMP or TT method is superior for ACL reconstruction in terms of both stability and function of knee [1, 5–9, 12, 16–21]. The most important finding of our study was that the use of AMP method resulted in a significantly lower and deeper placement of the femoral tunnel, and a shorter tunnel length compared to the TT method. However, there was no statistical difference in terms of clinical function and knee joint stability between the AMP method and TT method.

In our study there was no statistically significant difference in the Lysholm score, the IKDC score and the Tegner score between the AMP group and TT group at last follow-up. Similarly,previous retrospective studies [1, 6, 7, 19, 20] have not definitively demonstrated a resultant clinical superiority in knee joint function with AMP technique. And, the prospective randomized comparative study of Hussein M et al. [16] and meta-analysis of Riboh JC et al. [12] both demonstrated that there is no statistical difference between the two groups on knee function. However,the retrospective cohort study of Kilinc BE et al. [21] demonstrated that ACL reconstruction with AMP method was better than with the TT technique in term of clinical function. The meta-analysis of Chen H et al. [17] also demonstrated that with the AM technique was better than that with the TT technique in terms of functional recovery of the knee.

Table 2 Clinical function score between two groups

	Pre-operative			Last follow-up		
	AMP group	TT group	*P* value	AMP group	TT group	*P* value
Lysholm score (Mean ± SD,range)	45.9 ± 6.6(24–70)	45.4 ± 6.2(23–67)	.729	93.3 ± 5.0(75–97)	91.6 ± 6.5(68–97)	.123
IKDC score (Mean ± SD,range)	35.7 ± 6.3(15–55)	36.1 ± 6.6(18–55)	.703	89.5 ± 8.8(50–97)	87.4 ± 10.0(50–95)	.273
Tegner score (Mean ± SD,range)	5.0 ± 1.0(1–7)	5.0 ± 1.1 (1–6)	.778	6.8 ± 1.4 (2–8)	6.3 ± 1.4 (2–8)	.081

AMP:Anteromedial portal, *TT*:Transtibial, *IKDC*: International Knee Documentation Committee

Table 3 Clinical function score between pre-operative and post-operative

	AMP group			TT group		
	Pre-operative	Last follow-up	*P* value	Pre- operative	Last follow-up	*P* value
Lysholm score (Mean ± SD,range)	45.9 ± 6.6(24–70)	93.3 ± 5.0(75–97)	<.01	45.4 ± 6.2(23–67)	91.6 ± 6.5(68–97)	<.01
IKDC score (Mean ± SD,range)	35.7 ± 6.3(15–55)	89.5 ± 8.8 (50–97)	<.01	36.1 ± 6.6(18–55)	87.4 ± 10.0(50–95)	<.01
Tegner score (Mean ± SD,range)	5.0 ± 1.0(1–7)	6.8 ± 1.4 (2–8)	<.01	5.0 ± 1.1 (1–6)	6.3 ± 1.4 (2–8)	<.01

AMP:Anteromedial portal, *TT*:Transtibial *IKDC*: International Knee Documentation Committee

We found no statistically significant difference in the Lachman test, the Pivot-shift test and the KT-1000 measurement between the AMP group and TT group. Similarly,the retrospective study of Rezazadeh S et al. [1] demonstrated that anteroposterior and rotational stability did not differ statistically between two methods. And,the prospective randomized comparative study of Bohn MB et al. [18] also demonstrated that no significant difference in rotational stability walking, running, and pivoting was seen between two techniques at 1-year follow-up. However, Musahl V et al. [15] used a corpse-controlled study, and demonstrated that knee kinematics was closer to the intact knee with the AMP technique. The prospective randomized comparative study of Hussein M et al. [16] also demonstrated that anteroposterior and rotational stability of the knee was better with the AMP technique. The meta-analysis of Chen H et al. [17] and Riboh JC et al. [12] both demonstrated that with the AM technique were better than that with the TT technique in terms of postoperative stability.

TT method has the advantages of a simpler operation with shorter operation time, small incision and parallel tibial-femoral tunnel allowing for easy graft passage [23]. However, the most important drawback is that due to the limitations of the tibial tunnel, it is difficult to accurately locate the femoral tunnel in the anatomical ACL footprint, and the femoral tunnel is often located near the top of the intercondylar notch [23]. This is deemed a major factor for failure of ACL reconstruction [2]. In addition with this method, the surgeon may compromise the tibial tunnel in order to achieve the required femoral tunnel location [23, 24]. This can then result in short tibial tunneling that affects the fixation of the graft at the tibial end [24]. The AMP method not only makes it easier to locate the femoral tunnel in the ACL anatomical footprint, it also enables a more oblique femoral tunnel [25], reduces tunnel widening and can help retain residual ACL fibers [23]. But the AMP approach can result in a shorter femoral tunnel [25] and difficulty passing graft material through the tunnel [23]. Technical requirements are high and there is a greater risk of posterior breach in the condylar cortex or damage to the posterior articular cartilage and common peroneal nerve [23, 26].

Table 4 Knee joint stability assessment

	AMP group (*n* = 56)	TT group (*n* = 48)	*P* value
Lachman test			.630
Negative	44	36	
1+	12	11	
2+	0	1	
3+	0	0	
Pivot-shift test			.146
Negative	44	32	
1+	12	14	
2+	0	2	
3+	0	0	
KT 1000 (Mean ± SD,range,mm)	1.5 ± 0.9 (1–4)	1.6 ± 0.8 (1–5)	.455

AMP Anteromedial portal, *TT* Transtibial

The length of the femoral tunnel measured in this study was statistically significantly shorter with the AMP approach compared to TT method. A shorter femoral tunnel (less than 25 mm) makes the femoral tendon - bone effective healing length shorter, and leading to the smaller the healing strength [14]. However, the results of this paper and Shin YS et al. [9] show that the mean length of femoral tunnel prepared by AMP method, although shorter, is still greater than 30 mm, and none of the femoral tunnel lengths were shorter than 25 mm. Larson AI et al. [8] used a corpse-controlled study, and their results also show AMP group average femoral tunnel length greater than 30 mm. Osti M et al. [5] also demonstrate an average femoral tunnel length above 30 mm but suggest caution, as the AMP group($n = 32$) did have a higher, though not statistically significant proportion(6%) with a femoral tunnel shorter than 25 mm. The corpse-controlled study of Bedi A et al. [13] showed that 41.7% of the femoral tunnel lengths in the AMP group ($n = 12$) were shorter than 25 mm and with the knee flexed to 120 °, the mean length of the femoral tunnel prepared by the AMP method was 21.3 mm.

In this paper, the femoral tunnel location was evaluated using CT-based three-dimensional reconstruction and the quadrant method described by Bernard M et al. [22]. Tunnel location in our study was significantly a deeper, lower and more anatomical with the AMP

Table 5 Tunnel parameters

	AMP group	TT group	*P* value
Tunnel length (Mean ± SD,range,mm)	37.3 ± 3.9 (28–46)	42.0 ± 4.8 (32–55)	<.01
Tunnel position			
Depth ratio (Mean ± SD,range,%)	20.3 ± 2.0 (17–23)	22.1 ± 2.1 (19–26)	<.01
Height ratio (Mean ± SD,range,%)	33.3 ± 1.8 (30–36)	30.2 ± 1.7 (27–33)	<.01

AMP:Anteromedial portal, *TT*:Transtibial

technique than with the TT method. Similarly, Osti M et al. [5] although a non randomized study, showed that tunnel location was significantly lower with the AMP technique but there was no statistically significant difference in depth between the two methods. Larson AI et al. [8] and Gadikota HR et al. [11] used a corpse-controlled study, and both demonstrated the location of femoral tunnel was significantly lower and deeper. In addition to, the meta-analysis of Riboh JC et al. [12] also demonstrated that more anatomic graft placement with AMP method. The deeper and lower the femoral tunnel, the more inclined the graft, which not only maintains the anteroposterior stability, but also the rotational stability. The evidence suggests overall that the AMP approach better locates the femoral tunnel in an anatomical footprint [6, 7, 11, 12, 19], with a deeper and lower tunnel location that is potential superior for maintaining the stability of the knee. This should translate clinically into better outcomes on knee stability testing. However, our study was not able to demonstrate this difference to statistical significance in term of knee stability testing.

Our studies strengths include a prospective randomized design, with one surgeon performing the procedures to reduce operative variability and the use of CT-based three-dimensional reconstruction as a recognized and reliable method of assessing femoral tunnel location. Our study includes larger group sizes than the majority of other studies, and extends the evidence whether length and position of femoral tunnel, knee stability and clinical functional outcomes are superior in AMP method.

The limitations include a relatively short follow-up time, with a mean around 25 months. It is therefore not possible to comment on differences in stability or function that may or may not be apparent over a longer timeframe. Although larger than most studies on this topic, the sample size is still relatively small, and thus may not be able to demonstrate significant differences between the groups. In addition, as reflective of the population most affected by these types of ACL injury, the population assessed is young and predominantly male, without other concurrent injuries or osteoarthritis and therefore findings may not apply to those patients that fall outside of these characteristics. For future directions a prospective randomized trial with larger sample size and longer term follow up is required. An assessment of other aspects such as operative times, costs and complications including graft failure rates would also be informative in recommending a particular method.

Our current study demonstrated that the AMP approach provides a deeper, lower and more anatomically placed femoral tunnel location compared to TT method. AMP technique produces a shorter tunnel, which surgeons performing this procedure should be mindful of. Those undergoing AMP repair were not proven statistically significant in term of function and stability of knee, and as such the AMP approach cannot be conclusively declared the superior method.

Conclusion

The use of AMP method resulted in a significantly lower and deeper placement of the femoral tunnel, and a shorter tunnel length compared to the TT technique. However, there was no statistical difference in terms of clinical function and knee joint stability between the AMP method and TT method.

Abbreviations

ACL: Anterior cruciate ligament; AMP: Anteromedial portal; BMI: Body mass index; IKDC: International Knee Documentation Committee; TT: Transtibial

Acknowledgements

Thanks are due to Kun Shan for valuable discussion.

Funding

All authors have not received grant support or research funding.

Authors' contributions

YH G and PZ G conceived and designed the study; and YH G analysed the data. YH G wrote the paper; YH G and PZ G reviewed and edited the manuscript. All authors read and approved the manuscript.

Consent for publication

Not applicable.

Competing interests

The authors declare no competing interests.

Author details

[1]Qingdao University Medical College, Qingdao, China. [2]Department of Orthopaedic Surgery, Qindao University Medical College Affiliated Yantai Yuhuangding Hospital, Yantai, Shandong, People's Republic of China.

References

1. Rezazadeh S, Ettehadi H, Vosoughi AR. Outcome of arthroscopic single-bundle anterior cruciate ligament reconstruction: anteromedial portal technique versus transtibial drilling technique. Musculoskelet Surg. 2016;100: 37–41.
2. Marchant BG, Noyes FR, Barber-Westin SD, et al. Prevalence of nonanatomical graft placement in a series of failed anterior cruciate ligament reconstructions. Am J Sports Med. 2010;38:1987–96.
3. Kopf S, Forsythe B, Wong AK, et al. Transtibial ACL reconstruction technique fails to position drill tunnels anatomically in vivo 3D CT study. Knee Surg Sports Traumatol Arthrosc. 2012;20:2200–7.
4. Noh JH, Roh YH, Yang BG, et al. Femoral tunnel position on conventional magnetic resonance imaging after anterior cruciate ligament reconstruction in young men: transtibial technique versus anteromedial portal technique. Arthroscopy. 2013;29:882–90.
5. Osti M, Krawinkel A, Ostermann M, et al. Femoral and tibial graft tunnel parameters after transtibial, anteromedial portal, and outside-in single-bundle anterior cruciate ligament reconstruction. Am J Sports Med. 2015;43: 2250–8.
6. Azboy I, Demirtas A, Gem M, et al. A comparison of the anteromedial and transtibial drilling technique in ACL reconstruction after a short-term follow-up. Arch Orthop Trauma Surg. 2014;13:963–9.
7. Sukur E, Akman YE, Senel A, et al. Comparing Transtibial and anteromedial drilling techniques for single-bundle anterior cruciate ligament reconstruction. Open Orthop J. 2016;10:481–9.
8. Larson AI, Bullock DP, Pevny T. Comparison of 4 femoral tunnel drilling techniques in anterior cruciate ligament reconstruction. Arthroscopy. 2012; 28:972–9.
9. Shin YS, Ro KH, Jeon JH, et al. Graft-bending angle and femoral tunnel length after single-bundle anterior cruciate ligament reconstruction: comparison of the transtibial, anteromedial portal and outside-in techniques. Bone Joint J. 2014; 96-B:743–751.
10. Yau WP, Fok AW, Yee DK. Tunnel positions in transportal versus transtibial anterior cruciate ligament reconstruction: a case-control magnetic resonance imaging study. Arthroscopy. 2013;29:1047–52.
11. Gadikota HR, Sim JA, Hosseini A, et al. The relationship between femoral tunnels created by the transtibial, anteromedial portal, and outside-in techniques and the anterior cruciate ligament footprint. Am J Sports Med. 2012;40:882–8.
12. Riboh JC, Hasselblad V, Godin JA, et al. Transtibial versus independent drilling techniques for anterior cruciate ligament reconstruction: a systematic review, meta-analysis, and meta-regression. Am J Sports Med. 2013;41:2693–702.
13. Bedi A, Raphael B, Maderazo A, et al. Transtibial versus anteromedial portal drilling for anterior cruciate ligament reconstruction: a cadaveric study of femoral tunnel length and obliquity. Arthroscopy. 2010;26:342–50.
14. Greis PE, Burks RT, Bachus K, et al. The influence of tendon length and fit on the strength of a tendon-bone tunnel complex. A biomechanical and histologic study in the dog. Am J Sports Med. 2001;29:493–7.
15. Musahl V, Plakseychuk A, VanScyoc A, et al. Varying femoral tunnels between the anatomical footprint and isometric positions: effect on kinematics of the anterior cruciate ligament-reconstructed knee. Am J Sports Med. 2005;33:712–8.
16. Hussein M, van Eck CF, Cretnik A, et al. Prospective randomized clinical evaluation of conventional single-bundle, anatomic single-bundle, and anatomic double-bundle anterior cruciate ligament reconstruction: 281 cases with 3- to 5-year follow-up. Am J Sports Med. 2012;40:512–20.
17. Chen H, Tie K, Qi Y, et al. Anteromedial versus transtibial technique in single-bundle autologous hamstring ACL reconstruction: a meta-analysis of prospective randomized controlled trials. J Orthop Surg Res. 2017;12:167–79.
18. Bohn MB, Sorensen H, Petersen MK, et al. Rotational laxity after anatomical ACL reconstruction measured by 3-D motion analysis: a prospective randomized clinical trial comparing anatomic and nonanatomic ACL reconstruction techniques. Knee Surg Sports Traumatol Arthrosc. 2015;23: 3473–81.
19. Tasdemir Z, Gulabi D, Saglam F, et al. Does the anteromedial portal provide clinical superiority compared to the transtibial portal in anterior cruciate ligament reconstruction in nonprofessional athletes in short-term follow-up? Acta Orthop Traumatol Turc. 2015;49:483–91.
20. Franceschi F, Papalia R, Rizzello G, et al. Anteromedial portal versus transtibial drilling techniques in anterior cruciate ligament reconstruction: any clinical relevance? A retrospective Comparative Study Arthroscopy. 2013;29:1330–7.
21. Kilinc BE, Kara A, Oc Y, et al. Transtibial vs anatomical single bundle technique for anterior cruciate ligament reconstruction: a retrospective cohort study. Int J Surg. 2016;29:62–9.
22. Bernard M, Hertel P, Hornung H, et al. Femoral insertion of the ACL. Radiographic quadrant method Am J Knee Surg. 1997;10:14–21.
23. Robin BN, Jani SS, Marvil SC, et al. Advantages and disadvantages of Transtibial, anteromedial portal, and outside-in femoral tunnel Drilling in Single-Bundle Anterior Cruciate Ligament Reconstruction: a systematic review. Arthroscopy. 2015;31:1412–7.
24. Heming JF, Rand J, Steiner ME. Anatomical limitations of transtibial drilling in anterior cruciate ligament reconstruction. Am J Sports Med. 2007;35: 1708–15.
25. Lee DH, Kim HJ, Ahn HS, et al. Comparison of femoral tunnel length and obliquity between Transtibial, anteromedial portal, and outside-in surgical techniques in single-bundle anterior cruciate ligament reconstruction: a meta-analysis. Arthroscopy. 2016;32:142–50.
26. Otani M, Nozaki M, Kobayashi M, et al. Comparative risk of common peroneal nerve injury in far anteromedial portal drilling and transtibial drilling in anatomical double-bundle ACL reconstruction. Knee Surg Sports Traumatol Arthrosc. 2012;20:838–43.

26

Balloon kyphoplasty and additional anterior odontoid screw fixation for treatment of unstable osteolytic lesions of the vertebral body C2

Anna Voelker*, Nicolas H. von der Hoeh and Christoph-Eckhard Heyde

Abstract

Background: Unstable osteolytic lesions of the occipitocervical junction are rare and may occur in hematological malignancy or vertebral hemangioma, among others. Different case reports have been published about vertebroplasty for treatment of spinal metastases of the upper cervical spine. Only few cases concern balloon kyphoplasty of C2. We present a consecutive case series including four patients with an osteolytic lesion of the dens axis and describe a technical note for balloon kyphoplasty of C2 and an additional anterior odontoid screw fixation.

Methods: Four consecutive patients with an osteolytic lesion of the vertebral body of C2 were treated by anterior balloon kyphoplasty and additional anterior odontoid screw fixation of the dens axis. The radiological imaging showed a lytic process of the vertebral body C2 with no vertebral collapse but involvement of more than 50% of the vertebral body in all patients.

Results: Two cases of potentially unstable osteolytic lesions of C2 by myeloma, one case with metastatic osteolytic lesion of C2 by adenocarcinoma of the colon and one patient with vertebral hemangioma located in C2 were presented to our clinic. In all cases, surgical treatment with an anterior balloon kyphoplasty of C2 and an additional anterior, bicortical odontoid screw placement was performed. Control x-rays showed sufficient osteosynthesis and cement placement in the vertebral body C2.

Discussion: Anterior balloon kyphoplasty and anterior odontoid screw placement is a safe treatment option for large osteolytic lesions of C2. The additional odontoid screw placement has the advantage of providing more stabilization and may prevent late complications, like odontoid fractures. For patients with potentially unstable or large osteolytic lesions of the dens without spinal cord compression or neurological symptoms we recommend the placement of an anterior odontoid screw when performing a balloon kyphoplasty. Level of evidence: - IV: retrospective or historical series.

Keywords: Osteolytic lesion C2, Metastasis dens, Anterior odontoid screw, Balloon kyphoplasty C2, Myeloma lesion dens axis, Cervical spine

* Correspondence: anna.voelker@medizin.uni-leipzig.de
University Hospital Leipzig, Department of Orthopedic, Trauma and Plastic Surgery, Liebigstrasse 20, 04103 Leipzig, Germany

Background

Metastatic lesions of the cervical spine are rare, especially at the occipitocervical junction (C0-C2). Metastatic spread occurs predominately at the thoracic and lumbal spine because of the better blood supply. Less than 1% of spinal metastasis occur at the craniocervical junction [1].

Nowadays, improved cancer treatment and longer life expectancy of tumor patients lead to an increasing number of this medical condition.

Most patients present with symptoms of heavy neck pain and a reduction of cervical motion. Neurological deficits are rare.

Myeloma is the most common underlying disease that leads to osteolytic lesions of the spine.

Bone destruction due to lytic lesions and generalized osteopenia may result in collapse of the vertebra [2]. Hence, pathological fracture of the vertebra body with neurological deficits, based on spinal cord compression, is the feared complication [2].

Literature describes different treatment options for treatment of C2 metastasis. Non- operative therapy includes immobilization, chemo- and external beam radiation therapy [3]. A variety of surgical procedures were published, including posterior instrumentation [4], open vertebroplasty by anterior approach [5–7], vertebroplasty by anterolateral approach either conventionally or percutaneously [8, 9], transoral vertebroplasty [10, 11], open dorsal vertebroplasty of the dens axis [12] and balloon kyphoplasty [13] .

One case report described balloon kyphoplasty and anterior screw fixation in a pathological fracture of the dens, induced by renal cell carcinoma [14]. Another case report described the treatment of a pathological fracture involving the odontoid process with radiofrequence thermoablation, cement augmentation and odontoid screw fixation [15]. Furthermore, Terraux et al. published a case report about balloon kyphoplasty and anterior screw fixation of odontoid fractures in two elderly patients [16]. Blondel et al. published a case series about anterolateral kyphoplasty in the management of cervical metastasis, including one case with a pathological fracture of C2 treated with kyphoplasty and an anterior screw [17]. In special cases unconventional procedures have been described. Bourgli used bone cement filling around a screw from C3 to odontoid in a case with anterior body collapse of C2 and a C1/C2 instability [18].

So far, no publication on balloon kyphoplasty and anterior odontoid screw fixation can be found for treatment of potentially unstable osteolytic lesions of C2.

We demonstrate a technical note for balloon kyphoplasty of C2 in combination with an anterior odontoid screw in two cases of osteolytic lesions in C2 by myeloma, in one case with metastatic osteolytic lesion by adenocarcinoma of the colon and in one case of large osteolytic process in C2 by hemangioma.

Methods

Four Patients with unstable osteolytic lesion of the dens axis were treated with balloon kyphoplasty of C2 and an additional anterior, bicortical odontoid screw placement. All patients were presented to our clinic with neck pain. Imaging including x-ray, Computed tomography scan (CT-Scan) and Magnetic resonance imaging (MRI) of the cervical spine was performed. The definition of spinal instability was calculated by the Spine Instability Neoplastic Score (SINS). The radiological imaging showed a lytic process of the vertebral body C2 with no vertebral collapse but more than 50% involvement of the vertebral body in all patients. Surgical procedures were performed in the manner as described below.

Technical note of balloon kyphoplasty of C2 and an additional anterior, bicortical odontoid screw placement

General anesthesia was performed with orotracheal intubation. The patient was placed on a radiolucent table in supine position with padding under the shoulders to induce reclination of the neck. Extension of the cervical spine was achieved by positioning the head in a horseshoe head rest. We used a gauze bandage in-between the jaw of the patient to obtain adequate AP view.

Two c-arm X-ray units were used, one in anterior-posterior, and one in lateral view (Fig. 1).

After a free K-wire placement on the skin, to simulate the trajectory for the screw placement a unilateral transverse skin incision was made on the right side at the C5 level. The platysma was cut in longitudinal direction, as was the superficial cervical fascia. Atraumatic preparation was performed along the medial border of the sternocleidomastoid muscle to the middle cervical fascia. We approached the anterior surface of the spine after opening the middle cervical fascia and made a blunt dissection medial to the carotid artery, and lateral to the esophagus and trachea.

The inferior edge of the C2 vertebral body was palpated and a K-wire was drilled centrally into the odontoid process bicortically under biplanar fluoroscopy, using a cannulated drill bit system (2,7 mm) to prepare the screw hole bicortically.

Following this, a second K-wire was placed on the anterior, inferior edge of C2, next to the screw hole in the area of the osteolytic lesion, to prepare the kyphoplasty working canal. Under fluoroscopy guidance, the K-wire was drilled in oblique and cranial direction into the osteolytic lesion, without penetrating the dorsal cortical bone of C2. Step by step, a cannulated drill bit system enlarged the entry point and the canal of the kyphoplasty trocar (2,7 mm and 3,5 mm drill bit). After removal of the second K-wire, the Jamshidi-Needle (*Kyphon*, Medtronic, USA) was placed into the osteolytic lesion under fluoroscopy guidance. A biopsy was

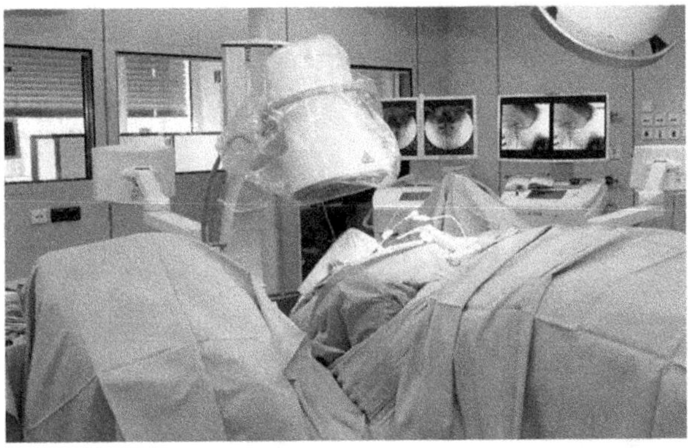

Fig. 1 This picture shows the set-up in the OR with two c-arm X-ray units for anterior-posterior view, as well as for lateral view of the dens axis

performed with the hand drill for histopathologic investigation. Thereupon, the balloon was placed into the body of C2 through the working cannula and was expanded with contrast. (Fig. 2). Subsequently, the balloon was deflated, removed and the cavity was filled with cement, using the *Kyphon* cement fillers (Fig. 3). We used polymethylmethacrylate (PMMA) cement with high primary viscosity to prevent cement leakage. The used cement volume varied from case to case between 1,5 to 2,5 ml. Lastly, a cannulated 4.0 mm self-tapping screw was placed bicortically over the first K-wire. All single steps were performed with biplanar fluoroscopy guidance (Fig. 3). Example radiation exposure: area dose c-arm number one: 128,1 cGy*cm2; area dose c-arm number two: 95,7 cGy*cm2.

X-ray documentation showed satisfactory filling of the osteolytic lesion with cement and a good central screw placement. A soft collar was placed post operatively and the patient was monitored in the intensive care unit for 24 h after prompt extubation.

Results

Case 1: A 76-year-old woman was presented to our clinic with severe neck pain and paresthesia in the left hand. Next to the multiple osteolytic lesions of the whole spine, CT-scan and MRI showed an unstable osteolytic lesion in C2 (16 mm × 11 mm × 15 mm) (Fig. 4) and an osteolytic lesion of C7 with destruction of the pedicle and with a spinal stenosis. First, we performed dorsal stabilization C5-Th2 with laminectomy of C7, based on mild neurological deficits in the left hand. The histopathological investigation confirmed suspected myeloma (Durie/Salmon Classification Stage III, Karnofsky Performance Score: 60%). Balloon kyphoplasty and anterior screw fixation of C2 was performed 2 weeks later. The patient recovered well. Neck pain diminished post operatively and x-rays showed good placement of the odontoid screw and cement in C2. Some cement leakage was detected posteriorly, however without neurological symptoms (Fig. 5). A soft collar was worn for 2 weeks postoperative. After wound healing, the patient was treated systemically by hematologist.

Case 2: An 82-year-old female patient with known myeloma (Durie/Salmon Classification Stage III, Karnofsky Performance Score: 70%) was presented in our outpatient clinic by her treating radiologist because of an osteolytic lesion in C2 (14 mm × 11 mm × 16 mm) (Fig. 6). The patient had a history of mild neck pain. The osteolytic lesion was detected during myeloma CT-scan staging. A MRI of the entire spine showed no further osteolytic lesions.

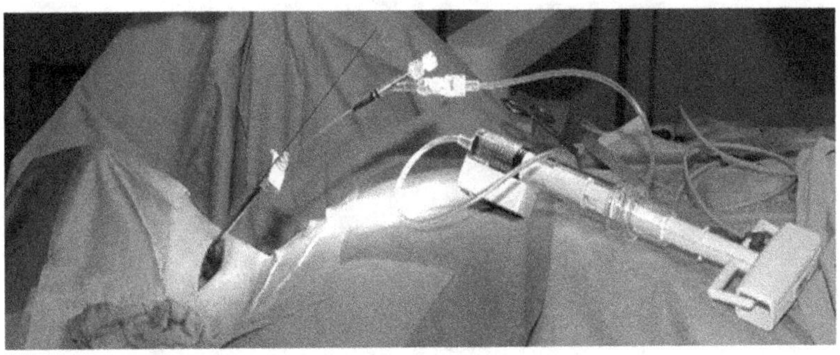

Fig. 2 Shows the unilateral anterior transverse approach on the right side of the patient's neck. K-wire is placed for anterior odontoid screw placement and the balloon for kyphoplasty into the dens axis

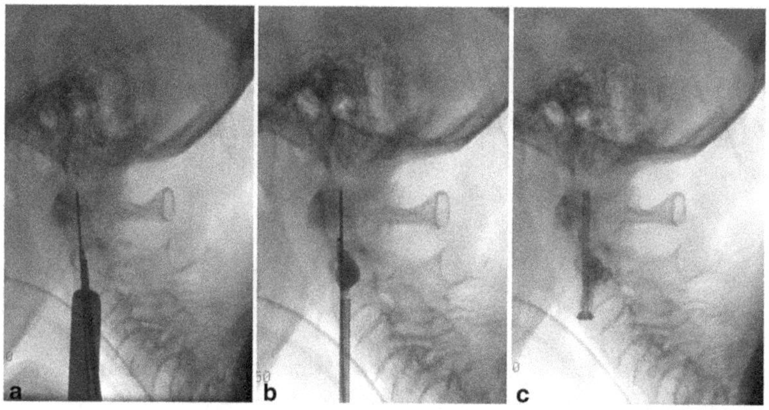

Fig. 3 Shows step- by- step procedure under lateral fluoroscopic guidance. Picture A shows the placed K-wire in the odontoid process and the placed trocar for balloon kyphoplasty. Picture B shows the filled balloon within the osteolytic lesion of C2 and picture C shows the result after cement application in the osteolytic lesion, as well as the placed bicortical anterior odontoid screw

Surgery was performed in the same manner with balloon kyphoplasty of the osteolytic lesion of C2 and placement of an additional odontoid screw (Fig. 7). A soft collar was worn for 2 weeks after surgery. The patient recovered well. X-rays showed sufficient osteosynthesis and cement placement in C2. Further treatment of the myeloma was conducted by the hematologist.

Case 3: A 78-year old man with a known history of adenocarcinoma of the colon (Karnofsky Performance Score: 60%) complained about a short history of severe neck pain. CT-scan of the cervical spine showed a large osteolytic process in the vertebra body of C2 (13,6 mm × 20 mm × 20,9 mm) (Fig. 8). MRI of the total spine ruled out further osteolytic lesions. Surgery with balloon kyphoplasty and additional odontoid screw was performed without complications. Following wound healing, radiotherapy of the dens axis was introduced (2,5 Gy five to six times per week, total dose 30 Gy).

Case 4: A 76-year old patient was presents to our clinic with a known osteolytic process inside the vertebra body of the dens axis (12,9 mm × 20,2 mm, 21 mm) (Fig. 9) by multiple hemangioma of the spine. In the patient's history, an unstable osteolytic lesion of Th12 was stabilized with a screw-rod instrumentation. Radiological imaging with CT-scan and MRI of the cervical spine was done and surgery with balloon kyphoplasty and additional odontoid screw placement was performed. Control x-rays showed sufficient osteosynthesis and cement placement in the vertebral body C2 (Fig. 9). A soft collar was worn for 2 weeks after surgery.

Discussion

Metastases, including osteolytic lesions of the craniocervical junction, are rare entities. Literature describes a variety of treatment procedures. The aim of treatment is to maintain stability for pain relief and to improve patients' quality of life.

Chemotherapy and radiotherapy are useful options for conservative treatment.

Local radiotherapy of symptomatic bone lesions in myeloma patients reduce pain, yet it takes time until symptom relief sets in. Lee et al. reported the time span

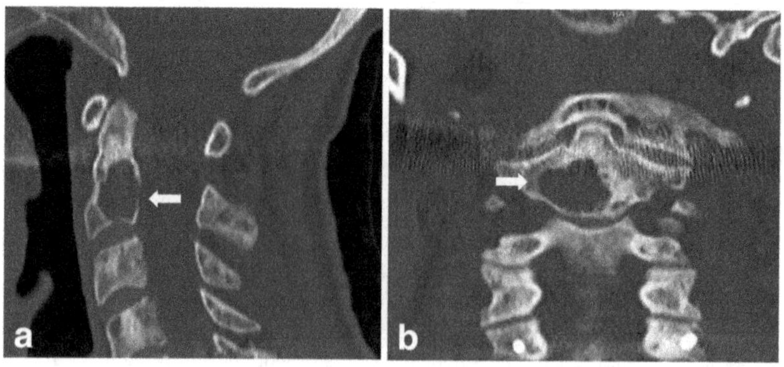

Fig. 4 CT-scan in lateral (**a**) and coronal (**b**) view with instable osteolytic lesion (arrows) in the base of C2 (16 mm × 11 mm × 15 mm) (Case 1)

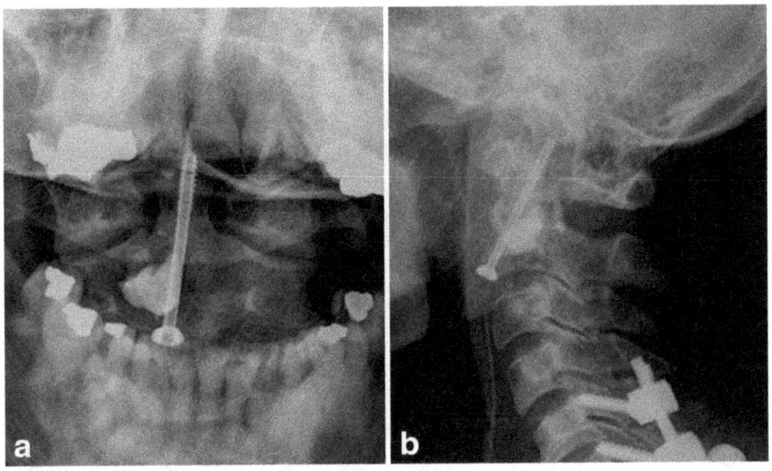

Fig. 5 The postoperative x-ray shows cement in the base of C2 after balloon kyphoplasty and anterior odontoid screw (coronal view (**a**) and lateral view (**b**). Slight posterior cement leakage after kyphoplasty. Additional posterior instrumentation C5 to Th2 and laminectomy of C7 were performed for osteolytic lesion of C7 with compressed spinal cord (Case 1)

for symptom relief to be between 1 and 67 days (average time is 7 days) [19]. The study however does not describe improvement of bone stability through radiotherapy. Rief et al. showed that stability of bone occurred in one third of patients with osteolytic metastases of the thoracic and lumbar spine over a 6-month period after radiotherapy [20].

Rades et al. determined that multi-fraction radiotherapy shows a significantly better remineralization of the bone, than single fraction radiotherapy [21]. Remineralization begins 2 to 3 weeks after radiotherapy and the process continues to up to 2 months [22].

Treatment with radiotherapy is limited for patients with acute pain and in case of pathological fractures, because of the long duration of symptom relief and time needed for remineralization of the bone.

Different surgical therapies for cervical spinal metastases have been published. In general, patients with low risk myeloma have at least a 50% chance of surviving more than 10 years nowadays due to improved treatment [23]. One of our patients with myeloma was diagnosed initially on the basis of a biopsy taken from the tumor mass in C7 during the first surgery. The other patient had a known history of myeloma with a Durie/Salmon Classification Stage III and a Karnofsky Performance Score of 70%. The patient with known history of adenocarcinoma of the colon had a Karnofsky Performance Score of 60%. Goals of treatments of spinal metastasis are the pain reduction as well the upholding of the quality of life [24]. These were the reasons our decisions to operate was based on in all three patients with suspected tumor or known tumor disease.

For pathological fractures or large osteolytic lesions of the thoracic or lumbal spine vertebroplasty or balloon kyphoplasty are established procedures. Both techniques lead to adequate pain relief. In 1987 Galibert et al.

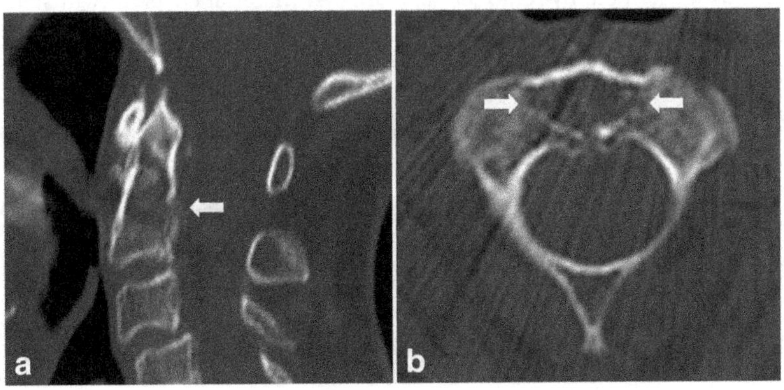

Fig. 6 CT-scan in lateral (**a**) and axial view (**b**) of patient no. 2. A large osteolytic lesion in C2 (14 mm × 11 mm × 16 mm) is seen in the middle of the base and partially in the area of the odontoid process (arrows) (Case 2)

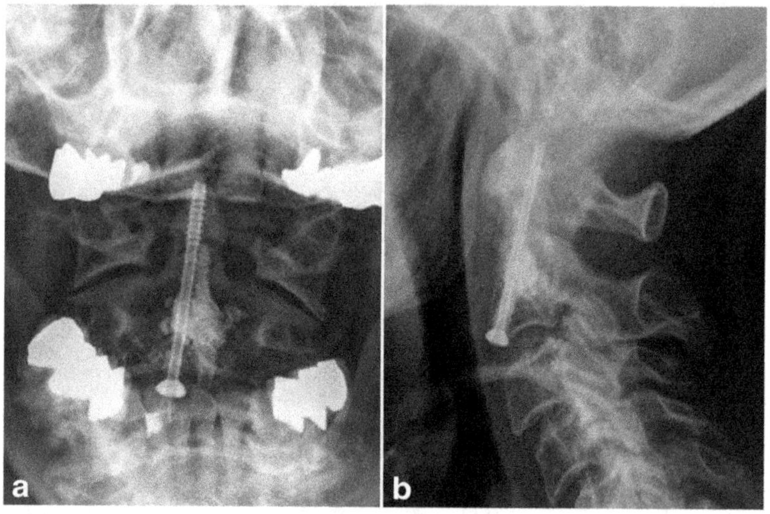

Fig. 7 X-ray of the dens (**a**) and the lateral (**b**) cervical spine of the first patient shows favorable cement filling of the osteolytic lesion, in the base of the dens and the additional anterior odontoid screw (Case 2)

published a case series of seven patients describing percutaneous acrylic vertebroplasty as a then new treatment in vertebral hemangioma instead of radiotherapy alone [25].

Khan et al. performed a pooled analysis of published case series of vertebral augmentation. Twenty-three studies, including balloon kyphoplasty and/ or vertebroplasty were evaluated. In all cases significant decrease in pain occurred shortly after the procedure. No difference in the extent of pain reduction between both procedures was found [26].

Only few studies about vertebroplasty and kyphoplasty in metastatic lesions of the dens axis were published.

Some case reports account for transoral approach for vertebroplasty of metastatic tumors in the upper cervical spine (C1 or C2), with or without combination of posterior stabilization. Patients treated transorally complained about pharyngeal discomfort and pain. Neck pain was reduced postoperatively [11, 27].

A CT guided percutaneous vertebroplasty technique of the upper cervical spine was described by Guo et al. [22]. They used a translateral approach between the carotid sheath and the vertebral artery for hemangiomas or metastatic lesions at C1-C3 in fifteen patients. Pain reduction could be achieved in all patients. Two patients had anterior cement leakage of the vertebra body. No vessel damage and no neurological symptoms occurred.

Kyphoplasty of C2 and C5 in a case of cervical metastases was published by Druschel et al. For this procedure, the typical anterior approach to the ventral cervical spine was used, like in the osteosynthesis of odontoid fractures [13]. Pain reduction after the procedure was good.

A meta-analysis comparing percutaneous vertebroplasty and balloon kyphoplasty for the treatment of single level vertebral compression fractures, carried out by Wang et al., showed balloon kyphoplasty to be superior. Balloon kyphoplasty has a higher volume of injected cement, better short- term pain relief, as well as a lower cement leakage rate than vertebroplasty. Longer operation time and higher material costs notwithstanding [28].

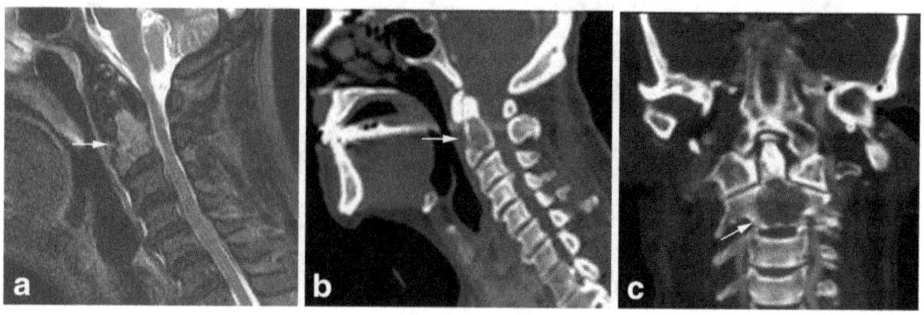

Fig. 8 MRI of the cervical spine (**a**) shows a metastatic lesion in the vertebral body of C2 without spinal cord compression. The CT-scan in lateral and frontal view shows an osteolytic lesion (arrow) in the base of C2 (13,6 mm × 20 mm × 20,9 mm) in the same patient (**b** and **c**) (Case 3)

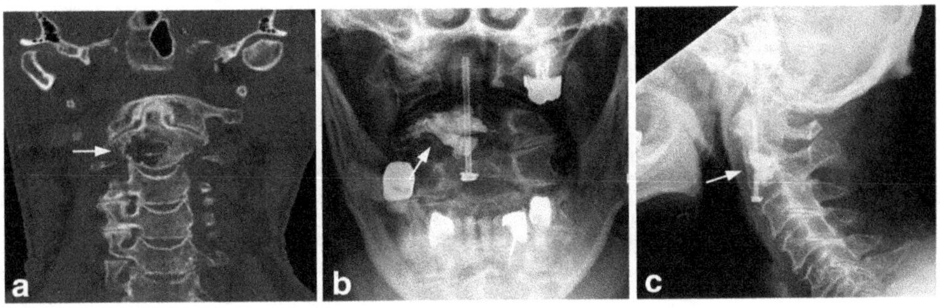

Fig. 9 CT-scan of the upper cervical spine in lateral view with osteolytic lesion of C2 (arrow) of patient with vertebral hemangioma (**a**). Postoperative x-rays show a good filling of osteolytic lesion and the additional anterior odontoid screw (**b** and **c**) (Case 4)

In our opinion the balloon kyphoplasty forms a more regular cavity and it is possible that some bone trabeculae are pressed against the wall through which it might be reinforced. On the other hand, ballooning should be performed carefully to ensure that the wall is not fractured. Additionally, the volume of the cement can be estimated due to the used volume for the balloon. The known lower cement leakage rate in balloon kyphoplasty is the main reason why we use this technique. Furthermore, the cavity created by the balloon leads to more application of cement and therefore to more stability of the vertebra body. In all four cases the main osteolysis was in the body of C2. Therefore, all screws had a good grip in the odontoid.

The complication rate after vertebroplasty and kyphoplasty in metastatic spinal diseases, as specified in literature, is about 4%. A systematic review about vertebroplasty and kyphoplasty for spinal metastases of C1 – C7 showed an asymptomatic cement leakage in 16% of the treated patients. About 4% of the patients had symptomatic complications, mainly mild odynophagia, occipital neuralgia, and one case with acute cerebellar and occipital infarction [29].

Another established method is combining a vertebroplasty of spinal osteolytic lesions associated with hema tologic malignancies with radiation therapy to synergize the effects of both procedures on pain reduction and to minimize recurrence of local pain [30].

Occipitocervical posterior stabilization and, if necessary, decompression, is the treatment of choice in cases of kyphosis, instability and/ or collapse of the vertebra, as well as narrowing of neurological structures and neurological deficits in metastatic diseases of the upper cervical spine [4].

Anterior screw fixation is one of the common procedures in the operative management of type II odontoid fractures next to posterior C1/C2 stabilization and fusion. It provides stability, good fusion rates and preserves C1/C2 motion [31].

In our opinion, an additional anterior screw placement in the odontoid process provides more augmentation of the C2 vertebra.

Gumpert et al. demonstrated a demineralization at the cement surface after kyphoplasty for calcium phosphate cement, as a sign of remodeling of the cancellous bone [32]. This may pose a risk for subsequent pathological fracture after kyphoplasty. Vertebral fractures were also noticed after kyphoplasty in osteoporotic fractures of the lumbal spine [33]. We used PMMA cement for the kyphoplasties in our cases.

Odontoid fractures are the most common spine fractures in patients older than 80 years. Considering myeloma incidence increasing with age [34], most of these patients present a higher risk of traumatic dens fracture. A further aspect is the known osteoporosis in older women. Two of our patients were females over 70 years of age at the time of treatment. It is to be assumed, that both patients also suffer from osteoporosis.

As a result, we recommend an additional stabilization with an anterior odontoid screw, in case of kyphoplasty of metastatic lesions of the dens axis.

Conclusion

Although the treatment of metastatic lesions of the dens is palliative, the life span of these patients increases due to better systemic therapy. Preserving functionality and reducing pain should be the ambition of treatment. Next to conservative treatment, surgical therapy may be necessary in cases of lytic lesions of the dens.

Our experience showed that balloon kyphoplasty and additional anterior odontoid screw fixation can be a good choice for treating patients with potentially unstable or large osteolytic lesions of the dens without spinal cord compression or neurological symptoms.

Abbreviations

CT-Scan: Computed tomography scan; Gy: Gray (unit); MRI: Magnetic resonance imaging; PMMA cement: Polymethylmethacrylate cement; SINS: Spine instability neoplastic score

Funding

There is no funding source.

Authors' contributions

AV wrote the manuscript of this article and was involved in the acquisition of the data. NvdH was involved in the design of the study and the acquisition of the data. He reviewed the article. CH initiated the project and reviewed the manuscript critically. All authors read and approved the final manuscript.

Consent for publication

All patients were informed about the publication and signed a consent for publication.

Competing interests

The authors declare that they have no competing interests.

References

1. Moulding HD, Bilsky MH. Metastases to the craniovertebral junction. Neurosurgery. 2010;66(3 Suppl):113–8.
2. Molloy S, Lai M, Pratt G, Ramasamy K, Wilson D, Quraishi N, et al. Optimizing the management of patients with spinal myeloma disease. Br J Haematol. 2015;171(3):332–43.
3. Bilsky MH, Shannon FJ, Sheppard S, Prabhu V, Boland PJ. Diagnosis and management of a metastatic tumor in the atlantoaxial spine. Spine. 2002; 27(10):1062–9.
4. Fehlings MG, David KS, Vialle L, Vialle E, Setzer M, Vrionis FD. Decision making in the surgical treatment of cervical spine metastases. Spine. 2009; 34(22 Suppl):S108–17.
5. Dorman JK. Vertebroplasty of the C2 vertebral body and dens using an anterior cervical approach: technical case report. Neurosurgery. 2010;67(4): E1143. 6; discussion E6
6. Shetty SR, Ganigi PM, Mandanna BK. Open C2 Vertebroplasty: case report, technique, and review of literature. Asian J Neurosurgery. 2017;12(4):710–4.
7. Baker JF, Shafqat A, Devitt A, McCabe JP. Stabilization of metastatic lesions affecting the second cervical vertebra. J Craniovertebral Junction Spine. 2015;6(2):56–9.
8. Sun G, Wang LJ, Jin P, Liu XW, Li M. Vertebroplasty for treatment of osteolytic metastases at C2 using an anterolateral approach. Pain Physician. 2013;16(4):E427–34.
9. Mont'Alverne F, Vallee JN, Cormier E, Guillevin R, Barragan H, Jean B, et al. Percutaneous vertebroplasty for metastatic involvement of the axis. AJNR Am J Neuroradiol. 2005;26(7):1641–5.
10. Martin JB, Gailloud P, Dietrich PY, Luciani ME, Somon T, Sappino PA, et al. Direct transoral approach to C2 for percutaneous vertebroplasty. Cardiovasc Intervent Radiol. 2002;25(6):517–9.
11. Papp Z, Marosfoi M, Szikora I, Banczerowski P. Treatment of C-2 metastatic tumors with intraoperative transoral or transpedicular vertebroplasty and occipitocervical posterior fixation. J Neurosurg Spine. 2014;21(6):886–91.
12. Guerre P, Krober M. Open dorsal vertebroplasty of the axis. Arch Orthop Trauma Surg. 2011;131(5):591–6.
13. Druschel C, Schaser KD, Melcher I, Haas NP, Disch AC. Minimally invasive combined anterior kyphoplasty for osteolytic C2 and C5 metastases. Arch Orthop Trauma Surg. 2011;131(7):977–81.
14. Blondel B, Litre F, Graillon T, Adetchessi T, Dufour H, Fuentes S. Metastatic odontoid fracture management by anterior screw fixation and kyphoplasty. Neuro-Chirurgie. 2013;59(4–5):191–4.
15. Zwolak P, Krober M. Acute neck pain caused by atlanto-axial instability secondary to pathologic fracture involving odontoid process and C2 vertebral body: treatment with radiofrequency thermoablation, cement augmentation and odontoid screw fixation. Arch Orthop Trauma Surg. 2015; 135(9):1211_5.
16. Terreaux L, Loubersac T, Hamel O, Bord E, Robert R, Buffenoir K. Odontoid balloon kyphoplasty associated with screw fixation for type II fracture in 2 elderly patients. J Neurosurg Spine. 2015;22(3):246–52.
17. Blondel B, Adetchessi T, Demakakos J, Pech-Gourg G, Dufour H, Fuentes S. Anterolateral kyphoplasty in the management of cervical spinal metastasis. Orthop Traumatol, Surg Res. 2012;98(3):341–5.
18. Bourghli A, Luc S, Obeid I, Guerin P, Gille O, Vital JM, et al. Management of a major atlanto-axial instability secondary to a lytic lesion of C2. Eur Spine J. 2015;24(1):180–4.
19. Lee JW, Lee JE. Local radiotherapy for palliation in multiple myeloma patients with symptomatic bone lesions. Radiation Oncol J. 2016;34(1):59–63.
20. Rief H, Heinhold M, Bruckner T, Schlampp I, Forster R, Welzel T, et al. Quality of life, fatigue and local response of patients with unstable spinal bone metastases under radiation therapy--a prospective trial. Radiat Oncol. 2014;9:133.
21. Rades D, Schild SE, Abrahm JL. Treatment of painful bone metastases. Nat Rev Clin Oncol. 2010;7(4):220–9.
22. Guo WH, Meng MB, You X, Luo Y, Li J, Qiu M, et al. CT-guided percutaneous vertebroplasty of the upper cervical spine via a translateral approach. Pain Physician. 2012;15(5):E733–41.
23. Hanbali A, Hassanein M, Rasheed W, Aljurf M, Alsharif F. The evolution of prognostic factors in multiple myeloma. Adv Hematol. 2017;2017:4812637.
24. Delank KS, Wendtner C, Eich HT, Eysel P. The treatment of spinal metastases. Dtsch Arztebl Int. 2011;108(5):71–9. quiz 80
25. Galibert P, Deramond H, Rosat P, Le Gars D. Preliminary note on the treatment of vertebral angioma by percutaneous acrylic vertebroplasty. Neuro-Chirurgie. 1987;33(2):166–8.
26. Khan OA, Brinjikji W, Kallmes DF. Vertebral augmentation in patients with multiple myeloma: a pooled analysis of published case series. AJNR Am J Neuroradiol. 2014;35(1):207–10.
27. Anselmetti GC, Manca A, Montemurro F, Tutton S, Chiara G, Battistella M, et al. Vertebroplasty using transoral approach in painful malignant involvement of the second cervical vertebra (C2): a single-institution series of 25 patients. Pain Physician. 2012;15(1):35–42.
28. Wang H, Sribastav SS, Ye F, Yang C, Wang J, Liu H, et al. Comparison of percutaneous Vertebroplasty and balloon Kyphoplasty for the treatment of single level vertebral compression fractures: a meta-analysis of the literature. Pain Physician. 2015;18(3):209–22.
29. De la Garza-Ramos R, Benvenutti-Regato M, Caro-Osorio E. Vertebroplasty and kyphoplasty for cervical spine metastases: a systematic review and meta-analysis. Int J Spine Surg. 2016;10:7.
30. Masala S, Anselmetti GC, Marcia S, Massari F, Manca A, Simonetti G. Percutaneous vertebroplasty in multiple myeloma vertebral involvement. J Spinal Disord Tech. 2008;21(5):344–8.
31. Mazur MD, Mumert ML, Bisson EF, Schmidt MH. Avoiding pitfalls in anterior screw fixation for type II odontoid fractures. Neurosurg Focus. 2011;31(4):E7.
32. Gumpert R, Bodo K, Spuller E, Poglitsch T, Bindl R, Ignatius A, et al. Demineralization after balloon kyphoplasty with calcium phosphate cement: a histological evaluation in ten patients. Eur Spine J. 2014;23(6):1361–8.
33. Fribourg D, Tang C, Sra P, Delamarter R, Bae H. Incidence of subsequent vertebral fracture after kyphoplasty. Spine. 2004;29(20):2270–6. discussion 7
34. Wildes TM, Campagnaro E. Management of multiple myeloma in older adults: Gaining ground with geriatric assessment. J Geriatr Oncol. 2017;8(1):1–7.

Outcomes of simultaneous high tibial osteotomy and anterior cruciate ligament reconstruction in anterior cruciate ligament deficient knee with osteoarthritis

Cheng Jin[1], Eun-Kyoo Song[2], Quan-He Jin[2], Nam-Hun Lee[2] and Jong-Keun Seon[2*]

Abstract

Background: We aimed to evaluate clinical and radiological results after simultaneous open-wedge high tibial osteotomy (HTO) and anterior cruciate ligament (ACL) reconstruction in patients with ACL deficiency combined with medial uni-compartmental osteoarthritis (OA) and varus deformity.

Methods: This retrospective study was performed using data collected from 2005 to 2011 on a total of 24 patients who were diagnosed with ACL injury and medial unicompartmental OA with varus deformity, and who subsequently underwent simultaneous open-wedge HTO and arthroscopic ACL reconstruction. The mean follow-up duration was 5.2 years. For clinical outcomes, we evaluated Lysholm score, Tegner activity score, range of motion, Lachmann test, and pivot-shift test, and for radiological outcomes, we evaluated the degree of varus deformity, progression of medial OA, tibial posterior slope, anterior instability, and postoperative complication.

Results: There were no limitations in range of motion found in any cases. Three patients showed progressive osteoarthritis on the medial compartment. The mechanical femorotibial angle was significantly corrected from varus 7.0 degrees to valgus 1.2 degrees, and the tibial posterior slope was not significantly changed. The Lysholm and Tegner activity scores were significantly improved after surgery (from 58 to 94 points on the Lysholm scale and from 4.0 to 5.3 points on the Tegner activity scale). Although the Lachman test and the pivot-shift test showed significant improvements after surgery, instability greater than Gr II was observed in three patients on the Lachman test and in four patients on the pivot-shift test. The side-to-side difference improved from 9.6 mm to 4.2 mm postoperatively as assessed using a Telos® arthrometer. There were no cases of nonunion or fixation loss.

Conclusions: Simultaneous open-wedge HTO and ACL reconstruction in patients with ACL injury with medial compartmental OA showed satisfactory functional outcomes and postoperative activity level scores. However, some patients showed residual instability and progression of OA.

Keywords: Knee, High tibial osteotomy, Anterior cruciate ligament reconstruction

* Correspondence: seonbell@jnu.ac.kr
[2]Center for Joint Disease, Chonnam National University Hwasun Hospital, Hwasun, South Korea
Full list of author information is available at the end of the article

Background

Anterior laxity in anterior cruciate ligament (ACL) deficient knees is a precursor to degenerative osteoarthritis (OA) [1, 2]. The risk of developing radiologically evident OA of at least Kellgren- Lawrence grade 2 is reported to be five-fold higher in the setting of anterior laxity than in uninjured knees [1, 3]. For patients with concomitant varus deformity, ACL reconstruction may restore the stability of the knee, but it cannot prevent the progression of medial compartmental OA [4, 5]. Furthermore, varus alignment adds an adduction moment while patients are walking [6]. This adduction moment force translates to varus thrust on the knee joint during the heel strike [6, 7]. This may stress the reconstructed ACL graft, causing early failure. The success of valgus high tibial osteotomy (HTO) in treating unicompartmental OA in young adults encouraged the authors to attempt the procedure in knees with ACL injuries in order to restore stability and prevent the progression of OA [8–10]. Such a procedure should theoretically unload the medial compartment and decrease the stress on the newly reconstructed ACL graft. However, such a procedure may also increase the risk of morbidity and delay the rehabilitation from the ACL reconstruction. Further, valgus HTO is known to increase the posterior slope of the proximal tibia, which may further accentuate the stress on the reconstructed graft [11, 12]. The indications and benefits of this combined surgery therefore remain unclear in the literature. Variability in pathology, the follow-up period, and clinical scores used for evaluation makes comparisons between the available data difficult [13].

The aim of our study was to evaluate radiological and functional outcomes in patients with ACL deficient knees and medial unicompartmental OA undergoing simultaneous ACL reconstruction and HTO.

Methods

The institutional review board (Chonnam National University Hospital) approved this retrospective study prior to the commencement of this study. We reviewed the records of all patients who underwent simultaneous ACL reconstruction and HTO from 2005 to 2011 and got the written consents from the patients. The inclusion criterion for the study was an ACL deficient knee with varus deformity (more than 5 degrees) on full-leg length standing radiography as well as radiographically-proven (X-ray or MRI) isolated medial unicompartmental osteoarthritis (≥ Kellgren-Lawrence Gr I) with a minimum follow-up period of 3 years. Other ligamentous laxities, degenerative arthritis of the lateral compartment, tears of the lateral meniscus, inflammatory knee arthritis, and a follow-up period shorter than 3 years were regarded as exclusion criteria.

Two senior authors operated on all patients. Diagnostic arthroscopies were carried out prior to ACL reconstruction and osteotomy in all cases. Cartilage defects on the medial side were dealt with using micro-fractures (eight cases) when it is necessary. Partial meniscectomies (nine cases) or meniscal repair (five cases) were performed whenever deemed necessary by the surgeon. Quadrupled hamstring autografts were harvested from the ipsilateral side in all cases. After the drilling of a femoral tunnel through the outside-in technique using an ACL guide (Linvatec, Largo, FL, USA), medial opening biplanar high tibial osteotomy was performed as described in the literature [14]. The starting point of osteotomy on the medial side was shifted more distally than typically described to allow enough space for the tibial tunnel. The osteotomy was opened to the point at which the mechanical axis passed through the 62.5% point of the tibial plateau. This was fixed with two Aescula plates (Medysey, Seoul, Korea), non-locking plates with rectangular metal wedges. To maintain the tibial slope, the anterior plate was smaller than the posterior plate. A cancellous bone chip allograft was performed when the tibial opening was larger than 10 mm. This was followed by the drilling of a tibial tunnel. The graft was then passed through both the femoral and tibial tunnels and secured using a closed loop Endobutton (Smith & Nephew, Andover, MA, USA) or an adjustable loop TightRope (Arthrex, Naples, FL) on the femoral side and an interference screw on the tibial side. The tibial attachment was further secured using a spiked washer and a cortical screw. Range of motion exercises were begun as soon as possible. Knees were kept in a range of motion brace for 4 weeks. Toe touch partial weight bearing was allowed for the first 4 weeks after surgery, after which progressive tolerable weight bearing was encouraged.

An independent orthopedic fellow who was not directly involved in patient management collected all data. Preoperative and postoperative radiological and clinical records were evaluated. Range of motion, Lyslohm scores, Tegner activity scores, pivot-shift test, and Lachman tests were estimated in the clinical records. A Telos® device (Austin & Associates, Fallston, MD, US) was used to evaluate stress tests. Anterior laxities were evaluated in 30-degree flexion with 15Lb anterior stresses using the Telos device by side to side difference compared with a normal contralateral knee. The anterior-posterior and lateral radiographs were screened for the progression of osteoarthritis and for changes in posterior slope. Lastly, full-leg length standing radiographs taken preoperatively and 3 months postoperatively were assessed for preoperative and postoperative lower limb alignment.

Table 1 Preoperative and postoperative clinical and radiological results

	Preoperative	Final follow-up	*P*-value
Mechanical axis (in degree)	7.0 ± 2.3	−1.2 ± 1.4	< 0.001
Tegner activity score	4.0 ± 1.1	5.3 ± 0.9	< 0.001
Lysholm score	58.5 ± 12.0	94.0 ± 5.9	< 0.001
Anterior laxity on Telos stress radiography (in mm)	9.6 ± 2.8	4.2 ± 2.6	< 0.001
Posterior slope	9.1 ± 1.4	10.2 ± 2.3	0.092
Range of motion	137.3 ± 6.2	136.5 ± 6.0	0.691

-; valgus

Statistical analysis

All variables are expressed as means +/− standard deviations. The difference between preoperative and postoperative values was assessed using a paired-t test for continuous variables and a Chi-square test for categorical variables. A p value less than .05 was considered to be significant. SPSS software version 22 (IBM, Armonk, NY, USA) was used for all analysis.

Results

Our records yielded 24 patients that satisfied the inclusion criterion, consisting of 20 males and four females. The average age of our patients was 40.2 years (range, 29–52 years). The mean follow-up period was 5.2 years (range, 3–9 years). None of the patients required conversion to arthroplasty.

Table 1 presents the preoperative and final postoperative clinical and radiological outcomes of our study. At the final follow up, none of the patients had any range of motion (ROM) limitations. Clinical scores improved in all cases to pre-injured levels. The mechanical axis was corrected from preoperative varus 7.0 to a mean of valgus 1.2 degrees. None of the patients showed significant changes (more than three degrees from preoperative values) in posterior slope.

Clinically, anterior laxity was improved in all patients except for three who showed grade 2 laxity on the Lachman test and four who had a positive pivot-shift test (Table 2). Stress radiography confirmed the clinical findings of improved laxity, with a significant decrease in side-to-side difference in anterior laxity compared to preoperative values.

At the final follow-up, three patients showed progression of medial unicompartmental osteoarthritis (Table 3, Fig. 1). Two of them had medial meniscal damage and one had full thickness cartilage defect on medial femoral chondyle at the time of index surgery.

Three patients complained of hyperesthesia in the antero-lateral part of the proximal tibia and one patient had pain in the incision site. There was no case of nonunion of the osteotomy site. No other major complications were noted in our series.

Discussion

The most important finding of our study was that simultaneous ACL reconstruction and valgus HTO showed relatively good clinical and radiological outcomes in ACL deficient knees with osteoarthritis. However, some patients showed a moderate degree of instability or a progression of OA in spite of ACL reconstruction. Further studies are warranted to clearly define a patient subgroup that would benefit from the combined procedure.

Patients with combined laxity and medial compartmental OA tend to be young and therefore retaining their natural knee is a priority [15]. With the aim of restoring the laxity and alignment of the knee, many authors have suggested a combined ACL reconstruction and valgus osteotomy procedure [8–10]. Consistent with the results previously published by most authors, we found that none of our cases required conversion to total knee arthroplasty over a mid-term follow-up of an average of 5 years [8–10, 12, 16]. This substantiates the role of the combined procedure in such knees.

Most previous authors reported improved functional scores following combined surgery. We had a similar experience as we found Lysholm scores and Tegner activity scores to be significantly better after the operation

Table 2 Improvement of anterior instability based on Lachman and pivot shift test

Grade	Lachman test		P-value	Pivot-shift test		P-value
	Preoperative	Final follow-up		Preoperative	Final follow-up	
0	0	14	< 0.001	0	15	< 0.001
I	3	7		9	5	
II	14	3		11	4	
III	7	0		4	0	

Table 3 Progression of osteoarthritis on medial compartment

Grade	Preoperative	Final follow-up	P-value
I	10	8	0.682
II	9	10	
III	5	6	
IV	0	0	

than they were before the operation [8–10, 16–18]. All patients subjectively reported better stability of the knee. Despite these encouraging results, six patients (25%) showed progressive medial compartmental osteoarthritis on serial radiographs. Similarly, four patients (17%) had a positive pivot shift test, three of whom also had a positive grade 2 Lachman test. Complication rates in the literature are variably defined. In line with our experience, Zaffanigni et al. [19] reported 22% progression in medial compartmental OA after a 6.5-year follow-up. In contrast, Dejour et al. [20] found no difference in the OA rate preoperatively vs. postoperatively in a retrospective study.

A similar discrepancy exists in the rate of anterior laxity. Lattermann reported that 31% of patients developed graft insufficiency [8]. Consistent with our results, Schuster et al. [21] reported graft insufficiency in 18% of patients. However, others have described a 0% rate of graft insufficiency following the combined procedure [22]. Finally, contrary to our results, Dean et al. [23] conducted a systemic review and identified knee stiffness as the most common complication. We observed no loss of movement in any patient. These differences between reports may be the result of the use of different surgical techniques as well as differences in preoperative patient conditions, timings of the surgeries, rehabilitation protocols, and/or follow-up periods. The published data is heterogeneous regarding each of the above parameters, making comparisons difficult. Such wide differences in complication rates highlight the currently inadequate understanding of the true pathological nature of ACL deficiency with unicompartmental OA. It further stresses the need for future studies to define indications for the combined procedure. In addition, the combined procedure is a complex technique that requires meticulous preoperative planning, skilled intraoperative techniques, and an aggressive postoperative rehabilitation protocol.

Changes in tibial slope following high tibial osteotomy are well known to occur and may affect the stresses on a reconstructed graft [11]. We observed no significant differences between preoperative and postoperative values. However, despite maintenance of the slope in all cases, we observed graft insufficiency in 17% of cases, indicating that a non-mechanical mechanism may be involved in preventing graft healing. Consistent with our experience, Schuster et al. hypothesized that severe osteoarthritic changes and an associated catabolic intra-articular milieu may play a role in insufficient graft integration or compromise graft functionality [18].

There are a few limitations to our study. First, it is a retrospective study and is therefore subject to the associated usual biases. Secondly, the sample size is too small

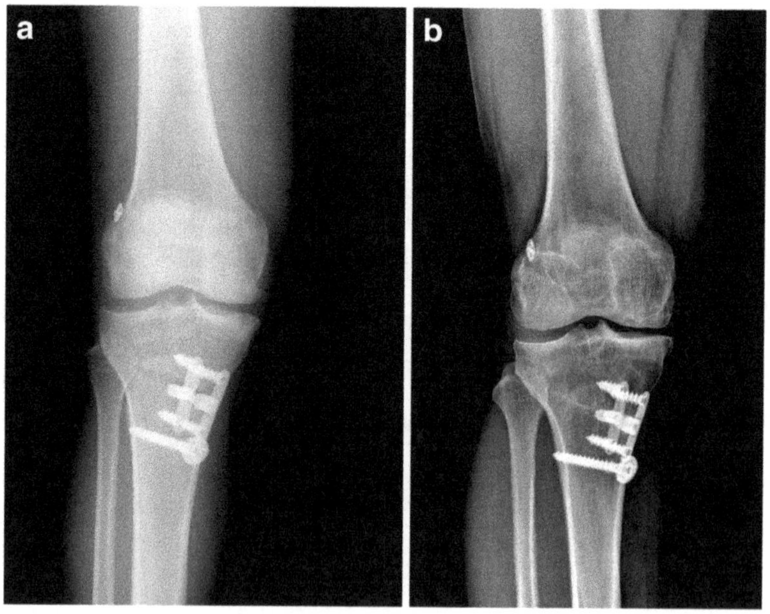

Fig. 1 **a** Immediate operative knee x-ray showing medial compartment osteoarthritis following ACL reconstruction and valgus high tibial osteotomy. **b** Knee x-ray taken three years following ACL reconstruction and valgus high tibial osteotomy that shows the progression of arthritis of medial compartment

to draw any definitive conclusions about the outcomes of this combined procedure. Thirdly, we carried out abrasion chondroplasty in the same setting, and as its role on ACL healing is still debatable, it may act as a confounding factor. The last limitation was that the majority of our patients were male and only four patients were female. Despite these limitations, our study strongly indicates a need for caution when choosing patients and performing combined ACL reconstruction and valgus HTO surgery, because of the possibility of a high complication rate.

Conclusions

Simultaneous open wedge HTO and ACL reconstruction showed satisfactory correction angles and improved knee joint function, delaying the need for arthroplasty. However, this combined procedure should be undertaken with caution, as it is associated with a high rate of laxity and the progression of osteoarthritis.

Abbreviations

ACL: Anterior cruciate ligament; HTO: High tibial osteotomy; OA: Osteoarthritis; ROM: Range of motion

Acknowledgements

The authors thank all clinical researchers involved in the research we included in this article. This study was not supported by any company or grant.

Authors' contributions

CJ Analysis of data and writing manuscript. EKS Make concepts and design of study. QHJ Data collection and analysis. NHL Analysis of data and writing manuscript. JKS Make concepts and design of study. Review and correction of draft manuscript. All authors have read and approved the manuscript and agreed it for submission to publish in this journal.

Consent for publication

Not applicable.

Competing interests

The authors declare that they have no competing interests.

Author details

[1]Department of Orthopedic Surgery, Chinese People's Armed Police Force, Zhejiang Corps Hospital, Jiaxing 314000, China. [2]Center for Joint Disease, Chonnam National University Hwasun Hospital, Hwasun, South Korea.

References

1. Ajuied A, Wong F, Smith C, Norris M, Earnshaw P, Back D, et al. Anterior cruciate ligament injury and radiologic progression of knee osteoarthritis: a systematic review and meta-analysis. Am J Sports Med. 2014;42:2242–52.
2. Lohmander LS, Englund PM, Dahl LL, Roos EM. The long-term consequence of anterior cruciate ligament and meniscus injuries: osteoarthritis. Am J Sports Med. 2007;35:1756–69.
3. Øiestad BE, Engebretsen L, Storheim K, Risberg MA. Knee osteoarthritis after anterior cruciate ligament injury: a systematic review. Am J Sports Med. 2009;37:1434–43.
4. Shelbourne KD, Benner RW. Isolated anterior cruciate ligament reconstruction in the chronic ACL-deficient knee with degenerative medial arthrosis. J Knee Surg. 2007;20:216–22.
5. Shelbourne KD, Stube KC. Anterior cruciate ligament (ACL)-deficient knee with degenerative arthrosis: treatment with an isolated autogenous patellar tendon ACL reconstruction. Knee Surg Sports Traumatol Arthrosc. 1997;5:150–6.
6. Marriott K, Birmingham TB, Kean CO, Hui C, Jenkyn TR, Giffin JR. Five-year changes in gait biomechanics after concomitant high tibial osteotomy and ACL reconstruction in patients with medial knee osteoarthritis. Am J Sports Med. 2015;43:2277–85.
7. Noyes FR, Schipplein OD, Andriacchi TP, Saddemi SR, Weise M. The anterior cruciate ligament-deficient knee with varus alignment: an analysis of gait adaptations and dynamic joint loadings. Am J Sports Med. 1992;20:707–16.
8. Lattermann C, Jakob RP. High tibial osteotomy alone or combined with ligament reconstruction in anterior cruciate ligament deficient knees. Knee Surg Sports Traumatol Arthrosc. 1996;4:32–8.
9. Neuschwander DC, Drez D Jr, Paine RM. Simultaneous high tibial osteotomy and ACL reconstruction for combined genu varum and symptomatic ACL tear. Orthopedics. 1993;16:679–84.
10. Noyes FR, Barber SD, Simon R. High tibial osteotomy and ligament reconstruction in varus angulated, anterior cruciate ligament-deficient knees: a two- to seven-year follow-up study. Am J Sports Med. 1993;21:2–12.
11. LaPrade RF, Oro FB, Ziegler CG, Wijdicks CA, Walsh MP. Patellar height and tibial slope after opening-wedge proximal tibial osteotomy: a prospective study. Am J Sports Med. 2010;38:160–70.
12. Laprade RF, Spiridonov SI, Nystrom LM, Jansson KS. Prospective outcomes of young and middle-aged adults with medial compartment osteoarthritis treated with a proximal tibial opening wedge osteotomy. Arthroscopy. 2012;28:354–64.
13. Li Y, Zhang H, Zhang J, Li X, Song G, Feng H. Clinical outcome of simultaneous high tibial osteotomy and anterior cruciate ligament reconstruction for medial compartment osteoarthritis in young patients with anterior cruciate ligament-deficient knees: a systematic review. Arthroscopy. 2015;31:507–19.
14. Kim KJ, Song EK, Seon JK, Seol JH. Biomechanical study of the fixation plates for opening wedge high tibial osteotomy. Knee Surg Relat Res. 2015;27:181–6.
15. Øiestad BE, Holm I, Aune AK, Gunderson R, Myklebust G, Engebretsen L, et al. Knee function and prevalence of knee osteoarthritis after anterior cruciate ligament reconstruction: a prospective study with 10 to 15 years of follow-up. Am J Sports Med. 2010;38:2201–10.
16. Mancuso F, Hamilton TW, Kumar V, Murray DW, Pandit H. Clinical outcome after UKA and HTO in ACL deficiency: a systematic review. Knee Surg Sports Traumatol Arthrosc. 2016;24:112–22.
17. Floerkemeier S, Staubli AE, Schroeter S, Goldhahn S, Lobenhoffer P. Outcome after high tibial open-wedge osteotomy: a retrospective evaluation of 533 patients. Knee Surg Sports Traumatol Arthrosc. 2013;211:170–80.
18. Schuster P, Schulz M, Mayer P, Schlumberger M, Immendoerfer M, Richter J. Open-wedge high tibial osteotomy and combined abrasion/microfracture in severe medial osteoarthritis and varus malalignment: 5-year results and arthroscopic findings after 2 years. Arthroscopy. 2015;31:1279–88.
19. Zaffagnini S, Bonanzinga T, Grassi A, Marcheggiani Muccioli GM, Musiani C, Raggi F, et al. Combined ACL reconstruction and closing-wedge HTO for varus angulated ACL-deficient knees. Knee Surg Sports Traumatol Arthrosc. 2013;21:934–41.

Permissions

All chapters in this book were first published in MD, by BioMed Central; hereby published with permission under the Creative Commons Attribution License or equivalent. Every chapter published in this book has been scrutinized by our experts. Their significance has been extensively debated. The topics covered herein carry significant findings which will fuel the growth of the discipline. They may even be implemented as practical applications or may be referred to as a beginning point for another development.

The contributors of this book come from diverse backgrounds, making this book a truly international effort. This book will bring forth new frontiers with its revolutionizing research information and detailed analysis of the nascent developments around the world.

We would like to thank all the contributing authors for lending their expertise to make the book truly unique. They have played a crucial role in the development of this book. Without their invaluable contributions this book wouldn't have been possible. They have made vital efforts to compile up to date information on the varied aspects of this subject to make this book a valuable addition to the collection of many professionals and students.

This book was conceptualized with the vision of imparting up-to-date information and advanced data in this field. To ensure the same, a matchless editorial board was set up. Every individual on the board went through rigorous rounds of assessment to prove their worth. After which they invested a large part of their time researching and compiling the most relevant data for our readers.

The editorial board has been involved in producing this book since its inception. They have spent rigorous hours researching and exploring the diverse topics which have resulted in the successful publishing of this book. They have passed on their knowledge of decades through this book. To expedite this challenging task, the publisher supported the team at every step. A small team of assistant editors was also appointed to further simplify the editing procedure and attain best results for the readers.

Apart from the editorial board, the designing team has also invested a significant amount of their time in understanding the subject and creating the most relevant covers. They scrutinized every image to scout for the most suitable representation of the subject and create an appropriate cover for the book.

The publishing team has been an ardent support to the editorial, designing and production team. Their endless efforts to recruit the best for this project, has resulted in the accomplishment of this book. They are a veteran in the field of academics and their pool of knowledge is as vast as their experience in printing. Their expertise and guidance has proved useful at every step. Their uncompromising quality standards have made this book an exceptional effort. Their encouragement from time to time has been an inspiration for everyone.

The publisher and the editorial board hope that this book will prove to be a valuable piece of knowledge for researchers, students, practitioners and scholars across the globe.

List of Contributors

Joon Ho Wang
Department of Orthopaedic Surgery, Samsung Medical Center, Sungkyunkwan University School of Medicine, Seoul 06351, South Korea Department of Health Sciences and Technology, SAIHST, Sungkyunkwan
University, Seoul 06351, South Korea Department of Medical Device Management and Research, SAIHST, Sungkyunkwan University, Seoul 06351, South Korea

Do Kyung Lee
Department of Orthopaedic Surgery, Konyang University Hospital, 158, Gwanjeodong-ro, Seo-gu, Daejeon, South Korea

Sung Taek Chung and Byung Hoon Lee
Department of Orthopaedic Surgery, Kang-Dong Sacred Heart Hospital, Hallym University Medical Center, Gil-dong, Seoul 134-701, South Korea

Felix Dyrna and Andreas Voss
Department of Orthopaedic Sports Medicine, Technical University, Munich, Germany

Leo Pauzenberger, Elifho Obopilwe, Augustus D. Mazzocca and Cory Edgar
Department of Orthopaedic Surgery, University of Connecticut, Farmington, CT, USA

Alessandro Castagna
Department of Shoulder and Elbow IRCCS Humanitas Institute, Milan, Italy

Philipp R. Heuberer, Brenda Laky and Werner Anderl
St. Vincent Shoulder and Sports Clinic Vienna, Baumgasse 20A, 1030 Vienna, Austria

Georg Brandl, Leo Pauzenberger and Bernhard Kriegleder
St. Vincent Shoulder and Sports Clinic Vienna, Baumgasse 20A, 1030 Vienna, Austria
Austrian Research group for Regenerative and Orthopedic Medicine (AURROM), Vienna, Austria

Patrick Stephan and Gerjon Hannink
Orthopaedic Research Laboratory, Radboud University Medical Center, Nijmegen, The Netherlands

Maarten A. Röling, Nina M. C. Mathijssen and Rolf M. Bloem
Department of Orthopaedics, Reinier de Graaf Groep, Delft, The Netherlands

H. Y. Chen and K. Sutherland
Bureau of Health Information, Level 11, 67 Albert Avenue, Chatswood, NSW 2067, Australia

I. A. Harris
Whitlam Orthopaedic Research Centre, Ingham Institute for Applied Medical Research, South Western Sydney Clinical School, University of NSW, High St, Kensington, NSW 2052, Australia

J-F. Levesque
Bureau of Health Information, Level 11, 67 Albert Avenue, Chatswood, NSW 2067, Australia
Centre for Primary Health Care and Equity, University of NSW, Sydney, NSW, Australia
Agency for Clinical Innovation, Level 4, 67 Albert Avenue, Chatswood, NSW 2067, Australia

Liang-Tseng Kuo
Department of Orthopedic Surgery, Division of Sports Medicine, Chang Gung Memorial Hospital, 6, Sec West, Chia-Pu Rd, Puzih, Chiayi 61363, Taiwan
Centre for Evidence-Based Medicine, Chang Gung Memorial Hospital, Chiayi, Taiwan
Chang Gung University of Science and Technology, Chiayi, Taiwan

Pei-An Yu and Chi-Lung Chen
Department of Orthopedic Surgery, Division of Sports Medicine, Chang Gung Memorial Hospital, 6, Sec West, Chia-Pu Rd, Puzih, Chiayi 61363, Taiwan

Wei-Hsiu Hsu
Department of Orthopedic Surgery, Division of Sports Medicine, Chang Gung Memorial Hospital, 6, Sec West, Chia-Pu Rd, Puzih, Chiayi 61363, Taiwan
College of Medicine, Chang Gung University, Taoyuan, Taiwan

Ching-Chi Chi
Centre for Evidence-Based Medicine, Chang Gung Memorial Hospital, Chiayi, Taiwan
College of Medicine, Chang Gung University, Taoyuan, Taiwan
Department of Dermatology, Chang Gung Memorial Hospital, Linkou, 5, Fuxing St, Guishan Dist, Taoyuan 33305, Taiwan

Katarina Friberger Pajalic and Aleksandra Turkiewicz
Department of Clinical Sciences Lund, Orthopaedics, Clinical Epidemiology
Unit, Faculty of Medicine, Lund University, Remissgatan 4, 221 85 Lund, Sweden

Martin Englund
Department of Clinical Sciences Lund, Orthopaedics, Clinical Epidemiology
Unit, Faculty of Medicine, Lund University, Remissgatan 4, 221 85 Lund, Sweden
Clinical Epidemiology Research & Training Unit, Boston University School of Medicine, Boston, MA, USA

Bing Wang, Guohua Lü and Lei Kuang
Department of Spine Surgery, The Second Xiangya Hospital of Central South University, Changsha City, China

Yoon-Ho Kwak, Sahnghoon Lee, Myung Chul Lee and Hyuk-Soo Han
Seoul National University Hospital, Seoul, Republic of Korea

Zhen-Yu Jia, Chen Zhang, Chen-chen Xue, Tian-ze Liu, Xuan Huang and Wei-Dong Xu
Department of Orthopedics, Changhai Hospital, Second Military Medical University, Shanghai, China

Shi-qi Cao
Department of Joint Surgery and Sports Medicine, Changzheng Hospital, Shanghai, China

Theresa Diermeier, Sepp Braun, Andreas B. Imhoff and Knut Beitzel
Department of Orthopaedic Sports Medicine, Technical University Munich, Ismaninger Str. 22, 81675 Munich, Germany

Robert A. Arciero
Department of Orthopaedic Surgery, University of Connecticut, 263 Farmington Ave, Farmington, CT 06030, USA

Florian B. Imhoff and Bastian Scheiderer
Department of Orthopaedic Sports Medicine, Technical University Munich, Ismaninger Str. 22, 81675 Munich, Germany
Department of Orthopaedic Surgery, University of Connecticut, 263 Farmington Ave, Farmington, CT 06030, USA

Joscha Schnell and Alejandro Magaña
Department of Mechanical Engineering, Institute for Machine Tools and Industrial Management, Technical University Munich, Boltzmannstr. 15, 85748 Garching, Munich, Germany

Walter Ryan Smith, Parke William Hudson and Brent Andrew Ponce
Department of Orthopaedic Surgery, University of Alabama at Birmingham, 1313 13 St. South, Birmingham, AL 35205, USA

Sakthivel Rajan Rajaram Manoharan
Department of Orthopaedic Surgery, University of Alabama at Birmingham, FOT 950, 20 Street South, Birmingham, AL 35294, USA

Emma Dunphy
E-Health Unit, Research Department of Primary Care and Population Health, Upper Third Floor UCL Medical School (Royal Free Campus), Rowland Hill Street, NW3 2PF, London, UK
Homerton University Hospital NHS Trust, Homerton Row E96SR, London, UK

Fiona L. Hamilton
E-Health Unit, Research Department of Primary Care and Population Health, Upper Third Floor UCL Medical School (Royal Free Campus), Rowland Hill Street, NW3 2PF, London, UK

Irena Spasić
School of Computer Science & Informatics, Cardiff University, Queens Building, 5 The Parade, Cardiff CF24 3AA, UK

Kate Button
School of Healthcare Sciences, Cardiff University, Eastgate House, Newport Road, Cardiff CF24 0AB, UK
Cardiff & Vale University Health Board, Health Park, Cardiff CF14 4XW, UK

Stefan Rahm, Karl Wieser, David E. Bauer, Felix WA Waibel, Dominik C. Meyer, Christian Gerber and Sandro F. Fucentese
Orthopaedic Department, Balgrist University Hospital, University of Zurich, Forchstrasse 340, CH-8008 Zurich, Switzerland

Nicholas Pergaminelis and Jesse Renouf
Orthopaedic Department, Western Health, Footscray, VIC 3011, Australia
The University of Melbourne, Parkville, VIC, Australia

Camdon Fary and Oren Tirosh
Orthopaedic Department, Western Health, Footscray, VIC 3011, Australia

Phong Tran
Orthopaedic Department, Western Health, Footscray, VIC 3011, Australia
The University of Melbourne, Parkville, VIC, Australia
Australian Institute for Musculoskeletal Science (The University of Melbourne and Western Health), St. Albans, VIC, Australia

Hai Wang, Guixing Qiu, Jianguo Zhang and Jianxiong Shen
Department of Orthopaedic Surgery, Peking Union Medical College Hospital, Peking Union Medical College and Chinese Academy of Medical Sciences, No. 1 Shuaifuyuan, Beijing 100730, China

Zheping Zhang
Department of Orthopaedic Surgery, Beijing Puren Hospital, Beijing, China

Simon Roner, Fabio Carrillo and Philipp Fuernstahl
Computer Assisted Research and Development Group, Balgrist University
Hospital, University of Zurich, Forchstrasse 340, 8008 Zurich, Switzerland

Lazaros Vlachopoulos, Andreas Schweizer and Ladislav Nagy
Department of Orthopaedics, Balgrist University Hospital, University of Zurich, Zurich, Switzerland

Theresa Diermeier, Elmar Herbst, Sepp Braun, Emine Saracuz, Andreas Voss, Andreas B. Imhoff and Andrea Achtnich
Research performed at the Department for Orthopaedic Sports Medicine, Klinikum rechts der Isar, TU Munich, Germany Department of Orthopaedic Sports Medicine, Klinikum rechts der Isar, TU Munich, Ismaninger Str. 22, 81675 Munich, Germany

Y. Akamatsu, H. Kobayashi, M. Tsuji, S. Nejima, K. Kumagai and T. Saito
Department of Orthopaedic Surgery, Yokohama City University, School of Medicine, 3-9, Fukuura, Kanazawa-ku, Yokohama 236-0004, Japan

Chun-Hao Fan
Sports Medicine Center, Chang Gung Memorial Hospital at Chia Yi, Chia Yi, Taiwan

Pei-An Yu and Robert Wen-Wei Hsu
Sports Medicine Center, Chang Gung Memorial Hospital at Chia Yi, Chia Yi, Taiwan
Department of Orthopaedic Surgery, Chang Gung Memorial Hospital at Chia Yi, No 6 West section, Chia Pu Road, Puzih, Chia Yi Hsien 613, Taiwan

Chi-Lung Chen, Liang-Tseng Kuo and Wei-Hsiu Hsu
Sports Medicine Center, Chang Gung Memorial Hospital at Chia Yi, Chia Yi, Taiwan
Department of Orthopaedic Surgery, Chang Gung Memorial Hospital at Chia Yi, No 6 West section, Chia Pu Road, Puzih, Chia Yi Hsien 613, Taiwan
School of Medicine, Chang Gung University, Tao-Yuan, Taiwan

Qining Yang
Department of Orthopaedics, The Second Affiliated Hospital of Soochow
University, Sanxiang Road No.1055, Suzhou 215004, Jiangsu, China
Department of joint orthopaedic surgery, Jinhua hospital of Zhejiang University (Jinhua municipal central hospital), Jinhua, Zhejiang 321000, People's Republic of China

Yongwei Zhou
Department of joint orthopaedic surgery, Jinhua hospital of Zhejiang University (Jinhua municipal central hospital), Jinhua, Zhejiang 321000, People's Republic of China

Youjia Xu
Department of Orthopaedics, The Second Affiliated Hospital of Soochow University, Sanxiang Road No.1055, Suzhou 215004, Jiangsu, China
Department of Orthopedics, 2nd Affiliated Hospital of Soochow University, Sanxiang Road No.1055, Suzhou, Jiangsu 215000, People's Republic of China

Bijal Desai, Veeral Desai and Amr Saleh
Faculty of Health Sciences, McMaster University, Hamilton, ON, Canada

Shivani Shah
Schulich School of Medicine and Dentistry, Western University, London, ON, Canada

Archita Srinath
Faculty of Medicine, University of Toronto, Toronto, ON, Canada

Andrew Duong
Department of Surgery, Division of Orthopaedic Surgery, McMaster University, Hamilton, ON, Canada

Sheila Sprague, Mohit Bhandari and Nicole Simunovic
Department of Health Research Methods, Evidence, and Impact (HEI), Division of Orthopaedic Surgery, McMaster University, Hamilton, ON, Canada
Department of Surgery, Division of Orthopaedic Surgery, McMaster University, Hamilton, ON, Canada

Alexander Barié, Michael Köpf, Ayham Jaber and Babak Moradi
Clinic for Orthopedics and Trauma Surgery, Center for Orthopedics, Trauma Surgery and Spinal Cord Injury, Heidelberg University Hospital, Schlierbacher Landstrasse 200a, 69118 Heidelberg, Germany

Jürgen Huber and Nikolaus Alexander Streich
Center for Joint Surgery and Sport Injuries, Sportopaedie Heidelberg, Clinic St. Elisabeth Heidelberg, Max Reger Strasse 5-7, 69121 Heidelberg, Germany

Holger Schmitt
Center for Orthopedics and Sports Trauma Surgery, Atos Clinic Heidelberg, Bismarckstraße 9-15, 69115 Heidelberg, Germany

Pengzhou Gai
Department of Orthopaedic Surgery, Qindao University Medical College Affiliated Yantai Yuhuangding Hospital, Yantai, Shandong, People's Republic of China

Yunhang Geng
Qingdao University Medical College, Qingdao, China
Department of Orthopaedic Surgery, Qindao University Medical College Affiliated Yantai Yuhuangding Hospital, Yantai, Shandong, People's Republic of China

Anna Voelker, Nicolas H. von der Hoeh and Christoph-Eckhard Heyde
University Hospital Leipzig, Department of Orthopedic, Trauma and Plastic Surgery, Liebigstrasse 20, 04103 Leipzig, Germany

Cheng Jin
Department of Orthopedic Surgery, Chinese People's Armed Police Force, Zhejiang Corps Hospital, Jiaxing 314000, China

Eun-Kyoo Song, Quan-He Jin, Nam-Hun Lee and Jong-Keun Seon
Center for Joint Disease, Chonnam National University Hwasun Hospital, Hwasun, South Korea

Index

www.ingramcontent.com/pod-product-compliance
Lightning Source LLC
LaVergne TN
LVHW080733210926
848485LV00003B/548